Target Organ Toxicology Series

Toxicology of the Gastrointestinal Tract

TARGET ORGAN TOXICOLOGY SERIES

Series Editors

A. Wallace Hayes, John A. Thomas, and Donald E. Gardner

TOXICOLOGY OF THE GASTROINTESTINAL TRACT
Shayne C. Gad, editor, 384 pp., 2007

IMMUNOTOXICOLOGY AND IMMUNOPHARMACOLOGY,
THIRD EDITION
*Robert Luebke, Robert House, and Ian Kimber,
editors, 676 pp., 2007*

TOXICOLOGY OF THE LUNG, FOURTH EDITION
Donald E. Gardner, editor, 696 pp., 2006

TOXICOLOGY OF THE PANCREAS
Parviz M. Pour, editor, 720 pp., 2005

TOXICOLOGY OF THE KIDNEY, THIRD EDITION
Joan B. Tarloff and Lawrence H. Lash, editors, 1200 pp., 2004

OVARIAN TOXICOLOGY
Patricia B. Hoyer, editor, 248 pp., 2004

CARDIOVASCULAR TOXICOLOGY, THIRD EDITION
Daniel Acosta, Jr., editor, 616 pp., 2001

NUTRITIONAL TOXICOLOGY, SECOND EDITION
Frank N. Kotsonis and Maureen A. Mackey, editors, 480 pp., 2001

TOXICOLOGY OF SKIN
Howard I. Maibach, editor, 558 pp., 2000

NEUROTOXICOLOGY, SECOND EDITION
Hugh A. Tilson and G. Jean Harry, editors, 386 pp., 1999

TOXICANT–RECEPTOR INTERACTIONS: MODULATION OF SIGNAL
TRANSDUCTIONS AND GENE EXPRESSION
Michael S. Denison and William G. Helferich, editors, 256 pp., 1998

(Continued)

Target Organ Toxicology Series

Toxicology of the Gastrointestinal Tract

Edited by

Shayne C. Gad

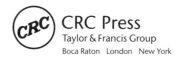

CRC Press
Taylor & Francis Group
Boca Raton   London   New York

CRC Press is an imprint of the
Taylor & Francis Group, an informa business

CRC Press
Taylor & Francis Group
6000 Broken Sound Parkway NW, Suite 300
Boca Raton, FL 33487-2742

© 2007 by Taylor & Francis Group, LLC
CRC Press is an imprint of Taylor & Francis Group, an Informa business

No claim to original U.S. Government works
Printed in the United States of America on acid-free paper
10 9 8 7 6 5 4 3 2 1

International Standard Book Number-10: 0-8493-2793-8 (Hardcover)
International Standard Book Number-13: 978-0-8493-2793-3 (Hardcover)

Library of Congress Cataloging-in-Publication Data

Toxicology of the gastrointestinal tract / Shayne C. Gad, editor.
        p. ; cm. -- (Target organ toxicology series)
    "A CRC title."
    Includes bibliographical references and index.
    ISBN-13: 978-0-8493-2793-3 (alk. paper)
    ISBN-10: 0-8493-2793-8 (alk. paper)
    1. Gastrointestinal system--Pathophysiology. 2. Toxicology. I. Gad, Shayne C.,
1948- II. Series. [DNLM: 1. Gastrointestinal Tract--drug effects. 2. Gastrointestinal
Tract--physiology. 3. Intestinal Absorption--drug effects. WI 102 T675 2006] I. Title.
II. Series.

RC802.T692 2006
616.3'3061--dc22   2006023250

Visit the Taylor & Francis Web site at
http://www.taylorandfrancis.com

and the CRC Press Web site at
http://www.crcpress.com

Dedication

To Spunky Dustmop Gad (1993–2006), the world's only published Lhasa Apso and a good friend and partner in raising my children through all the years it was just us. You will always be missed.

Preface

Toxicology of the Gastrointestinal Tract focuses on the specifics of the toxicology of the gastrointestinal tract — on adverse effects of xenobiotic agents and pharmaceuticals on the structure and function of the tract. Starting with an overview of basic aspects of structure and function, the chapters proceed to take focused looks at specific issues. This book is also concerned with a critical appraisal of what we have come to know about the interactions of chemicals and drugs with this critical organ system and the experimental methods and attempts to identify those regions of research that should prove productive for our future efforts.

Within these two broad objectives, the volume focuses on a number of specific areas of intestinal research. These areas reflect the increasing awareness and documentation of the multiple roles of the multiple components of the GI tract, starting with its well recognized and major roles of nutrient absorption and service as a protective barrier. In addition, emphasis is given to the expanding body of knowledge that relates to the intestines as major metabolic and immunologic organs involved in the synthesis and degradation of both natural and foreign substances. A further dimension is the inclusion of focused overviews of the function and dysfunction of human absorptive processes and the effects on these processes of microbial flora and specific classes of toxicants that target the GI tract.

Editor

Shayne C. Gad, Ph.D., DABT has been the principal of Gad Consulting Services since 1994. He has more than 30 years of broad-based experience in the fields of toxicology, drug and device development, document preparation, and statistics and risk assessment. Before 1994, he served as director of toxicology and pharmacology for Synergen in Boulder, Colorado, director of medical affairs at Becton, Dickinson in Research Triangle Park, North Carolina, and senior director of product safety and pharmacokinetics at G.D. Searle in Skokie, Illinois. Dr. Gad is a past president of the American College of Toxicology, a board certified toxicologist (DABT), and a fellow of the Academy of Toxicological Sciences. He is also a member of the Society of Toxicology, Teratology Society, Society of Toxicological Pathologies, Biometrics Society, and the American Statistical Association.

Dr. Gad has published 29 books and more than 300 chapters, papers, and abstracts in toxicology and other areas of interest. He has contributed to and has personal experience with investigational new drug (IND) applications (he successfully filed more than 64), NDA, PLA, ANDA, 510(k), IDE, and PMS preparation, and has broad experience with the design, conduct, and analysis of preclinical and clinical safety and pharmacokinetic studies for drugs, devices, and combination products. He is also a retired Navy captain with extensive operational experience at sea and overseas.

Contributors

William J. Brock
Brock Scientific Consulting, LLC
Montgomery Village, Maryland

Florence G. Burleson
BRT-Burleson Research
  Technologies, Inc.
Morrisville, North Carolina

Gary R. Burleson
BRT-Burleson Research
  Technologies, Inc.
Morrisville, North Carolina

Shayne C. Gad
Gad Consulting Services
Cary, North Carolina

Robin C. Guy
Robin Guy Consulting, LLC
Toxicology and Product Safety
  Assessment
Lake Forest, Illinois

David W. Hobson
H&H Scientific Services LLP
Boerne, Texas

Valerie L. Hobson
Texas Tech University
Department of Psychology
Lubbock, Texas

Henry I. Jacoby
Product Safety Labs, Inc.
Dayton, New Jersey

Robert W. Kapp, Jr.
BioTox
Lutherville, Maryland

Claire L. Kruger
ENVIRON International
Arlington, Virginia

Joseph V. Rodricks
ENVIRON International
Arlington, Virginia

Charles Spainhour
Clarks Summit, Pennsylvania

Allison A. Yates
ENVIRON International
Arlington, Virginia

Table of Contents

1 Introduction: The Gastrointestinal Tract as Barrier and as Absorptive and Metabolic Organ

Shayne C. Gad

CONTENTS

INTRODUCTION

Toxicology of the Gastrointestinal Tract, a volume of the Target Organ Toxicology Series, focuses on the specifics of the toxicology of the gastrointestinal tract — the adverse effects on its structure and function. Starting with an overview of basic aspects of structure and function, the chapters provide focused looks at specific issues. This book also provides a critical appraisal of what we have known about the interactions of chemical and drugs with organ systems and experimental methods and attempts to define regions of research that should prove productive for our future efforts.

Within these two broad objectives, the volume focuses on a number of specific areas of gastrointestinal tract research. These areas of research reflect the increasing awareness and documentation of the multiple roles of the many components of the gastrointestinal tract including the well recognized and major roles of nutrient absorption and barrier penetratation. In addition, emphasis is given to the expanding body of knowledge that relates to the intestines as major metabolic and immunologic organs involved in the synthesis and degradation of both natural and foreign substances. A further dimension is the inclusion of several discussions aimed directly at the function and dysfunction of human absorptive processes and the effects of microbial flora on these processes.

The gastrointestinal (GI) tract is one of the three great pathways into and out of the body; the other two being the skin and the respiratory tract. The GI tract is the great highway through the body and much more. Like the other two pathways, it is also a major metabolic organ and a major interface of the environment with the immune/lymphatic system.

A wide range of approaches and methodologies have been employed to evaluate the maturation and functions of the gastrointestinal tract. Because of their unusual morphologies, the mouth, intestines, and stomach can be examined *in vivo* and *in vitro* by a variety of techniques, each providing different kinds of relevant information and understanding. Sacs, loops, rings, and cells have provided ample data to reveal the importance of the GI tract as a barrier and absorptive organ and also as a highly active major metabolic tissue. Examination of the development of intestinal enzymes and metabolic pathways reveals an understanding of nutrient active transport and metabolism as well as metabolism of foreign substances. The relatively large mass of this organ system provides additional significance to its metabolic roles in the homeostasis of the organism as a whole.

Since ingestion is a major route of exposure to foreign substances, significant research involving the absorption and metabolism of these substances is needed. In addition, the effects of foreign substances on normal intestinal functions constitute an area of research requiring further attention. Currently, more Americans are affected by serious diseases of the gastrointestinal tract than any other system except the cardiovascular system; this provides emphasis for the increasing concern for understanding possible environmental contributions to gastrointestinal disease.

STRUCTURE

The GI tract or alimentary canal (Figure 1.1) is a continuous tube that extends from the mouth to the anus through the ventral body cavity. Organs of the gastrointestinal tract include the mouth, most of the pharynx, esophagus, stomach, small intestine, and large intestine. The length of the GI tract taken from an adult cadaver is about 9 m (30 ft). In a living person, it is much shorter because the muscles along the walls of GI tract organs are in a state of tonus (sustained contraction). It should be noted that the associated digestive organs are the teeth, tongue, salivary glands, liver, gallbladder, and pancreas.

The GI tract contains and processes food from the time it is eaten until it is digested and absorbed or eliminated. In portions of the GI tract, muscular contractions in the wall physically break down the food by repetitive mixing. The contractions for mixing also help to dissolve foods by mixing them with fluids

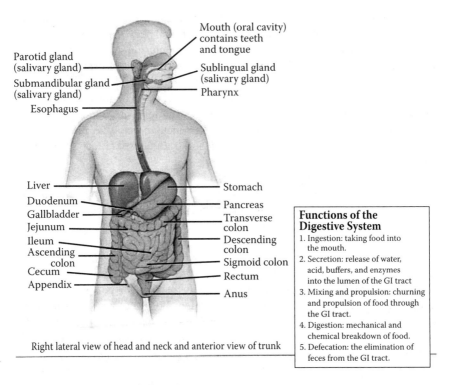

Parotid gland (salivary gland)
Submandibular gland (salivary gland)
Esophagus

Mouth (oral cavity) contains teeth and tongue
Sublingual gland (salivary gland)
Pharynx

Liver
Duodenum
Gallbladder
Jejunum
Ileum
Ascending colon
Cecum
Appendix

Stomach
Pancreas
Transverse colon
Descending colon
Sigmoid colon
Rectum
Anus

Functions of the Digestive System
1. Ingestion: taking food into the mouth.
2. Secretion: release of water, acid, buffers, and enzymes into the lumen of the GI tract
3. Mixing and propulsion: churning and propulsion of food through the GI tract.
4. Digestion: mechanical and chemical breakdown of food.
5. Defecation: the elimination of feces from the GI tract.

Right lateral view of head and neck and anterior view of trunk

FIGURE 1.1 Gastrointestinal tract.

secreted into the tract. Enzymes secreted by accessory structures and cells that line the tract break down the food chemically. Wave-like contractions of the smooth muscle in the wall of the GI tract propel the food along the tract, from the esophagus to the anus. The digestive system performs six basic processes:

Ingestion — This process involves taking foods and liquids into the mouth (eating).

Secretion — Each day, cells within the walls of the tract and accessory digestive organs secrete a total of about 7 liters of water, acid, buffers, and enzymes into the lumen of the tract.

Mixing and propulsion — Alternating contraction and relaxation of smooth muscle in the walls of the GI tract mix food and secretions and propel them toward the anus. This capability of the GI tract to mix and move material along its length is termed motility.

Digestion — Mechanical and chemical processes break down ingested food into small molecules. In mechanical digestion, the teeth cut and grind food before it is swallowed, and then smooth muscles of the stomach and small intestine churn the food. As a result, food molecules become dissolved and thoroughly mixed with digestive enzymes. In chemical digestion, the large carbohydrate, lipid, protein, and nucleic acid molecules in food are split into smaller molecules by hydrolysis. Digestive enzymes produced by the salivary glands, tongue, stomach, pancreas, and small intestine catalyze these catabolic reactions. A few substances in food can be absorbed without chemical digestion. These include amino acids, cholesterol, glucose, vitamins, minerals, and water.

Absorption — The entrance of ingested and secreted fluid, ions, and the small molecules that are products of digestion into the epithelial cells lining the lumen of the GI tract is called absorption. The absorbed substances pass into blood or lymph and circulate to cells throughout the body.

Defecation — Wastes, indigestible substances, bacteria, cells sloughed from the lining of the GI tract, and digested material that were not absorbed leave the body through the anus in a process called defecation. The eliminated material is termed feces.

The wall of the GI tract from the lower esophagus to the anal canal has the same basic, four-layered arrangement of tissues. The four layers of the tract, from deep to superficial, are the mucosa, submucosa, muscularis, and serosa.

MUCOSA

The mucosa or inner lining of the tract is a mucous membrane (as are the other surfaces of externally communicating body channels or orifices). It is composed of a layer of epithelium in direct contact with the contents of the tract, connective tissue, and a thin layer of smooth muscle.

The epithelium in the mouth, pharynx, esophagus, and anal canal is mainly nonkeratinized stratified squamous epithelium that serves a protective function. Simple columnar epithelium, which functions in secretion and absorption, lines the stomach and intestines. Neighboring simple columnar epithelial cells are firmly sealed to each other by tight junctions that restrict leakage between the cells. The rate of renewal of GI tract epithelial cells is rapid (5 to 7 days.) Located among the absorptive epithelial cells are exocrine cells that secrete mucus and fluid into the lumen of the tract, and several types of endocrine cells, collectively called enteroendocrine cells, that secrete hormones into the bloodstream.

The lamina propria is areolar connective tissue containing many blood and lymphatic vessels, which are the routes by which nutrients absorbed into the tract reach the other tissues of the body. This layer supports the epithelium and binds it to the muscularis mucosae. The lamina propria also contains the majority of the cells of the mucosa-associated lymphatic tissue (MALT). These prominent lymphatic nodules contain immune system cells that protect against disease. MALT is present all along the GI tract, especially in the tonsils, small intestine, appendix, and large intestine, and it contains about as many immune cells as are present in all the rest of the body. The lymphocytes and macrophages in MALT mount immune responses against microbes such as bacteria that may penetrate the epithelium. It should be noted that current ICH and FDA guidance suggests examination of the MALT tissues when evaluating potential immunotoxicity.

A thin layer of smooth muscle fibers called the muscularis mucosae throws the mucous membrane of the stomach and small intestine into many small folds that increase the surface area for digestion and absorption. Movements of the muscularis mucosae ensure that all absorptive cells are fully exposed to the contents of the gastrointestinal tract.

SUBMUCOSA

The submucosa consists of areolar connective tissue that binds the mucosa to the muscularis. It contains many blood and lymphatic vessels that receive absorbed food molecules. Also located in the submucosa is the submucosal plexus or plexus of Meissner, an extensive network of neurons. The neurons are part of the enteric nervous system (ENS), the "brain of the gut." The ENS consists of about 100 million neurons in two plexuses that extend the entire length of the tract. The submucosal plexus contains sensory and motor enteric neurons, plus parasympathetic and sympathetic postganglionic neurons that innervate the mucosa and submucosa. Enteric nerves in the submucosa regulate movements of the mucosa and vasoconstriction of blood vessels. Because its neurons also innervate secretory cells of mucosal and submucosal glands, the ENS is important in controlling secretions by the GI tract. The submucosa may also contain glands and lymphatic tissue.

MUSCULARIS

The muscularis of the mouth, pharynx, and superior and middle parts of the esophagus contains skeletal muscle that produces voluntary swallowing. Skeletal muscle also forms the external anal sphincter that permits voluntary control of defecation. Throughout the rest of the tract, the muscularis consists of smooth muscle that is generally found in two sheets: an inner sheet of circular fibers and an outer sheet of longitudinal fibers. Involuntary contractions of the smooth muscle help break down food physically, mix it with digestive secretions, and propel it along the tract. Between the layers of the muscularis is a second plexus of the enteric nervous system — the myenteric plexus or plexus of Auerbach. The myenteric plexus contains enteric neurons, parasympathetic ganglia, parasympathetic postganglionic neurons, and sympathetic postganglionic neurons that innervate the muscularis. This plexus mostly controls tract motility, in particular the frequency and strength of contraction of the muscularis.

SEROSA

The serosa is the superficial layer of those portions of the GI tract that are suspended in the abdominopelvic cavity. It is a serous membrane composed of areolar connective tissue and simple squamous epithelium. As we will see shortly, the esophagus, which passes through the mediastinum, has a superficial layer called the adventitia composed of areolar connective tissue. Inferior to the diaphragm, the serosa is also called the visceral peritoneum; it forms a portion of the peritoneum, which we examine in detail next.

The peritoneum is the largest serous membrane of the body; it consists of a layer of simple squamous epithelium (mesothelium) with an underlying supporting layer of connective tissue. The peritoneum is divided into the parietal peritoneum, which lines the wall of the abdominopelvic cavity, and the visceral peritoneum, which covers some of the organs in the cavity and is their serosa. The slim space between the parietal and visceral portions of the peritoneum is called the peritoneal cavity, which contains serous fluid. In certain diseases, the peritoneal cavity may become distended by the accumulation of several liters of fluid, a condition called ascites. As we will see, some organs lie on the posterior abdominal wall and are covered by peritoneum only on their anterior surfaces. Such organs, including the kidneys and pancreas, are said to be retroperitoneal.

Unlike the pericardium and pleurae that smoothly cover the heart and lungs, the peritoneum contains large folds that weave between the viscera. The folds bind the organs to each other and to the walls of the abdominal cavity. They also contain blood vessels, lymphatic vessels, and nerves that supply the abdominal organs.

The greater omentum, the largest peritoneal fold, drapes over the transverse colon and coils of the small intestine like a "fatty apron." Because the greater omentum is a double sheet that folds back upon itself, it is a four-layered structure. From attachments along the stomach and duodenum, the greater omentum extends downward anterior to the small intestine, then turns and extends upward and attaches to the transverse colon. The greater omentum normally contains a considerable amount of adipose tissue. Its adipose tissue content can greatly expand with weight gain, giving rise to the characteristic "beer belly" seen in some overweight individuals. The many lymph nodes of the greater omentum contribute macrophages and antibody-producing plasma cells that help combat and contain infections of the GI tract.

The falciform ligament attaches the liver to the anterior abdominal wall and diaphragm. The liver is the only digestive organ attached to the anterior abdominal wall.

The lesser omentum arises as two folds in the serosa of the stomach and duodenum, and it suspends the stomach and duodenum from the liver. It contains some lymph nodes.

Another fold of the peritoneum called the mesentery is fan-shaped and binds the small intestine to the posterior abdominal wall. It extends from the posterior abdominal wall to wrap around the small intestine and then returns to its origin, forming a twice-mixed solution and move the luminal contents along the tract.

Peritonitis

Peritonitis is an acute inflammation of the peritoneum. A common cause of the condition is contamination of the peritoneum by infectious microbes that can result from accidental or surgical wounds in the abdominal wall or from perforation or rupture of abdominal organs. If, for example, bacteria gain access to the peritoneal cavity through an intestinal perforation or rupture of the appendix, they can produce an acute, life-threatening form of peritonitis. A less serious form of peritonitis can result from the continual contact of inflamed peritoneal surfaces.

The mouth, also referred to as the oral or buccal cavity, is formed by the cheeks, hard and soft palates, and tongue. Forming the lateral walls of the oral cavity are the cheeks — muscular structures covered externally by skin and internally by nonkeratinized stratified squamous epithelium. The anterior portions of the cheeks end at the lips.

The lips or labia are fleshy folds surrounding the opening of the mouth. They are covered externally by skin and internally by a mucous membrane. There is a transition zone where the two kinds of covering tissue meet. This portion of the lips is nonkeratinized, and the color of the blood in the underlying blood vessels is visible through the transparent surface layer. The inner surface of each lip is attached to its corresponding gum by a midline fold of mucous membrane called the labial frenulum.

The orbicularis oris muscle and connective tissue lie between the skin and the mucous membrane of the oral cavity. During chewing, contraction of the buccinator muscles in the cheeks and orbicularis oris muscle in the lips helps keep food between the upper and lower teeth.

The vestibule of the oral cavity is a space bounded externally by the cheeks and lips and internally by the gums and teeth. The oral cavity proper is a space that extends from the gums and teeth to the fauces, the opening between the oral cavity and the pharynx or throat.

The hard palate — the anterior portion of the roof of the mouth — is formed by the maxillae and palatine bones, is covered by mucous membrane, and forms a bony partition between the oral and nasal cavities. The soft palate that forms the posterior portion of the roof of the mouth is an arch-shaped muscular partition between the oropharynx and nasopharynx that is lined by mucous membrane.

Hanging from the free border of the soft palate is a conical muscular process called the uvula. During swallowing, the soft palate and uvula are drawn superiorly, closing off the nasopharynx and preventing swallowed foods and liquids from entering the nasal cavity. Lateral to the base of the uvula are two muscular folds that run down the lateral sides of the soft palate. Anteriorly, the palatoglossal arch extends to the side of the base of the tongue; posteriorly, the palatopharyngeal arch extends to the side of the pharynx. The palatine tonsils are situated between the arches, and the lingual tonsils are situated at the base of the tongue. At the posterior border of the soft palate, the mouth opens into the oropharynx through the fauces.

SALIVARY GLANDS

A salivary gland is any cell or organ that releases a secretion called saliva into the oral cavity. Ordinarily, the glands secrete only enough saliva to keep the mucous membranes of the mouth and pharynx moist and to cleanse the mouth and teeth. When food enters the mouth, however, secretion of saliva increases, and it lubricates, dissolves, and begins the chemical breakdown of the food.

The mucous membrane of the mouth and tongue contains many small salivary glands that open directly or indirectly via short ducts to the oral cavity. These glands include labial, buccal, and palatal glands in the lips, cheeks, and palate, respectively, and lingual glands in the tongue, all of which make a small contribution to saliva. However, most saliva is secreted by the major salivary glands that lie beyond the oral mucosa. Their secretions empty into ducts that lead to the oral cavity.

There are three pairs of major salivary glands: the parotid, submandibular, and sublingual glands. The parotid glands are located inferior and anterior to the ears, between the skin and the masseter muscle. Each secretes saliva into the oral cavity via a parotid duct that pierces the buccinator muscle to open into the vestibule opposite the second maxillary (upper) molar tooth. The submandibular glands are found beneath the base of the tongue in the posterior part of the floor of the mouth. Their ducts, the submandibular ducts, run under the mucosa on either side of the midline of the floor of the mouth and enter the oral cavity proper lateral to the lingual frenulum. The sublingual glands are superior to the submandibular glands. Their ducts, the lesser sublingual ducts, open into the floor of the mouth in the oral cavity proper.

Composition and Functions of Saliva

Chemically, saliva is 99.5% water and 0.5% solutes. Among the solutes are ions, including sodium, potassium, chloride, bicarbonate, and phosphate. Also present are some dissolved gases and various organic substances, including urea and uric acid, mucus, immunoglobulin A (IgA), the bacteriolytic enzyme lysozyme, and salivary amylase, a digestive enzyme that acts on starch.

Each major salivary gland supplies different proportions of ingredients to saliva. The parotid glands contain cells that secrete a serous liquid containing salivary amylase. Because the submandibular glands contain cells similar to those found in the parotid glands plus some mucous cells, they secrete a fluid that contains amylase but is thickened with mucus. The sublingual glands contain mostly mucous cells, so they secrete a much thicker fluid that contributes only a small amount of amylase to the saliva.

The water in saliva provides a medium for dissolving foods so that they can be tasted and digestive reactions can begin. Chloride ions in the saliva activate salivary amylase. Bicarbonate and phosphate ions buffer acidic foods that enter the mouth; as a result, saliva is only slightly acidic (pH 6.35 to 6.85). Urea and uric acid are found in saliva because salivary glands (like the sweat glands of the skin) help remove waste molecules from the body. Mucus lubricates the food so it can easily be moved about in the mouth, formed into a ball, and swallowed. IgA is a secreted type of antibody that prevents attachment of microbes so they cannot penetrate the epithelium. The lysozyme enzyme kills bacteria. Even though these substances help protect the mucous membrane from infection and the teeth from decay, they are not present in large enough quantities to eliminate all oral bacteria.

TONGUE

The tongue is an accessory digestive organ composed of skeletal muscle covered with mucous membrane. Together with its associated muscles, it forms the floor of the oral cavity. The tongue is divided into symmetrical lateral halves by a median septum that extends its entire length, and it is attached inferiorly to the hyoid bone, styloid process of the temporal bone, and mandible. Each half of the tongue consists of an identical complement of extrinsic and intrinsic muscles.

The extrinsic muscles of the tongue that originate outside the tongue and insert into connective tissues in the tongue include the hyoglossus, genioglossus, and styloglossus muscles. The extrinsic muscles move the tongue from side to side and in and out to maneuver food for chewing, shape the food into a rounded mass, and force the food to the back of the mouth for swallowing. They also form the floor of the mouth and hold the tongue in position. The intrinsic muscles originate in and insert into connective tissue within the tongue. They alter the shape and size of the tongue for speech and swallowing. The intrinsic muscles include the longitudinalis superior, longitudinalis inferior, transversus linguae, and verticalis linguae muscles. The lingual frenulum, a fold of mucous membrane in the midline of the undersurface of the tongue, is attached to the floor of the mouth and aids in limiting the movement of the tongue posteriorly. If the lingual frenulum is abnormally short or rigid — a condition called ankyloglossia — eating and speaking are impaired such that the person is said to be "tongue-tied."

The dorsum (upper surface) and lateral surfaces of the tongue are covered with papillae (projections of the lamina propria covered with keratinized epithelium). Many papillae contain taste buds, the receptors for taste. Fungiform papillae are mushroom-like elevations distributed among the filiform papillae that are more numerous near the tip of the tongue. They appear as red dots on the surface of the tongue, and most of them contain taste buds. Vallate papillae are arranged in an inverted V shape on the posterior surface of the tongue; all of them contain taste buds. Foliate papillae are located in small trenches on the lateral margins of the tongue but most of their taste buds degenerate in early childhood. Filiform papillae are pointed, thread-like projections distributed in parallel rows over the anterior two thirds of the tongue. Although filiform papillae lack taste buds, they contain receptors for touch and increase friction between the tongue and food, making it easier for the tongue to move food in the oral cavity. Lingual glands in the lamina propria secrete both mucus and a watery serous fluid that contains the lingual lipase enzyme that acts on triglycerides.

Pharynx

When food is first swallowed, it passes from the mouth into the pharynx, a funnel-shaped tube that extends from the internal nares to the esophagus posteriorly and to the larynx anteriorly. The pharynx is composed of skeletal muscle and lined by mucous membrane. Whereas the nasopharynx functions only in respiration, both the oropharynx and laryngopharynx have digestive as well as respiratory functions. Swallowed food passes from the mouth into the oropharynx and laryngopharynx, the muscular contractions of which help propel food into the esophagus and then into the stomach.

The movement of food from the mouth into the stomach is achieved by the act of swallowing or deglutition. Deglutition is facilitated by saliva and mucus and involves the mouth, pharynx, and esophagus. Swallowing occurs in three stages: (1) the voluntary stage in which the bolus is passed into the oropharynx; (2) the pharyngeal stage, which is the involuntary passage of the bolus through the pharynx into the esophagus; and (3) the esophageal stage, which is the involuntary passage of the bolus through the esophagus into the stomach.

Swallowing starts when the bolus is forced to the back of the oral cavity and into the oropharynx by the movement of the tongue upward and backward against the palate; these actions constitute the voluntary stage of swallowing. With the passage of the bolus into the oropharynx, the involuntary pharyngeal stage of swallowing begins. The respiratory passageways close, and breathing is temporarily interrupted. The bolus stimulates receptors in the oropharynx that send impulses to the deglutition center in the medulla oblongata and lower pons of the brain stem. The returning impulses cause the soft palate and uvula to move upward to close off the nasopharynx, and the larynx is pulled forward and upward under the tongue. As the larynx rises, the epiglottis moves backward and downward and seals off the rima glottidis. The movement of the larynx also pulls the vocal cords together, further sealing off the respiratory tract, and widens the opening between the laryngopharynx and esophagus. The bolus passes through the laryngopharynx and enters the esophagus in 1 to 2 seconds. The respiratory passageways then reopen, and breathing resumes.

Esophagus

The esophagus is a collapsible muscular tube that lies posterior to the trachea. It is about 25 cm (10 in.) long. The esophagus begins at the inferior end of the laryngopharynx and passes through the mediastinum anterior to the vertebral column. It pierces the diaphragm through an opening called the esophageal hiatus, and ends in the superior portion of the stomach. Sometimes, part of the stomach protrudes above the diaphragm through the esophageal hiatus. This condition is termed hiatal hernia.

Histology

The mucosa of the esophagus consists of nonkeratinized stratified squamous epithelium, lamina propria (areolar connective tissue), and a muscularis muscosae (smooth muscle). Near the stomach, the mucosa of the esophagus also contains mucous glands. The stratified squamous epithelium associated with the lips, mouth, tongue, oropharynx, laryngopharynx, and esophagus affords considerable protection against abrasion and wear and tear from food particles that are chewed, mixed with secretions, and swallowed. The submucosa contains areolar connective tissue, blood vessels, and mucous glands. The muscularis of the superior third of the esophagus is skeletal muscle, the intermediate third is skeletal and smooth muscle, and the inferior third is smooth muscle.

The superficial layer is known as the adventitia rather than the serosa. Because the areolar connective tissue of this layer is not covered by mesothelium and because the connective tissue merges with the connective tissue of surrounding structures of the mediastinum through which it passes. The adventitia attaches the esophagus to surrounding structures.

The esophagus secretes mucus and transports food into the stomach. It does not produce digestive enzymes or carry on absorption. The passage of food from the laryngopharynx into the esophagus is regulated at the entrance to the esophagus by a circular band or ring of normally contracted muscle called the upper esophageal sphincter. It consists of the cricopharyngeus muscle attached to the cricoid cartilage. The elevation of the larynx during the pharyngeal stage of swallowing causes the sphincter to relax, and the bolus enters the esophagus. This sphincter also relaxes during exhalation.

During the esophageal stage of swallowing, peristalsis, a progression of coordinated contractions and relaxations of the circular and longitudinal layers of the muscularis, pushes the food bolus onward. (Peristalsis occurs in other tubular structures including other parts of the GI tract and the ureters, bile ducts, and uterine tubes; in the esophagus it is controlled by the medulla oblongata.) In the section of the esophagus just superior to the bolus, the circular muscle fibers contract, constricting the esophageal wall and squeezing the bolus toward the stomach. Meanwhile, longitudinal fibers inferior to the bolus also contract. The contractions shorten this inferior section and push its walls outward so it can receive the bolus. The contractions are repeated in a wave that pushes the food toward the stomach. Mucus secreted by esophageal glands lubricates the bolus and reduces friction. The passage of solid or semisolid food from the mouth to the stomach takes 4 to 8 seconds; very soft foods and liquids pass through in about 1 second.

Just superior to the diaphragm, the esophagus narrows slightly due to a maintained contraction of the muscularis at the lowest part of the esophagus. Known as the lower esophageal sphincter, this structure relaxes during swallowing and thus allows the bolus to pass from the esophagus into the stomach.

STOMACH

Anatomy

The stomach has four main regions: the cardia, fundus, body, and pylorus (Figure 1.2). The cardia surrounds the superior opening of the stomach. The rounded portion superior to and to the left of the cardia is the fundus. Inferior to the fundus is the large central portion called the body. The region of the stomach that connects to the duodenum is the pylorus; it has two parts, the pyloric antrum that connects to the body of the stomach and the pyloric canal that leads into the duodenum. When the stomach is empty, the mucosa lies in large folds, called rugae, that can be seen with the unaided eye. The pylorus communicates with the duodenum of the small intestine via the pyloric sphincter. The concave medial border of the stomach is called the lesser curvature, and the convex lateral border is called the greater curvature.

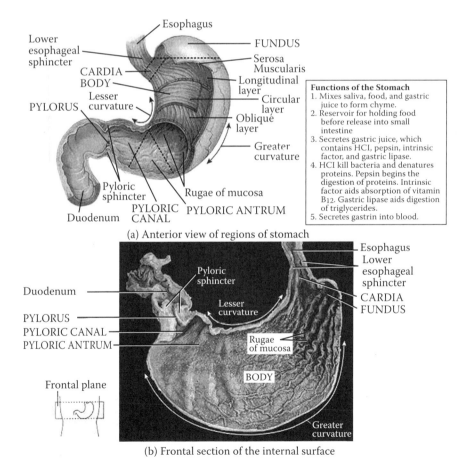

Functions of the Stomach
1. Mixes saliva, food, and gastric juice to form chyme.
2. Reservoir for holding food before release into small intestine
3. Secretes gastric juice, which contains HCl, pepsin, intrinsic factor, and gastric lipase.
4. HCl kill bacteria and denatures proteins. Pepsin begins the digestion of proteins. Intrinsic factor aids absorption of vitamin B_{12}. Gastric lipase aids digestion of triglycerides.
5. Secretes gastrin into blood.

(a) Anterior view of regions of stomach

(b) Frontal section of the internal surface

FIGURE 1.2 Four main regions of the stomach: cardia, fundus, body, and pylorus.

Histology

The stomach wall is composed of the same four basic layers as the rest of the GI tract, with certain modifications. The surface of the mucosa is a layer of simple columnar epithelial cells called surface mucous cells. The mucosa contains a lamina propria (areolar connective tissue) and a muscularis mucosae (smooth muscle). Epithelial cells extend down into the lamina propria, where they form columns of secretory cells called gastric glands that line many narrow channels called gastric pits. Secretions from several gastric glands flow into each gastric pit and then into the lumen of the stomach.

The gastric glands contain three types of exocrine gland cells that secrete their products into the stomach lumen: mucous neck cells, chief cells, and parietal cells. Both surface mucous cells and mucous neck cells secrete mucus. Parietal cells produce hydrochloric acid and the intrinsic factor needed for absorption of vitamin B_{12}. The chief cells secrete pepsinogen and gastric lipase. The secretions of the mucous, parietal, and chief cells form gastric juice (2000 to 3000 mL or roughly 2 to 3 qt.) per day. In addition, gastric glands include a type of enteroendocrine cell, the G cell, which is located mainly in the pyloric antrum and secretes gastrin hormone into the bloodstream. As we will see shortly, this hormone stimulates several aspects of gastric activity.

Three additional layers lie deep to the mucosa. The submucosa of the stomach is composed of areolar connective tissue. The muscularis has three layers of smooth muscle: an outer longitudinal layer, a middle circular layer, and an inner oblique layer. The oblique layer is limited primarily to the body of the stomach. The serosa is composed of simple squamous epithelium (mesothelium) and areolar connective tissue, and the portion of the serosa covering the stomach is part of the visceral peritoneum. At the lesser curvature of the stomach, the visceral peritoneum extends upward to the liver as the lesser omentum. At the greater curvature of the stomach, the visceral peritoneum continues downward as the greater omentum and drapes over the intestines.

SMALL INTESTINE

Anatomy

The small intestine is divided into three regions. The duodenum, the shortest region, is retroperitoneal. It starts at the pyloric sphincter of the stomach and extends about 25 cm until it merges with the jejunum. The jejunum is about 1 m long and extends to the ileum. Jejunum means "empty," which is how it is found at death. The final and longest region of the small intestine, the ileum, measures about 2 mm and joins the large intestine at the ileocecal sphincter.

Projections called circular folds are 10 mm (0.4 in.) permanent ridges in the mucosa. The circular folds begin near the proximal portion of the duodenum and end at about the midportion of the ileum; some extend all the way around the circumference of the intestine and others extend only part of the way around.

They enhance absorption by increasing surface area and causing the chyme to spiral rather than move in a straight line as it passes through the small intestine.

Histology

Even though the wall of the small intestine is composed of the same four coats that make up most of the GI tract, special features of both the mucosa and the submucosa facilitate the processes of digestion and absorption. The mucosa forms a series of finger-like villi, projections that are 0.5 to 1 mm long. The large number of villi (20 to 40 per square millimeter) vastly increases the surface area of the epithelium available for absorption and digestion and gives the intestinal mucosa a velvety appearance. Each villus has a core of lamina propria; embedded in this connective tissue are an arteriole, a venule, a blood capillary network, and a lacteal, which is a lymphatic capillary. Nutrients absorbed by the epithelial cells covering the villus pass through the wall of a capillary or a lacteal to enter blood or lymph, respectively.

The epithelium of the mucosa consists of simple columnar epithelium that contains absorptive cells, goblet cells, enteroendocrine cells, and Paneth's cells. The apical membranes of absorptive cells feature microvilli; each microvillus is a 10-mm long, cylindrical, membrane-covered projection that contains a bundle of 20 to 30 actin filaments.

The mucosa contains many deep crevices lined with glandular epithelium. Cells lining the crevices form the intestinal glands (crypts of Lieberkühn) and secrete intestinal juice. Many of the epithelial cells in the mucosa are goblet cells that secrete mucus. Paneth's cells, found in the deepest parts of the intestinal glands, secrete a bactericidal enzyme known as lysozyme and are capable of phagocytosis. They may have a role in regulating the microbial population in the intestines.

Three types of enteroendocrine cells, also in the deepest part of the intestinal glands, secrete hormones: secretin (by S cells), cholecystokinin (by CCK cells), and glucose-dependent insulinotropic peptide (by K cells). The lamina propria of the small intestine has an abundance of MALT. Solitary lymphatic nodules are most numerous in the distal part of the ileum. Groups of lymphatic nodules referred to as aggregated lymphatic follicles (Peyer's patches) are also present in the ileum. The muscularis mucosae consists of smooth muscle. The submucosa of the duodenum contains duodenal (Brunner's) glands that secrete an alkaline mucus that helps neutralize gastric acid in the chyme. Sometimes the lymphatic tissue of the lamina propria extends through the muscularis mucosae into the submucosa.

The muscularis of the small intestine consists of two layers of smooth muscle. The thinner outer layer contains longitudinal fibers; the thicker inner layer contains circular fibers. Except for a major portion of the duodenum, the serosa (or visceral peritoneum) completely surrounds the small intestine.

Large Intestine

The large intestine is the terminal portion of the GI tract and is divided into four principal regions. The overall functions of the large intestine are the completion of absorption, the production of certain vitamins, the formation of feces, and the expulsion of feces from the body.

Anatomy

The large intestine, which is about 1.5 m long and 6.5 cm in diameter, extends from the ileum to the anus. It is attached to the posterior abdominal wall by its mesocolon — a double layer of peritoneum. Structurally, the four major regions of the large intestine are the cecum, colon, rectum, and anal canal.

The opening from the ileum into the large intestine is guarded by a fold of mucous membrane called the ileocecal sphincter that allows materials from the small intestine to pass into the large intestine. Hanging inferior to the ileocecal valve is the cecum, a blind pouch about 6 cm long. Attached to the cecum is a coiled tube measuring about 8 cm in length called the appendix or vermiform appendix. The mesentery of the appendix or mesoappendix attaches the appendix to the inferior part of the mesentery ileum.

The open end of the cecum merges with a long tube called the colon, which is divided into ascending, transverse, descending, and sigmoid portions. Both the ascending and descending colon are retroperitoneal, whereas the transverse and sigmoid colon are not. The ascending colon ascends on the right side of the abdomen, reaches the inferior surface of the liver, and turns abruptly to the left to form the right colic flexure. The colon continues across the abdomen to the left side as the transverse colon. It curves beneath the inferior end of the spleen on the left side as the left colic flexure and passes inferiorly to the level of the iliac crest as the descending colon. The sigmoid colon begins near the left iliac crest, projects medially to the midline, and terminates as the rectum at about the level of the third sacral vertebra.

The rectum, the last 20 cm of the GI tract, lies anterior to the sacrum and coccyx. The terminal 2 to 3 cm of the rectum is called the anal canal. The mucous membrane of the anal canal is arranged in longitudinal folds called anal columns that contain a network of arteries and veins. The opening of the anal canal to the exterior, called the anus, is guarded by an internal anal sphincter of smooth muscle (involuntary) and an external anal sphincter of skeletal muscle. Normally these sphincters keep the anus closed except during the elimination of feces.

Histology

The wall of the large intestine differs from that of the small intestine in several respects. No villi or permanent circular folds are found in the mucosa, which consists of simple columnar epithelium, lamina propria (areolar connective tissue), and muscularis mucosae. The epithelium contains mostly absorptive and goblet cells. The absorptive cells function primarily in water absorption, whereas the goblet cells secrete mucus that lubricates the passage of the colonic contents. Both absorptive and goblet cells are located in long, straight, tubular intestinal glands that extend the full thickness of the mucosa. Solitary lymphatic nodules are also found in the lamina propria of the mucosa and may extend through the muscularis mucosae into the submucosa. The submucosa of the large intestine is similar to that found in the rest of the GI tract. The muscularis consists of an external layer of longitudinal smooth muscle and an internal layer of circular smooth muscle. Unlike other parts of the GI tract, portions of the longitudinal muscles are thickened, forming three conspicuous longitudinal barriers.

FUNCTION OF GI TRACT

Several minutes after food enters the stomach, gentle, rippling, peristaltic movements called mixing waves pass over the stomach every 15 to 25 seconds. These waves macerate food, mix it with secretions of the gastric glands, and reduce it to a soupy liquid called chyme. Few mixing waves are observed in the fundus (its primary function is storage). As digestion proceeds in the stomach, more vigorous mixing waves begin at the body of the stomach and intensify as they reach the pylorus. The pyloric sphincter normally remains almost but not completely closed. As food reaches the pylorus, each mixing wave forces several milliliters of chyme into the duodenum through the pyloric sphincter. Most of the chyme is forced back into the body of the stomach, where mixing continues. The next wave pushes the chyme forward again and forces a little more into the duodenum. These forward and backward movements of the gastric contents are responsible for most mixing in the stomach.

MECHANICAL AND CHEMICAL DIGESTION IN MOUTH

Mechanical digestion in the mouth results from chewing or mastication (pronounced mas-ti-KAY-shun = to chew): food is manipulated by the tongue, ground by the teeth, and mixed with saliva. As a result, the food is reduced to a soft, flexible, easily swallowed mass called a bolus (= lump). Food molecules begin to dissolve in the water in saliva, an important activity because enzymes can react with food molecules in a liquid medium only. Two enzymes, salivary amylase and lingual lipase, contribute to chemical digestion in the mouth. Salivary amylase initiates the breakdown of starch. Dietary carbohydrates are either monosaccharide and disaccharide sugars or complex polysaccharides.

Food may remain in the fundus about an hour without becoming mixed with gastric juice. During this time, digestion by salivary amylase continues. Soon, however, the churning action mixes chyme with acidic gastric juice, inactivating salivary amylase and activating lingual lipase, which starts to digest triglycerides into fatty acids and triglycerides.

Even though parietal cells secrete hydrogen ions (H^+) and chloride ions (Cl^-) separately into the stomach lumen, the net effect is secretion of hydrochloric acid (HCl). Proton pumps powered by H^+/K^+ ATPases actively transport H^+ into the

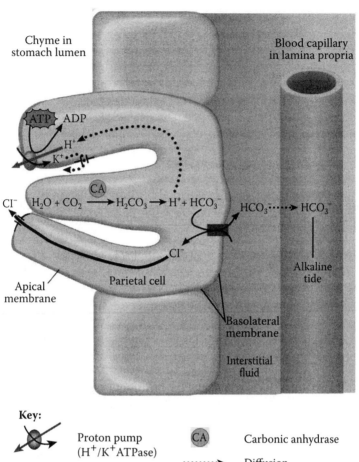

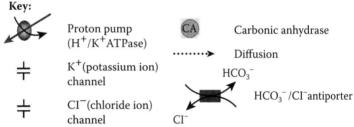

FIGURE 1.3 Transport of hydrogen ions into lumen and potassium ions into cells.

lumen while bringing potassium ions (K^+) into the cell (Figure 1.3). At the same time Cl^- and K^+ diffuse out through Cl and K channels in the apical membrane (next to the lumen). The carbonic anhydrase enzyme that is especially plentiful in parietal cells catalyzes the formation of carbonic acid (H_2CO_3) from water (H_2O) and carbon dioxide (CO_2). As carbonic acid dissociates, it provides a ready source of H^+ for the proton pumps but also generates bicarbonate ions (HCOO). As HCO_3 builds up in the cytosol, it exits the parietal cell in exchange for Cl via Cl^-/HCO_3^- antiporters in the basolateral membrane (next to the lamina propria). HCO_3^- diffuses into nearby blood capillaries. This "alkaline tide" of bicarbonate ions entering the bloodstream after a meal may be large enough to slightly elevate blood pH and make urine more alkaline.

The strongly acidic fluid of the stomach kills many microbes in food. HCl partially denatures proteins in food and stimulates the secretion of hormones that promote the flow of bile and pancreatic juice. Enzymatic digestion of proteins also begins in the stomach. The only proteolytic enzyme in the stomach is pepsin, which is secreted by chief cells. Because pepsin breaks certain peptide bonds between the amino acids making up proteins, a protein chain of many amino acids is broken down into smaller peptide fragments. Pepsin is most effective in the very acidic environment of the stomach (pH 2); it becomes inactive at higher pH.

Note that pepsin is secreted in an inactive form called pepsinogen; in this form, it cannot digest the proteins in the chief cells that produce it. Pepsinogen is not converted into active pepsin until it comes into contact with active pepsin molecules or hydrochloric acid secreted by parietal cells. The stomach epithelial cells are also protected from gastric juices by a 1- to 3-mm thick layer of alkaline mucus secreted by surface mucous cells and mucous neck cells.

Another enzyme of the stomach is gastric lipase, which splits the short-chain triglycerides in fat molecules found in milk into fatty acids and monoglycerides. This enzyme has a limited role in the adult stomach and operates best at a pH of 5 to 6. More important than either lingual lipase or gastric lipase is pancreatic lipase, an enzyme secreted by the pancreas into the small intestine.

Only a small amount of absorption occurs in the stomach because its epithelial cells are impermeable to most materials. However, mucous cells of the stomach absorb some water, ions, and short-chain fatty acids, as well as certain drugs (especially aspirin and other NSAIDs) and alcohol.

REGULATION OF GASTRIC SECRETION AND MOTILITY

Both neural and hormonal mechanisms control the secretion of gastric juice and the contraction of smooth muscles in the stomach wall. Events in gastric digestion occur in three overlapping phases: the cephalic, gastric, and intestinal phases.

Cephalic Phase

The cephalic phase of gastric digestion consists of reflexes initiated by sensory receptors in the head. Even before food enters the stomach, the sight, smell, taste, or thought of food initiates this reflex. The cerebral cortex and the feeding center in the hypothalamus send nerve impulses to the medulla oblongata. The medulla then transmits impulses to parasympathetic preganglionic neurons in the vagus nerves that stimulate parasympathetic postganglionic neurons in the submucosal plexus. In turn, impulses from parasympathetic postganglionic neurons stimulate the gastric glands to secrete pepsinogen, hydrochloric acid, and mucus into stomach chyme and gastrin into the blood. Impulses from parasympathetic neurons also increase stomach motility. Emotions such as anger, fear, and anxiety may slow digestion in the stomach because they stimulate the sympathetic nervous system, which inhibits gastric activity.

Gastric Phase

Once food reaches the stomach, sensory receptors in the stomach initiate both neural and hormonal mechanisms to ensure that gastric secretion and motility continue. This is the gastric phase of gastric digestion. Food of any kind distends (stretches) the stomach and stimulates stretch receptors in its walls. Chemoreceptors in the stomach monitor the pH of the stomach chyme. When the stomach walls are distended or pH increases because proteins have entered the stomach and glands and secreted some of the stomach acid, the stretch receptors and chemoreceptors are activated and a neural negative feedback loop is set in motion. From the stretch receptors and chemoreceptors, nerve impulses propagate to the submucosal plexus, where they activate parasympathetic and enteric neurons. The resulting nerve impulses cause waves of peristalsis and continue to stimulate the flow of gastric juice from parietal cells, chief cells, and mucous cells.

The peristaltic waves mix the food with gastric juice. When the waves become strong enough, a small quantity of chyme (about 10 to 15 mL) squirts past the pyloric sphincter into the duodenum. As the pH of the stomach chyme becomes more acidic again and the stomach walls are less distended because chyme has passed into the small intestine, a negative feedback cycle suppresses secretion of gastric juice. During the cephalic and gastric phases, digestion in the stomach is stimulated; during the intestinal phase, gastric juice secretion and gastric peristalsis are inhibited.

Hormonal negative feedback also regulates gastric secretions during the gastric phase. Partially digested proteins buffer H^+, thus increasing pH, and ingested food distends the stomach. Chemoreceptors and stretch receptors monitoring these changes stimulate parasympathetic neurons that release acetylcholine. In turn, acetylcholine stimulates secretion of the gastrin hormone by G cells, enteroendocrine cells in the mucosa of the pyloric antrum. (A small amount of gastrin is also secreted by enteroendocrine cells in the small intestine; additionally, some chemicals in food directly stimulate gastrin release.) Gastrin enters the bloodstream and finally reaches its target cells, the gastric glands.

Gastrin stimulates growth of the gastric glands and secretion of large amounts of gastric juice. It also strengthens contraction of the lower esophageal sphincter, increases motility of the stomach, and relaxes the pyloric and ileocecal sphincters (described later). Gastrin secretion is inhibited when the pH of gastric juice drops below 2.0 and is stimulated when the pH rises. This negative feedback mechanism helps provide an optimal low pH for the functioning of pepsin, the killing of microbes, and the denaturing of proteins in the stomach.

Acetylcholine released by parasympathetic neurons and gastrin secreted by G cells stimulate parietal cells to secrete more HCl in the presence of histamine. In other words, histamine, a paracrine substance released by mast cells in the lamina propria, acts on nearby parietal cells synergistically with acetylcholine and gastrin to enhance their effects. Receptors for all three substances are present in the plasma membranes of parietal cells. The histamine receptors on parietal cells are called H_2 receptors; they mediate different responses than do the H_1 receptors involved in allergic responses.

Intestinal Phase

The intestinal phase of gastric digestion is due to activation of receptors in the small intestine. While reflexes initiated during the cephalic and gastric phases stimulate stomach secretory activity and motility, those occurring during the intestinal phase have inhibitory effects that slow the exit of chyme from the stomach and prevent overloading of the duodenum with more chyme than it can handle. In addition, responses occurring during the intestinal phase promote the continued digestion of foods that have reached the small intestine. When chyme containing fatty acids and glucose leaves the stomach and enters the small intestine, it triggers enteroendocrine cells in the small intestinal mucosa to release into the blood two hormones that affect the stomach: secretin and cholecystokinin (CCK).

Regulation of Gastric Emptying

Gastric emptying, the periodic release of chyme from the stomach into the duodenum, is regulated by both neural and hormonal reflexes as follows:

1. Stimuli such as distention of the stomach and the presence of partially digested proteins, alcohol, and caffeine initiate gastric emptying.
2. These stimuli increase the secretion of gastrin and generate parasympathetic impulses in the vagus nerves.
3. Gastrin and nerve impulses stimulate contraction of the lower esophageal sphincter, increase motility of the stomach, and relax the pyloric sphincter.
4. The net effect of these actions is gastric emptying.

Neural and hormonal reflexes also help ensure that the stomach does not release more chyme than the small intestine can process. The neural reflex (or enterogastric reflex) and CCK inhibit gastric emptying as follows:

1. Stimuli such as distention of the duodenum and the presence of fatty acids, glucose, and partially digested proteins in the duodenal chyme inhibit gastric emptying.
2. These stimuli then initiate the enterogastric reflex. Nerve impulses propagate from the duodenum to the medulla oblongata where they inhibit parasympathetic stimulation and stimulate sympathetic activity in the stomach. The same stimuli also increase secretion of CCK.

3. Increased sympathetic impulses and CCK both decrease gastric motility.
4. The net effect of these actions is inhibition of gastric emptying.

Within 2 to 4 hours after a meal is eaten, the stomach has emptied its contents into the duodenum. Foods rich in carbohydrate spend the shortest time in the stomach; high protein foods remain somewhat longer, and emptying is slowest after a fat-laden meal containing large amounts of triglycerides. The reason for slower emptying after eating of triglycerides is that fatty acids in chyme stimulate release of CCK, which slows stomach emptying.

Vomiting or emesis is the forcible expulsion of the contents of the upper tract (stomach and sometimes duodenum) through the mouth. The strongest stimuli for vomiting are irritation and distension of the stomach; other stimuli include unpleasant sights, general anesthesia, dizziness, and certain drugs such as morphine and derivatives of digitalis. Nerve impulses are transmitted to the vomiting center in the medulla oblongata, and returning impulses propagate to the upper tract organs, diaphragm, and abdominal muscles. Vomiting involves squeezing the stomach between the diaphragm and abdominal muscles and expelling the contents through open esophageal sphincters. Prolonged vomiting, especially in infants and elderly people, can be serious because the loss of acidic gastric juice can lead to alkalosis (higher than normal blood pH).

From the stomach, chyme passes into the small intestine. Because chemical digestion in the small intestine depends on activities of the pancreas, liver, and gallbladder, we first consider the activities of these accessory digestive organs and their contributions to digestion in the small intestine.

Role and Composition of Bile

Each day, hepatocytes in the liver secrete 800 to 1000 mL (about a quart) of bile, a yellow, brownish, or olive-green liquid. Bile has a pH of 7.6 to 8.6 and consists mostly of water and bile acids, bile salts, cholesterol, a phospholipid called lecithin, bile pigments, and several ions.

Bile is partially an excretory product and partially a digestive secretion. Bile salts — sodium salts and potassium salts of bile acids (mostly cholic acid and chenodeoxycholic acid) play a role in emulsification, the breakdown of large lipid globules into a suspension of droplets about 1 µm in diameter, and in the absorption of lipids following their digestion. The tiny lipid droplets present a very large surface area that allows pancreatic lipase to more rapidly accomplish digestion of triglycerides. Cholesterol is made soluble in bile by bile salts and lecithin.

The principal bile pigment is conjugated bilirubin. The phagocytosis of aged red blood cells liberates iron, globin, and bilirubin (derived from heme). The iron and globin are recycled and some of the bilirubin is converted to conjugated bilirubin in which the bilirubin is attached to glucuronic acid molecules. Conjugated bilirubin is then secreted into the bile and is eventually broken down in the intestine. Stercobilin, one of its breakdown products, gives feces their normal brown color.

Regulation of Bile Secretion

After they have served their function as emulsifying agents, most bile salts are reabsorbed by active transport in the final segment of the small intestine (ileum) and enter portal blood flowing toward the liver. Although hepatocytes continually release bile, they increase production and secretion when the portal blood contains more bile acids; thus, as digestion and absorption continue in the small intestine, bile release increases. Between meals, after most absorption has occurred, bile flows into the gallbladder for storage because the sphincter of the hepatopancreatic ampulla closes off the entrance to the duodenum. After a meal, several neural and hormonal stimuli promote production and release of bile:

1. Parasympathetic impulses propagate along axons of the vagus nerve and stimulate the liver to increase bile production.
2. Fatty acids and amino acids in chyme entering the duodenum stimulate some duodenal enteroendocrine cells to secrete CCK into the blood. Acidic chyme entering the duodenum stimulates other enteroendocrine cells to secrete secretin into the blood.
3. CCK causes contraction of the wall of the gallbladder. This squeezes stored bile from the gallbladder into the cystic duct and through the common bile duct. CCK also causes relaxation of the sphincter of the hepatopancreatic ampulla and this allows bile to flow into the duodenum.
4. Secretin, which stimulates secretion of pancreatic juice rich in HCO_3, also stimulates the secretion of HCO_3^- by hepatocytes into bile.

Stretching of the stomach as it receives food and the buffering of gastric acids by proteins in food trigger the release of gastrin. Gastrin in turn promotes secretion of gastric juice and increases gastric motility so that ingested food becomes well mixed into a thick, soupy chyme. Reflux of the acidic chyme into the esophagus is prevented by tonic contraction of the lower esophageal sphincter, which is enhanced by gastrin.

The major stimulus for secretion of secretin is acidic chyme (high concentration of H^+) entering the small intestine. In turn, secretin promotes secretion of bicarbonate ions into pancreatic juice and bile. HCO_3^- acts to buffer (soak up) excess HCO_3. Besides these major effects, secretin inhibits secretion of gastric juice, promotes normal growth and maintenance of the pancreas, and enhances the effects of CCK. Overall, secretin causes buffering of acid in chyme that reaches the duodenum and slows production of acid in the stomach. Table 1.1 summarizes the hormones that control digestion.

Amino acids from partially digested proteins and fatty acids from partially digested triglycerides stimulate secretion of CCK by enteroendocrine cells in the mucosa of the small intestine. CCK stimulates secretion of pancreatic juice that is rich in digestive enzymes and ejection of bile into the duodenum, slows gastric emptying by promoting contraction of the pyloric sphincter, and produces satiety (feeling full to satisfaction) by acting on the hypothalamus in the brain. Like

TABLE 1.1
Major Hormones Controlling Digestion

Hormone	Stimulus and Site of Secretion	Actions
Gastrin	Distension of stomach, partially digested proteins and caffeine in stomach, and high pH of stomach chyme stimulate gastrin secretion by enteroendocrine G cells located mainly in mucosa of pyloric antrum of stomach	Major effects: Promotes secretion of gastric juice, increases gastric motility, and promotes growth of gastric mucosa Minor effects: Constricts lower esophageal sphincter; relaxes pyloric sphincter and ileocecal sphincter
Secretin	Acidic (high H^+ level) chyme that enters the small intestine stimulates secretion of secretin by enteroendocrine S cells in mucosa of duodenum	Major effects: Stimulates secretion of pancreatic juice and bile that are rich in bicarbonate ions Minor effects: Inhibits secretion of gastric juice, promotes normal growth and maintenance of pancreas, and enhances effects of CCK
CCK	Partially digested proteins (amino acids), triglycerides, and fatty acids that enter small intestine stimulate secretion of CCK by enteroendocrine CCK cells in mucosa of small intestine; CCK is also released in brain	Major effects: Stimulates secretion of pancreatic juice rich in digestive enzymes, causes ejection of bile from gallbladder and opening of sphincter of hepatopancreatic ampulla (sphincter of Oddi), induces satiety (feeling full to satisfaction) Minor effects: Inhibits gastric emptying, promotes normal growth and maintenance of pancreas, enhances effects of secretin

secretin, CCK promotes normal growth and maintenance of the pancreas; it also enhances the effects of secretin.

In addition to gastrin, secretin, and CCK, at least ten other so-called gut hormones are secreted by and have effects on the GI tract. They include motilin, substance P, and bombesin, all of which stimulate motility of the intestines. Vasoactive intestinal polypeptide (VIP) stimulates secretion of ions and water by the intestines and inhibits gastric acid secretion. Gastrin-releasing peptide stimulates release of gastrin; and somatostatin inhibits gastrin release. Some of these hormones are thought to act as local hormones, whereas others are secreted into the blood or even into the lumen of the GI tract. The physiological roles of these and other gut hormones are still under investigation.

Now that we have examined the sources of the main digestive enzymes and hormones, we can discuss the next part of the GI tract and continue the story of digestion and absorption. The major events of digestion and absorption occur in a long tube called the small intestine. Because most digestion and absorption of nutrients occur in the small intestine, its structure is specially adapted for these functions. Its length alone provides a large surface area for digestion and absorption, and that area is further increased by circular folds, villi, and microvilli. The small intestine begins at the pyloric sphincter of the stomach, coils through the central and inferior part of the abdominal cavity, and eventually opens into the large intestine. It averages 2.5 cm in diameter; its length is about 3 m in a living person and about 6.5 m in a cadaver due to the loss of smooth muscle tone after death.

Role of Intestinal Juice and Brush-Border Enzymes

Intestinal juice is a clear yellow fluid secreted in amounts of 1 to 2 liters a day. It contains water and mucus and is slightly alkaline (pH 7.6). Together, pancreatic and intestinal juices provide a liquid medium that aids the absorption of substances from chyme as they come in contact with the microvilli. The absorptive epithelial cells synthesize several digestive enzymes, called brush-border enzymes, and insert them into the plasma membranes of the microvilli. Thus, some enzymatic digestion occurs at the surfaces of the epithelial cells that line the villi rather than in the lumen exclusively, as occurs in other parts of the GI tract. Among the brush-border enzymes are four carbohydrate-digesting enzymes called a-dextrinase, maltase, sucrase, and lactase; protein-digesting enzymes called peptidases (aminopeptidase and dipeptidase); and two types of nucleotide-digesting enzymes, nucleosidases and phosphatases. Also, as cells slough off into the lumen of the small intestine, they break apart and release enzymes that help digest nutrients in the chyme.

Mechanical Digestion in Small Intestine

The two types of movements of the small intestine — segmentations and a type of peristalsis called a migrating motility complex (MMC) — are governed mainly by the myenteric plexus. Segmentations are localized, mixing contractions that occur in portions of intestine distended by a large volume of chyme. Segmentations mix chyme with the digestive juices and bring the particles of food into contact with the mucosa for absorption; they do not push the intestinal contents along the tract.

A segmentation starts with the contractions of circular muscle fibers in a portion of the small intestine, an action that constricts the intestine into segments. Next, muscle fibers that encircle the middle of each segment also contract, dividing each segment again. Finally, the fibers that first contracted relax, and each small segment unites with an adjoining small segment so that large segments are formed again. As this sequence of events repeats, the chyme sloshes back and forth. Segmentations occur most rapidly in the duodenum, about 12 times per minute, and progressively slow to about 8 times per minute in the ileum. This movement is similar to alternately squeezing the middle and then the ends of a capped tube of toothpaste.

After most of a meal has been absorbed, which lessens distention of the wall of the small intestine, segmentation stops and peristalsis begins. The type of peristalsis known as MMC that occurs in the small intestine begins in the lower portion of the stomach and pushes chyme forward along a short stretch of small intestine before dying out. The MMC slowly migrates down the small intestine, reaching the end of the ileum in 90 to 120 minutes; then another MMC begins in the stomach. Altogether, chyme remains in the small intestine for 3 to 5 hours.

Chemical Digestion in Small Intestine

Salivary amylase in the mouth converts starch (a polysaccharide) to maltose (a disaccharide), maltotriose (a trisaccharide), and a-dextrins (short-chain, branched fragments of starch with five to ten glucose units). In the stomach, pepsin converts proteins to peptides (small fragments of proteins), and lingual and gastric lipases convert some triglycerides into fatty acids, diglycerides, and monoglycerides. Thus, chyme entering the small intestine contains partially digested carbohydrates, proteins, and lipids. The completion of the digestion of carbohydrates, proteins, and lipids is a collective effort of pancreatic juice, bile, and intestinal juice in the small intestine.

Digestion of Carbohydrates

Although the action of salivary amylase may continue in the stomach for a while, the acidic pH of the stomach destroys salivary amylase and ends its activity. Thus, only a few starches are reduced to maltose by the time chyme leaves the stomach. Those starches not already broken down into maltose, maltotriose, and a-dextrins are cleaved by pancreatic amylase, an enzyme in pancreatic juice that acts in the small intestine. Although amylase acts on both glycogen and starches, it does not act on another polysaccharide, an indigestible plant fiber called cellulose. After amylase has split starch into smaller fragments, a brush-border enzyme called a-dextrinase acts on the resulting a-dextrins, clipping off one glucose unit at a time.

Ingested molecules of sucrose, lactose, and maltose (three disaccharides) are not acted on until they reach the small intestine. Three brush-border enzymes digest the disaccharides into monosaccharides. Sucrase breaks sucrose into a molecule of glucose and a molecule of fructose; lactase digests lactose into a molecule of glucose and a molecule of galactose; and maltase splits maltose and maltotriose into two or three molecules of glucose, respectively. Digestion of carbohydrates ends with the production of monosaccharides, as mechanisms exist for their absorption.

Lactose Intolerance

The mucosal cells of the small intestine of some people fail to produce enough lactase, an enzyme essential for the digestion of lactose. This results in a condition called lactose intolerance, in which undigested lactose in chyme retains fluid in the feces and bacterial fermentation of lactose results in the production of gases. Symptoms of lactose intolerance include diarrhea, gas, bloating, and abdominal cramps after consumption of milk and other dairy products. The severity of symptoms varies from relatively minor to sufficiently serious to require medical attention. Persons with lactose intolerance can take dietary supplements to aid in the digestion of lactose.

Digestion of Proteins

Protein digestion starts in the stomach, where proteins are fragmented into peptides by the action of pepsin. Enzymes in pancreatic juice — trypsin, chymotrypsin, carboxypeptidase, and elastase — continue to break proteins down into peptides. Although all these enzymes convert whole proteins into peptides, their actions differ somewhat because each splits peptide bonds between different amino acids. Trypsin, chymotrypsin, and elastase all cleave the peptide bond between a specific amino acid and its neighbor; carboxypeptidase breaks the peptide bond that attaches the terminal amino acid to the carboxyl (acid) end of the peptide. Protein digestion is completed by two peptidases in the brush border: aminopeptidase and dipeptidase. Aminopeptidase acts on peptides by breaking the peptide bond that attaches the terminal amino acid to the amino end of the peptide. Dipeptidase splits dipeptides into single amino acids.

Digestion of Lipids

The most abundant lipids in the diet are triglycerides consisting of a molecule of glycerol bonded to three fatty acid molecules. Enzymes that split triglycerides and phospholipids are called lipases. In adults, most lipid digestion occurs in the small intestine, although some occurs in the stomach through the action of lingual and gastric lipases. When chyme enters the small intestine, bile salts emulsify the globules of triglycerides into droplets about 11 μm in diameter. This increases the surface area exposed to pancreatic lipase, another enzyme in pancreatic juice. The enzyme hydrolyzes triglycerides into fatty acids and monoglycerides, the main end products of triglyceride digestion. Pancreatic and gastric lipases remove two of the three fatty acids from glycerol; the third remains attached to the glycerol, forming a monoglyceride.

Digestion of Nucleic Acids

Pancreatic juice contains two nucleases. Ribonuclease digests RNA and deoxyribonuclease digests DNA. The nucleotides that result from the action of the two nucleases are further digested by brush-border enzymes called nucleosidases and phosphatases into pentoses, phosphates, and nitrogenous bases. These products are absorbed via active transport.

Regulation of Intestinal Secretion and Motility

The most important mechanisms that regulate small intestinal secretion and motility are enteric reflexes that respond to the presence of chyme; vasoactive intestinal polypeptide also stimulates the production of intestinal juice. Segmentation movements depend mainly on intestinal distention, which initiates nerve impulses to the enteric plexuses and the central nervous system (CNS). Enteric reflexes and returning parasympathetic impulses from the CNS increase motility; sympathetic impulses decrease intestinal motility. Migrating motility complexes strengthen when most nutrients and water have been absorbed, that is, when the walls of the small intestine are less distended. With more vigorous peristalsis, the chyme moves along toward the large intestine as fast as 10 cm/sec. The first remnants of a meal reach the beginning of the large intestine in about 4 hr.

Absorption in Small Intestine

All the chemical and mechanical phases of digestion from the mouth through the small intestine are directed toward changing food into forms that can pass through the epithelial cells lining the mucosa and into the underlying blood and lymphatic vessels. These forms are monosaccharides (glucose, fructose, and galactose) from carbohydrates; single amino acids, dipeptides, and tripeptides from proteins; and fatty acids, glycerol, and monoglycerides from triglycerides. Passage of these digested nutrients from the gastrointestinal tract into the blood or lymph is called absorption.

Absorption of materials occurs via diffusion, facilitated diffusion, osmosis, and active transport. About 90% of all absorption of nutrients occurs in the small intestine; the other 10% occurs in the stomach and large intestine. Any undigested or unabsorbed material left in the small intestine passes on to the large intestine.

Absorption of Monosaccharides

All carbohydrates are absorbed as monosaccharides. The capacity of the small intestine to absorb monosaccharides is huge: an estimated 120 g/hr. As a result, all dietary carbohydrates that are digested normally are absorbed, leaving only indigestible cellulose and fibers in the feces. Monosaccharides pass from the lumen through the apical membrane via facilitated diffusion or active transport. Fructose, a monosaccharide found in fruits, is transported via facilitated diffusion; glucose and galactose are transported into epithelial cells of the villi via secondary active transport coupled to the active transport of Na^+. The transporter has binding sites for one glucose molecule and two sodium ions; unless all three sites are filled, neither substance is transported. Galactose competes with glucose to ride the same transporter. (Because both Na^+ and glucose or galactose move in the same direction, this is a symporter). The same type of Na^+ glucose symporter reabsorbs filtered blood glucose in the tubules of the kidneys. Monosaccharides then move out of the epithelial cells through their basolateral surfaces via facilitated diffusion and enter the capillaries of the villi.

Absorption of Amino Acids, Dipeptides, and Tripeptides

Most proteins are absorbed as amino acids via active transport processes that occur mainly in the duodenum and jejunum. About half of the absorbed amino acids are present in food; the other half come from proteins in digestive juices and dead cells that slough off the mucosal surface. Normally, 95 to 98% of the protein present in the small intestine is digested and absorbed. Several transporters carry different types of amino acids. Some amino acids enter epithelial cells of the villi via Na^+-dependent secondary active transport processes that are similar to the glucose transporter; other amino acids are actively transported by themselves. At least one symporter brings dipeptides and tripeptides together with H^+; the peptides then are hydrolyzed to single amino acids inside the epithelial cells. Amino acids move out of the epithelial cells via diffusion and enter capillaries of the villus. Both monosaccharides and amino acids are transported in the blood to the liver by way of the hepatic portal system. If not removed by hepatocytes, they enter the general circulation.

Absorption of Lipids

All dietary lipids are absorbed via simple diffusion. Adults absorb about 95% of the lipids present in the small intestine; due to their lower production of bile, newborn infants absorb only about 85% of lipids. As a result of their emulsification and digestion, triglycerides are broken down into monoglycerides and fatty acids. Recall that lingual and pancreatic lipases remove two of the three fatty acids from glycerol during digestion of a triglyceride; the other fatty acid remains attached to glycerol, thus forming a monoglyceride. The small amount of short-chain (fewer than 10 to 12 carbon atoms) fatty acids in the diet passes into the epithelial cells via simple diffusion and follows the same route taken by monosaccharides and amino acids into blood capillaries of villi.

Most dietary fatty acids, however, are long-chain types. They and monoglycerides reach the bloodstream by a different route and require bile for adequate absorption. Bile salts are amphipathic; they have both polar and nonpolar (hydrophobic) portions. They can form tiny spheres 2 to 10 nm in diameter called micelles that include 20 to 50 bile salt molecules. Because they are small and have polar portions of bile salt molecules at their surfaces, micelles can dissolve in the water of intestinal fluid. In contrast, partially digested dietary lipids can dissolve in the nonpolar central cores of micelles. It is in this form that fatty acids and monoglycerides reach the epithelial cells of the villi.

At the apical surfaces of the epithelial cells, fatty acids and monoglycerides diffuse into the cells, leaving the micelles behind in chyme. The micelles continually repeat this ferrying function. When chyme reaches the ileum, 90 to 95% of the bile salts are reabsorbed and returned by the blood to the liver. Salt secretion by hepatocytes into bile, reabsorption by the ileum, and resecretion into bile constitute the enterohepatic circulation. Insufficient bile salts, due either to obstruction of the bile ducts or removal of the gallbladder, can result in the loss of up to 40% of dietary lipids in feces due to diminished lipid absorption. Moreover, when lipids are not absorbed properly, the fat-soluble A, D, E, and K vitamins are not adequately absorbed.

Within the epithelial cells, many monoglycerides are further digested by lipase to glycerol and fatty acids. The fatty acids and glycerol are then recombined to form triglycerides that aggregate into globules along with phospholipids and cholesterol and become coated with proteins. These large (about 80 nm in diameter) spherical masses are called chylomicrons. The hydrophilic protein coats keep the chylomicrons suspended and prevent them from sticking to each other. Chylomicrons leave the epithelial cell via exocytosis. Because they are so large and bulky, chylomicrons cannot enter blood capillaries in the small intestine; instead, they enter the much leakier lacteals. From there they are transported by way of lymphatic vessels to the thoracic duct and enter the blood at the left subclavian vein.

Within 10 min after their absorption, about half the chylomicrons have already been removed from the blood as they pass through capillaries in the liver and adipose tissue. This removal is accomplished by the lipoprotein lipase enzyme in capillary endothelial cells that breaks down triglycerides in chylomicrons and other lipoproteins into fatty acids and glycerol. The fatty acids diffuse into hepatocytes and adipose cells and combine with glycerol during resynthesis of triglycerides. Two or three hours after a meal, few chylomicrons remain in the blood.

Absorption of Electrolytes

Many of the electrolytes absorbed by the small intestine come from gastrointestinal secretions; some are contained in ingested foods and liquids. Sodium ions are actively transported out of intestinal epithelial cells by sodium–potassium pumps (Na^+/K^+ ATPase) after they have moved into epithelial cells via diffusion and secondary active transport. Thus, most sodium ions in gastrointestinal secretions are reclaimed and not lost in the feces. Negatively charged bicarbonate, chloride, iodide, and nitrate ions can passively follow Na^+ or be actively transported. Calcium ions also are absorbed actively in a process stimulated by calcitriol. Other electrolytes such as iron, potassium, magnesium, and phosphate ions also are absorbed via active transport mechanisms.

Absorption of Vitamins

The fat-soluble A, D, E, and K vitamins are included with ingested dietary lipids in micelles and are absorbed via simple diffusion. Most water-soluble vitamins, such as most B vitamins and vitamin C, also are absorbed via simple diffusion. Vitamin B_{12}, however, combines with intrinsic factor produced by the stomach and the combination is absorbed in the ileum via an active transport mechanism.

Absorption of Water

The total volume of fluid that enters the small intestine each day (about 9.3 liters) comes from ingestion of liquids (about 2.3 liters) and from various gastrointestinal secretions (about 7.0 liters). The small intestine absorbs about 8.3 liters of the fluid; the remainder passes into the large intestine, where most of the remainder (about 0.9 liter) is also absorbed. Total water excretion in the feces is normally limited to a tenth of a liter per day.

All water absorption in the GI tract occurs via osmosis from the lumen of the intestines through epithelial cells and into blood capillaries. Because water can move across the intestinal mucosa in both directions, the absorption of water from the small intestine depends on the absorption of electrolytes and nutrients to maintain an osmotic balance with the blood. The absorbed electrolytes, monosaccharides, and amino acids establish a concentration gradient for water that promotes water absorption via osmosis. Table 1.2 summarizes the digestive activities of the pancreas, liver, gallbladder, and small intestine.

Mechanical Digestion in Large Intestine

The passage of chyme from the ileum into the cecum is regulated by the action of the ileocecal sphincter. Normally, the valve remains partially closed so that the passage of chyme into the cecum occurs slowly. Immediately after a meal, a gastroileal reflex intensifies ileal peristalsis and forces any chyme in the ileum into the cecum. The gastrin hormone also relaxes the sphincter. Whenever the cecum is distended, the degree of contraction of the ileocecal sphincter intensifies.

Movements of the colon begin when substances pass the ileocecal sphincter. Because chyme moves through the small intestine at a fairly constant rate, the time required for a meal to pass into the colon is determined by gastric emptying time. As food passes through the ileocecal sphincter, it fills the cecum and accumulates in the ascending colon.

One movement characteristic of the large intestine is haustral churning. In this process, the haustra remain relaxed and become distended as they fill up. When the distension reaches a certain point, the walls contract and squeeze the contents into the next haustrum. Peristalsis also occurs, although at a slower rate (3 to 12 contractions per minute) than in more proximal portions of the tract. A final type of movement is mass peristalsis, a strong peristaltic wave that begins at about the middle of the transverse colon and quickly drives the contents of the colon into the rectum. Because food in the stomach initiates this gastrocolic reflex in the colon, mass peristalsis usually takes place three or four times a day, during or immediately after a meal.

Chemical Digestion in Large Intestine

The final stage of digestion occurs in the colon through the activity of bacteria that inhabit the lumen. Mucus is secreted by the glands of the large intestine, but no enzymes are secreted. Chyme is prepared for elimination by the action of bacteria that ferment any remaining carbohydrates and release hydrogen, carbon dioxide, and methane gases. These gases contribute to flatus in the colon, termed flatulence when it is excessive. Bacteria also convert any remaining proteins to

TABLE 1.2
Digestive Activities in Pancreas, Liver, Gallbladder, and Small Intestine

Structure	Locations	Activity
Pancreas		Delivers pancreatic juice into duodenum via pancreatic duct
Liver		Produces bile (bile salts) necessary for emulsification and absorption of lipids
Gallbladder		Stores, concentrates, and delivers bile into duodenum via common bile duct
Small intestine		Major site of digestion and absorption of nutrients and water in GI tract
Mucosa/submucosa		
	Intestinal glands	Secrete intestinal juice
	Duodenal (Brunner's) glands	Secrete alkaline fluid to buffer stomach acids and mucus for protection and lubrication
	Microvilli	Microscopic membrane-covered projections of epithelial cells containing brush-border enzymes that increase surface area for digestion and absorption
Villi		Finger-like projections of mucosa that are sites of absorption of digested food and increase surface area for digestion and absorption
Circular folds		Folds of mucosa and submucosa that increase surface area for digestion and absorption
Muscularis		
	Segmentation	Alternating contractions of circular smooth muscle fibers that produce segmentation and resegmentation of sections of small intestine; mixes chyme with digestive juices and brings food into contact with mucosa for absorption
	Migrating motility complex	Type of peristalsis consisting of waves of contraction and relaxation of circular and longitudinal smooth muscle fibers passing length of small intestine; moves chyme toward ileocecal sphincter

amino acids and break down the amino acids into simpler substances: indole, skatole, hydrogen sulfide, and fatty acids. Some indole and skatole are eliminated in the feces and contribute to their odor; the rest is absorbed and transported to the liver where they are converted to less toxic compounds and excreted in the urine. Bacteria also decompose bilirubin to simpler pigments including the stercobilin that gives feces their brown color. Several vitamins needed for normal metabolism, including some B vitamins and vitamin K, are bacterial products that are absorbed in the colon.

Absorption and Feces Formation in Large Intestine

By the time chyme has remained in the large intestine 3 to 10 hours, it has become solid or semisolid because of water absorption and is called feces. Chemically, feces consist of water, inorganic salts, sloughed-off epithelial cells from the mucosa of the gastrointestinal tract, bacteria, products of bacterial decomposition, unabsorbed digested materials, and indigestible parts of food.

Although 90% of all water absorption occurs in the small intestine, the large intestine absorbs enough to make it an important organ in maintaining the body's water balance. Of the 0.5 to 1.0 liter of water that enters the large intestine, all but about 100 to 200 mL is absorbed via osmosis. The large intestine also absorbs ions including sodium and chloride and some vitamins.

Occult Blood

Occult blood is hidden; it is not detectable by the human eye. The main diagnostic value of occult blood testing is to screen for colorectal cancer. Two substances often examined for occult blood are feces and urine. Several types of products are available for at-home testing for hidden blood in feces. The tests are based on color changes when reagents are added to the feces. The presence of occult blood in urine may be detected at home by using dip-and-read reagent strips.

Defecation Reflex

Mass peristaltic movements push fecal material from the sigmoid colon into the rectum. The resulting distention of the rectal wall stimulates stretch receptors and this initiates a defecation reflex that empties the rectum. The defecation reflex occurs as follows. In response to distention of the rectal wall, the receptors send sensory nerve impulses to the sacral spinal cord. Motor impulses from the cord travel along parasympathetic nerves back to the descending colon, sigmoid colon, rectum, and anus. The resulting contraction of the longitudinal rectal muscles shortens the rectum, thereby increasing the pressure within it. This pressure, along with voluntary contractions of the diaphragm and abdominal muscles and parasympathetic stimulation opens the internal anal sphincter.

Diarrhea is an increase in the frequency, volume, and fluid content of the feces caused by increased motility of and decreased absorption by the intestines. When chyme passes too quickly through the small intestine and feces pass too quickly through the large intestine, there is not enough time for absorption. Frequent diarrhea can result in dehydration and electrolyte imbalances. Excessive motility may be caused by lactose intolerance, stress, and microbes that irritate the gastrointestinal mucosa.

Constipation is infrequent or difficult defecation caused by decreased motility of the intestines. Because the feces remain in the colon for prolonged periods, excessive water absorption occurs, and the feces become dry and hard. Constipation may be caused by poor habits (delaying defecation), spasms of the colon, insufficient fiber in the diet, inadequate fluid intake, lack of exercise, emotional stress, and certain drugs. A common treatment is a mild laxative such as milk of magnesia to induce defecation. However, many physicians maintain that laxatives are habit-forming, and that adding fiber to the diet, increasing the amount of exercise, and increasing fluid intake are safer ways of controlling this common problem.

Dietary Fiber

Dietary fiber consists of indigestible plant carbohydrates such as cellulose, lignin, and pectin found in fruits, vegetables, grains, and beans. Insoluble fiber that does not dissolve in water includes the woody or structural parts of plants such as the skins of fruits and vegetables and the bran coatings around wheat and corn kernels. Insoluble fiber passes through the GI tract largely unchanged but speeds the passage of material through the tract. Soluble fiber that dissolves in water forms a gel that slows the passage of material through the tract. It is found in abundance in beans, oats, barley, broccoli, prunes, apples, and citrus fruits.

REFERENCES

1. Guyton, A.C. and Hall, J.E., *Textbook of Medical Physiology*, 9th ed., W.B. Saunders, Philadelphia, 1996.
2. Hamm, A.W., *Histology*, 7th Ed., J.B. Lippincott Co., Philadelphia, 1974.
3. Kumer, V., Abbas, A.D., and Fausto, N., *Pathologic Basis of Disease*, 7th ed., Elsevier Saunders, Philadelphia, 2005.
4. Sodeman, W.A. and Sodeman, T.M., *Sodeman's Pathologic Physiology*, W.B. Saunders, Philadelphia, 1974.
5. Tortura, G.J. and Grabowski, S.R., The digestive system, in *Principles of Anatomy and Physiology*, John Wiley & Sons, New York, 2003, p. 852.

2 Methods for Analysis of Gastrointestinal Function

Robin C. Guy

CONTENTS

INTRODUCTION

The gastrointestinal (GI) tract is very complex. It performs numerous functions, many of which may be assessed through proven methodology. A number of the published tests for GI functionality are targeted for the human population, but many tests may also be utilized in laboratory animals. Numerous methods can assess GI functionality appropriate for preclinical testing *in vivo* and *in vitro*. GI functions include transit, absorption, digestion, secretion, microflora, immunity, and viscerosensitivity (abdominal pain). Specific tests and models for functional analyses are also mentioned in this chapter.

It is estimated that 60 to 70 million people are affected by all digestive diseases.[1] Fourteen million people required hospitalization for digestive-related diseases in 2002; of all inpatient hospitalization procedures, 6 million were for digestive diagnostic and therapeutic procedures. This chapter will primarily discuss non-clinical methods of analyses needed to assist in the interpretation of GI effects and models used for specific functionality assessments. Determination of the selection of a model is not a cut-and-dried process. For example, for *in vitro* analyses, numerous endogenous interactions are not possible. Homogenization of tissue, for instance, usually inactivates various messenger systems, as in the adenylate cyclase systems and ion channels, e.g., Ca^{2+} channels. However, *in vitro* studies can provide beneficial data.[2]

Many *in vivo* responses are affected by a variety of factors. Responses may be different in a variety of situations, for example, anesthetized versus unanesthetized animals, animals with open abdomens in surgical situations versus post-surgical animals, and fed versus fasted animals. For both *in vitro* or *in vivo* studies, tissues may release chemicals (e.g., prostaglandins, leukotrienes, enzymes) when activated, dissected, damaged, made ischemic, and exposed to unusual stress. As another example, myogenic activities of the GI muscles are affected by *in vitro* conditions as the frequency is reduced from uncoupling of higher frequency oscillators or from coupled oscillators originating from the same or different muscle layers. Any study conducted *in vitro* or *in vivo* must take a variety of factors into consideration and both qualitative and quantitative conclusions in addition to extrapolations should be drawn on a battery of studies, not on a single independent study. Additional factors to consider are reviewed by Daniel et al.[2]

TRANSIT

Transit (how materials mix and progress through the GI tract) is one of the main functions of the tract. Different areas have distinct functions. Transit is controlled primarily by three mechanisms: myogenic, neural, and chemical.[3] A myogenic mechanism is an electrical control activity (ECA) generated in the smooth muscle that affects resting membrane potential, frequency and periodic oscillations of membrane potential, and phase relationships in adjacent cells. Neural mechanisms concern control of the extrinsic and intrinsic nerves. Chemical mechanisms are various substances released from the nerves, cells, and glands. Transit occurs in the esophagus, stomach, small intestines, and colon.

GI motility may be studied in isolated single smooth muscle cell preparations that are widely available in a variety of species including guinea pigs, dogs, rabbits, and humans.[2] Cell lines for *in vitro* analyses of GI function and analyses are described in Zweibaum et al.[35] In addition, human intestinal smooth muscle cells have been shown to retain their sensitivity to stimuli for at least 6 days into culture.

ESOPHAGEAL TRANSIT

The motility of the esophagus is relatively easy to study in humans because it is readily accessible. Control of motility is more difficult to analyze because normal human tissue is not readily available. The human esophagus consists of striated muscle in the proximal one-third to one-half and smooth muscle in the remaining length.[4] In common laboratory animals, namely dogs, cats, rats, and mice, the esophagus is primarily composed of striated muscle. Many marsupials and some non-human primates have tissue in similar proportions to humans. The use of an appropriate laboratory animal model may be restrictive, but the North American opossum (Didelphys sp.) has been used as an animal model.[4] Additional animals used to study esophageal function include the Australian possum and non-human primates.

The movement of food in the esophagus has been shown to be inhibited by muscarinic blockers (antimuscarinic, anticholinergic).[5]

An esophagoscopy is a convenient method for the observation of the esophagus, especially the lower portion.[6] It is also useful for obtaining biopsy samples and cytologic brushings in cases of suspected cancer. Animals may need to be anesthetized to prevent discomfort through the procedure.

Intraluminal pressure studies of the esophagus are used to detect achalasia and motor disorders of the muscle tissue and sphincter. A thin catheter with pressure sensors imbedded in the wall is inserted into the esophagus. The outer end of the catheter is attached to a transducer that records pressure. The catheter records the duration and sequence of esophageal contractions, including assessments of the integrated muscle activities of the different types of muscle in the esophageal wall. In addition, *in vivo* studies in which pressure gauges have been surgically implanted at specific points along the esophagus to record findings have been conducted.[7]

Verapamil is a calcium channel blocker that was tested to determine its efficacy as a treatment for esophageal disorders.[8] In the baboon, verapamil inhibits the amplitude of esophageal contractions in the smooth muscle section of the esophagus and decreases the lower esophageal sphincter pressure. To determine this, baboons were fasted for 24 hours and then anesthetized with ketamine hydrochloride prior to placement in restraint chairs. An esophageal manometric catheter was inserted through the nose and into the stomach. The catheter was slowly pulled across the gastroesophageal junction until the distal sleeve sensor recorded lower esophageal sphincter pressure. Based on the design of the catheter, this placement resulted in the measurement of primary striated muscle activity and smooth muscle activity.

The rhesus monkey (*Macaca mulatta*) was used in manometric studies to compare data obtained from similar human studies.[9] A small triple-lumen catheter was constructed. Animals were fasted overnight and placed supine in restraining boxes. A pneumographic belt was placed around the chest or upper abdomen to record breathing. A disruption in the rhythmic respiratory waves indicated the act of swallowing. The catheter was placed through the mouth to the stomach. The catheter was then withdrawn at 0.5 to 1 cm increments to record pressure at each site. The study measured resting gastric pressure, gastroesophageal pressure gradient, the point of respiratory phase reversal, sphincter tone (inferior and superior esophageal sphincter), primary and secondary peristalsis (at the upper, middle, and lower third of the esophagus), and diffuse spasms. This study concluded that there were functional esophageal similarities in the macaque and human.

Myoelectric activity of the esophagus can also be recorded *in vivo* utilizing bipolar or monopolar electrodes.[7] This provides a more precise measurement of muscle activity than does pressure recording. The electrodes are sewn into the outside of the esophagus. The measurements indicate the sum of activities in the various muscle layers.

Motor activity can also be studied *in vitro*.[7] Strips of the esophageal muscle tissue are bathed in oxygenated physiologic solutions. These tissues are connected to force transducers. Chemicals of interest may be added to the solutions to determine their effect on motor function. In addition, intracellular microelectrodes may be used to determine the electrical activity of individual esophageal smooth muscle cells.[7]

Forceful reverse peristalsis occurs during emesis. Emesis can occur in dogs and cats and most of the time in monkeys, but not in rats, mice, or rabbits. Prolonged or repeated emesis may be responsible for alterations in normal electrolyte concentrations. Blood samples may be obtained to determine whether electrolytes have been affected.

GASTRIC EMPTYING

Gastric emptying is the process by which the contents of the stomach (chyme) are moved into the duodenum. Three types of movements occur in the full stomach: peristaltic waves, systolic contractions of the terminal antrum, and reduction of the size of the stomach. It has been determined that liquids leave the stomach earlier than solids, and smaller solid particles leave the stomach earlier than larger particles.[10,11]

At fasting, the intraluminal pressure in the stomach is equal to the intra-abdominal pressure.[10] In a study to determine the effects of pressure on a full stomach, pressure was recorded in a vagally innervated pouch of the fundus of the stomach of a dog.[10] The effects of gastric emptying may be measured by the x-ray of radio-opaque particles.[12] Beagle dogs were fasted for approximately 15 hours. Various sized radio-opaque particles (1 to 3 mm in diameter) were prepared and placed into size 000 gelatin capsules. The capsules were administered orally to the dogs (fasted or 5 minutes after a meal). Following administration of the capsule, the dogs were x-rayed every 2 to 3 minutes for the first 15 minutes, and every 15 minutes thereafter to determine the locations of the particles.

An assessment of the difference in the motility of large and small particles as well as liquids in the canine stomach was described.[11] A duodenal fistula was surgically implanted in the dogs. Cubes of beef liver labeled with ^{57}[Co]cyanocobalamine were fed to the dogs as the digestible solid food. Plastic spheres (7 mm) were fed as indigestible solid food. The liquid food was a dextrose solution tagged with polyethylene [1,2-^{3}H]glycol. Samples of the duodenal contents were aspirated through a tube inserted into the fistula at various time points. The radioactivity for each marker was determined. The effects of test material administered prior to feeding on the motility of different food particle size and consistency can be determined.

The effect of liquid nutrient loads on gastric emptying was assessed in the rhesus monkey, *Macaca mulatta*.[13] Intragastric cannulas (41 mm ID × 76 mm OD) were surgically implanted in the male monkeys in the stomach dorsal to the greater curvature. The end of the cannula was externalized by the left side of the spine and through the intercostal space at the level of the stomach. Canvas jackets were placed on the monkeys for protection. In addition, the exterior cannula was placed in a flexible steel cable that extended to the back of the cage so that infusions could be performed without handling the monkeys. The monkeys' movements were unrestricted. They were allowed to recover from surgery for 2 weeks before the gastric emptying experiments. Prior to the experiments, animals were fasted for 16 hours. In addition, to determine the status of the contents in the stomach 1 hour prior to the start of the study, 50 mL of isotonic saline (0.15 M NaCl) at 37°C was infused, then immediately withdrawn from the stomach. If the stomach was empty of any food contents, the studies were conducted. Test materials were administered to the monkeys followed by the liquid nutrient loading (100 mL) 30 minutes later. A marker consisting of non-nutritive phenol red dye was mixed with the test loads. Ten minutes later, the material remaining in the stomach was withdrawn and the stomach was repeatedly washed with saline until traces of the dye were no longer present. The volume of material remaining in the stomach was then determined by dye dilution spectrophotometry. This method may be used to determine the gastric inhibitory effect of a test material.

Other factors can affect transit time. Liquid gastric emptying time was delayed in diabetic hyperglycemic rats.[14] Intraperitoneal injections of a synthetic cholecystokinin slowed the gastric emptying of both liquid and solid food in rats.[15] In addition, electromechanical changes from canine fundal and antral smooth muscle preparations have been shown to have different responses to nerve stimulation which accounts for their physiologic responses *in vivo*.[16]

MOTILITY OF SMALL INTESTINE

The chyme that leaves the stomach is moved down into the duodenum. Once in the intestine, it moves slowly via short, weak propulsive movements to allow for digestion and absorption. In the dog, propulsive activity has been measured by injecting body-temperature isotonic saline into the upper small intestine at a pressure of 1 Hg.[10] The amount of time it takes for a specific volume of fluid to be transported is an indication of the intestinal motility. The rate of transport is affected by feeding, as the rate is reduced by 80%. This reduction is due to increased intestinal contractions that narrow the lumen, thereby increasing resistance to transport. The rate of transport is also affected by atonic conditions, where movement would be rapid since there is less resistance. Morphine and castor oil have also been shown to effect transit, and these could be used as positive controls. Morphine causes inhibitory neurons to be suppressed, thereby causing spasms in the duodenum. Morphine also increases phasic and tonic activities of the smooth muscles in the GI tract. These effects slow down transport and may cause increased absorption of water from the feces, which may lead to constipation. Castor oil (ricinoleic acid) causes a transient increased activity followed by a prolonged inhibition.[10]

Safety pharmacologic studies have been designed to determine the effects of drugs on the GI tract. Chapter 3 is devoted to this discussion. However, one study determines the GI propulsion effects of a drug and will be discussed briefly. In this study, the test article is administered to a rat. A 10% suspension of activated charcoal in aqueous methylcellulose is administered by oral gavage to the animal. The rats are then euthanized 30 minutes after receiving the charcoal suspension. The intestines are removed and laid out on moist paper. The distance that the charcoal traveled is evaluated and compared to control animals to determine increased or decreased transit.

Rats were used to examine small intestinal transit specifically.[17] Since gastric emptying is variable, intraduodenal injections were made for consistency. Male rats weighing approximately 200 to 300 kg were used. They underwent intraduodenal intubation 5 days prior to the study. Further details are described in detail in the manuscript. The procedure did not obstruct the duodenum or interfere with normal eating and drinking. A variety of treatments were used to alter intestinal propulsion. Drugs (0.5 mL) were administered 2 hours prior to killing the animals. The solution administered intraduodenally was Krebs 0.1 M phosphate buffer with 100 mg glucose, 2.0 mg polyethylene glycol, 0.5 mg phenol red, and 100 μC of chromium as the sodium salt of chromate ($NA_2^{51}CrO_4$). Control animals were killed at 0, 15, 30, and 60 minutes after the intraduodenal injections. To prevent the movement of ^{51}Cr during dissection and removal of the intestines, ligatures were placed at various points as soon as the animals were killed. In increasing magnitude of slowed propulsion, morphine sulfate (10 mg/kg intramuscularly with epinephrine), chlorisondamine chloride (ganglionic blocking agent, 8 mg/kg subcutaneously) and mecamylamine hydrochloride (ganglionic blocking agent, 10 mg/kg subcutaneously) had greater retarding effects on propulsion than other drugs. The leading edge traveled a shorter distance in the intestine than in the control animals. Accelerated propulsion was obtained by irradiation (whole body radiation, 1400 R at 75 R/minute).

Another study determined the effects of certain drugs on the motility of the rat small intestine and investigated whether motility affects small intestinal bacterial flora.[18] Under conditions of extreme stagnation of motility, significant bacterial overgrowth was found.

To determine effects on the myoelectric complex of the movement of the fasting intestine, unanesthetized dogs may be used.[10] Dogs are fasted for 12 hours before observations are performed. The dogs previously had surgically implanted electrodes placed in a row on the serosal surface of the gastric antrum and along the entire length of the small intestine. The leads from the electrodes are fed through to the surface of the body. Strain gauges may be sewn into muscle to determine movement. Catheters may be inserted into the lumen to measure pressure. After the animal has recovered from surgery, the electrical activity can then be monitored under a variety of test conditions. Contract medium can also be injected through the catheter so that cinefluorography can be utilized to observe the motility of the intestinal contents.

MOTILITY OF LARGE INTESTINE

Many of the preceding techniques can be used to track transit in the large intestine. However, the motility of the large intestine is not as regular and is more variable than that of the stomach and small intestine. As with the small intestine and the stomach, specific hormones and peptides may affect the motility in the colon. Stimulation of motility is produced by gastrin, cholecystokinin, substance P, and enkephalins, while motility is inhibited by glucagons, vasoactive intestinal polypeptide, and secretin.[5] A comparative anatomical study of the distal end of the colon was conducted in eight mammalian species.[19] Due to the extreme differences in the anatomy and physiology of the colon, there appears to be no ideal animal model for studies of the large intestine.[20] However, specific aspects of colonic motility have been investigated.

The motility in the large intestines was examined in the cat.[21] Highly sensitive semiconductor strain gage transducers were implanted extraluminally to detect colonic motility as it is affected by stimulation of areas of the central nervous system. Three transducers per animal were attached to the surface of the colon transversely. They were attached to the colon near the cecum, at the middle part of the colon, and at the sigmoid colon. The transducers did not appear to interfere with the spontaneous activity of the colon. Intraluminal transducers were also surgically placed in the colon through small antimesenteric incisions of the intestinal wall. Pressure was recorded by the intraluminal transducers by means of balloons filled with water, or by open ended tubes filled with saline.

The intraluminal balloons were sometimes observed to induce some degree of colonic activity. In addition, solid or semisolid fecal mass blocked the open-ended tubing on occasion. It was determined that for the feline colon, the extraluminal strain gage transducer was able to record the movements of various segments of the colon directly, while intraluminal recordings both with balloons or open ended tubes were only able to record activity in a specific area. Although the extraluminal transducer provided more sensitive readings, it was not able to differentiate between contractile activity in longitudinal and circular muscle layers. In the same study, it was determined that deep anesthesia was associated with decreased peristaltic motility, and minimal to no effects of nerve stimulation. However, light anesthesia produced artifacts and a muscle relaxing agent was needed.

Many drugs exert effects on the function of the large intestine.[20,22] These may be used to analyze or compare the motility of the colon or a colonic effect in *in vivo* or *in vitro* studies. The drugs cited should not be construed as a complete list or include drugs that affect the entire large intestine; that may not be the case with all of the drugs. Alpha-adrenergic drugs increase contractions in circular muscle, but inhibit contractions on the longitudinal muscle of the cat colon. Beta-agonists and dopamine cause inhibition of motility. The effects of atropine and other anticholenergics on motility vary, depending on the methodology; however, there may be a very small and brief inhibitory effect of atropine *in vivo*. *In vitro* studies with atropine showed no effect on the electromyogram or spontaneous contractions of the circular layer of the cat colon; however, it decreased spontaneous contractions of the longitudinal muscle layer. Substance P increases potent contractions of the circular muscle layer. Metenkephalin increases motility in the cat intestine. Bradykinin inhibits motility in both layers of the muscle *in vivo*, but at high concentrations *in vitro*, stimulates the longitudinal muscle layer. Cholecystokinin stimulates the circular muscle layers *in vivo*. Angiotensin increases the contractions in both layers *in vitro*. Morphine increases the intensity of the spike activity and prolongs the duration of slow waves in the cat colon *in vitro*. Gamma-aminobutyric acid induces a temporary relaxation in both layers of the guinea pig colon. As discussed for the small intestine, castor oil increases colonic activity.

Numerous cell lines for colonic function assays have been established and are described in Zweibaum, et al.[35]

SECRETIONS

Secretions in the GI tract include gastric acid, hormones, bile, enzymes, electrolytes, and mucus. Some examples of tests for the analyses of these secretions are listed below, although they do not constitute a complete list.

Gastric acid determination is a procedure to evaluate gastric secretion function by measuring the amount of acid secreted from the stomach.[23] This is the most widely practiced procedure in humans.[24] In humans, it is often used in conjunction with the gastric acid stimulation test, a procedure that measures gastric acid output after injection of a drug to stimulate gastric acid secretion. In fasted animals, a flexible tube is inserted through the mouth or nasogastrically to the stomach, with proper positioning confirmed by fluoroscopy or x-ray. After a short acclimation period, specimens are obtained every 15 minutes for a period of 90 minutes. The first two specimens are discarded to eliminate gastric contents that might be affected by the stress of the intubation process. The specimens are then analyzed for gastric acid. A gastric acid stimulation test may be conducted immediately after the last gastric sampling. Pentagastrin or a similar drug that stimulates gastric acid output is injected subcutaneously. Specimens are collected every 15 minutes for 1 hour and analyzed for gastric secretions.

The effects of intragastric acid and pH changes may be monitored by a disposable radiotelemetric pH sensor, the Heidelberg capsule.[12,25,26] Capsules were calibrated prior to the surgery and the calibration was checked after the completion of the study. In addition, gastric juices were aspirated through a stomach tube inserted orally and the accuracy of the pH readings from the capsule was assessed by measuring the pH with a conventional pH meter. In one study, a length of surgical suture was attached to the Heidelberg capsule and held in place to ensure that the capsule would remain in the stomach.[9] In this manner, the pH of the stomach could be monitored continuously throughout the study. In another study, the capsule was allowed to traverse through the GI tract for collection of pH data both in the stomach and the small intestine.[26]

The effects of gastrointestinal hormones on function of the GI tract have been examined. Gastric inhibitory peptide has an insulinotropic action that was studied in humans, dogs, and rats.[27] Gastric inhibitory peptide is normally released after ingestion of carbohydrates and fats and after intraduodenal infusions of amino acids. Dogs with indwelling venous catheters and gastric fistulas were utilized and were fed peptone meals to determine the responses of gastric inhibitory peptide and serum insulin and glucose levels. This study was able to detect gastric inhibitory peptide release due to the utilization of a sensitive radioimmunoassay method for measuring gastric inhibitory peptide. A gastrin-deficient mouse was genetically developed to investigate the role of this peptide hormone in the development and function of the stomach.[28] It was determined that gastrin is critical for the function of the acid secretory system.

Bile is secreted from the liver. It is stored in humans and some other animals in the gallbladder and released into the duodenum. If the functionality of the liver, gallbladder, or ducts is compromised, changes in blood chemistry values may be observed. Extrahepatic cholestasis occurs when the flow of bile is obstructed and bile acids leak into the plasma.[29] Other changes may be observed in bilirubin, enzymes, and electrolytes.

Testing for pancreatic exocrine function can be conducted via a variety of assays.[24] These include tests that quantify pancreatic secretion through gastroduodenal intubation, studies that assess exocrine function indirectly using an orally administered test substance, tests that measure fat or pancreatic enzyme activity in feces, and measurement of pancreatic serum enzyme activity. Pancreatic secretions contain enzymes and an alkaline fluid to help neutralize the acid entering the duodenum. In humans, cats, and dogs, the pancreas secretes primarily during digestion.[30] Rats, sheep, and rabbits are continuous feeders and their pancreas secretes continuously. The centroacinar cells and duct cells secrete the alkaline fluid, and secretion of this fluid is stimulated by secretin and cholecystokinin.[24,30–32] Any chemical that affects the function of these cells will affect the material in the GI tract. Pancreatic fluid may be collected from animals for analysis using a surgically placed duodenal fistula with a tube placed opposite the pancreatic duct. In addition, secretions of amylase can be measured from pancreatic lobule preparations from which the lobules were excised and incubated in a medium.[33]

Calcium is secreted primarily in the jejunum and ileum and is stimulated by mucosal sodium and somatostatin.[34]

Rat cell lines have been established. The effects of metabolic function of the IEC cell line from rat small intestines have been determined by *in vitro* studies.[35] The RCC rat colonic cell line was obtained from tumors induced chemically.[35] The RCC-5 cell line has lost its ability to produce mucus *in vitro*. Therefore, it is used for the study of hormonal, nutritional, and physical conditions necessary for mucus differentiation of colon cells.

GALL BLADDER, BILE DUCTS, AND PANCREAS

Myoelectric activity is important for proper functioning of the GI tract. Gall bladder filling and emptying and duodenal bile acid delivery during fasting are cyclically coordinated with myoelectric activity.[36] To determine this, dogs were surgically implanted with duodenal cannulae and eight bipolar electrodes placed from the duodenum to the terminal ileum. During continuous intravenous infusion of [^{14}C]taurocholic acid, fasting myoelectric activity and duodenal delivery of the taurocholic acid were recorded under different conditions. Therefore, monitoring these parameters may help expose functional changes related to gall bladder filling and emptying in addition to duodenal bile acid distribution.

A study was conducted to determine the effects of sphincter of Oddi obstruction due to topical administration of carbachol on the sphincter.[37] This study assayed functionality through measurements of sphincter of Oddi motility, transsphincter flow, pancreatic duct pressure, pancreatic exocrine secretion, plasma amylase levels, and pancreatic tissue damage. The Australian brush-tailed possum (*Trichosurus vulpecula*) was used due to the similarity of its pancreatic and bile ducts to human ducts.

The effects of bile duct cannulation on functional gastrointestinal transit time were studied in F-344-rats[38] subjected to surgery consisting of laparotomy with gut manipulation, sham bile duct cannulation, actual bile duct cannulation, or halothane anesthesia alone. Rats received radio-opaque barium sulfate orally. Radiographic images were made within 2 minutes and periodically to locate movement of the barium through the GI tract. It was determined that bile duct cannulation markedly slowed gastrointestinal motility.

ABSORPTION

Selection of an animal model of gastrointestinal absorption depends upon the specific function to be studied.[39] Differences in absorption of various species are reviewed based on function, anatomical variation, GI tract pH, flora, functional differences, absorption of inorganics and organics, and confounding variables. In a study of 38 organic compounds, more than a third appeared to be differently absorbed by animal models as compared to human subjects.[39]

Absorption can be affected by a variety of parameters.[40] When selecting a study design to assess absorption-related features of the GI tract, certain parameters need to be taken into consideration. The following parameters are likely to have a major effect on the kinetics of gastrointestinal absorption: vascularity, transit time, surface area, contents, enterohepatic cycling, and the chemical properties of the compound studied.

Fat malabsorption can be measured from fat in fecal samples.[24,41,42] Stool samples are pooled, mixed with water, and homogenized. A sample may then be analyzed by hydrolysis, extraction, and titration of the fatty acids. Steatorrhea is a condition where more fat in the stool is present than normal, an indication of decreased fat absorption. A coagulation test for the determination of prothrombin time is an indication of vitamin K absorption.[33] An increase in prothrombin time may also be due to steatorrhea. Fat malabsorption has also been determined in breath tests to detect $^{14}CO_2$ levels after ingestion of meals containing ^{14}C labeled fats or triglycerides[43–45] or in non-radioactive breath tests.[46]

One indication of altered carbohydrate absorption is an oral glucose tolerance test.[33] A fasting blood sample is obtained, followed by samples every 30 minutes for approximately 2 hours after oral administration of a known amount of glucose dissolved in water. High values may indicate diabetes mellitus. Breath tests are also available to evaluate carbohydrate malabsorption by evaluating H_2 after the administration of carbohydrates.[24] Lactose intolerance testing may also be utilized.[24]

Protein absorption analyses of fecal samples are not normally conducted, as amino acids are partially catabolized and reused for protein synthesis[33] and are metabolized by bacteria in the large intestine.

Iron may become malabsorbed if the duodenum is damaged, as iron normally is absorbed at this location.[33] A blood smear from an animal with deficient iron absorption shows hypochromia and microcytosis. Serum iron levels are low with malabsorption. Additional assays for absorption of iron are whole body counts and fecal recovery. In these studies, after an overnight fast, animals are given oral dosages of 10 mcg Ci ^{59}Fe. A whole body count is made 4 hours later. For fecal recovery, feces are collected and radioactivity counted until less than 1% of the administered dose appears.

Absorption may be measured *in situ*, as described in a study on cadmium.[47] Under surgical procedures, a loop of the small intestine was isolated and cadmium was injected intraluminally. The mesenteric venous (portal) blood coming from the loop was collected for 90 minutes and analyzed for cadmium.

Microbial Flora

Normally, the lower GI tract contains many organisms that assist with typical gastrointestinal functionality. An imbalance may be due to an infection or xenobiotics, and could cause the GI tract to have impaired activity. *Escherichia coli* enterotoxin-induced diarrhea has been shown to produce changes in intestinal absorption and permeability.[48] A simple rectal culture test can identify and isolate organisms. A cotton swab is gently inserted into the rectum, rotated, and withdrawn. A smear is placed on culture media and incubated. The culture is observed at regular intervals. Organisms can then be identified and isolated.

The small intestine may also be sampled for bacterial flora. One method is a needle aspiration of the intestines. Another method utilizes a double-lumen radio-opaque tube.[49] The tube is placed down the esophagus of a fasted animal and positioned in the mid-jejunum area. Aspirates are taken and the tube is withdrawn. Samples are then plated for both aerobic and anaerobic cultures.

Many intestinal bacteria are able to deconjugate bile acids.[49] This normally occurs in the large intestine; however, if the deconjugation takes place in the small intestine, absorption of [^{14}C]glycine occurs. The glycine, administered orally as ^{14}C-glycine-glycocholic acid, is completely metabolized and produces $^{14}CO_2$, which may be measured in the breath.

Urinalyses may also be performed to detect excessive growth of bacteria in the small intestines.[49] Analysis for the presence of indican (indoxyl sulfate) may be conducted. Indoles are produced by bacteria, particularly *Escherichia coli* and *Bacterroides*.

IMMUNE FUNCTION

The GI tract has ample immune function activity.[50,51] Alteration of immune modulating cells and gut tissues is linked to abnormal function of the GI tract. Mucosal tissues have glandular secretions that secrete on the epithelial surface. Most antibody activity in mucosal secretions is of secretory IgA, but other factors need to be taken into consideration during a local immune response, including cellular and humoral mechanisms. There are many types of mucosal tissues, including gut-associated lymphoid tissues (Peyer's patches and isolated lymphoid follicles), bronchus-associated lymphoid tissues. Other antibody cells include but are not limited to IgG, IgM, T-lymphocytes, natural killer cells, mast cells, macrophages, goblet cells, and precursor B-cells from Peyer's patches.

Changes in the number of mast cells have been observed in a variety of immune responses in different tissues including the GI tract.[52] Mast cells have been found to influence the immunologic, physiologic, and pathologic functions of the GI tract including normal functions of the stomach and intestine. Mast cell-deficient mice models have been identified (WBB6F1-W/W^v and WCB6F1-Sl/Sl^d). These animals may be used to assess numbers, phenotypic characteristics, and anatomical distribution of mast cells potentially participating in responses including mast cell degranulation.

Normal immune function of the intestines is absent in inflammatory bowel diseases including Crohn's disease. There are many models of inflammatory bowel disease, but less progress has been made with models for fibrotic lesions.[53] It is difficult to analyze for fibrosis *in vivo* because it is difficult to determine the difference between indirect effects caused by altered inflammation from direct effects. CD-1 and BALB/c mice were sedated weekly and intrarectal injections of trinitrobenzene sulfonic acid were administered.[54] Only a fraction of the animals developed severe fibrosis, and not all of those animals had persistent fibrosis after the intrarectal injections ceased.

Inflammatory mediators, particularly platelet activating factor, play an important role in the pathogenesis of necrotizing enterocolitis, a life threatening gastrointestinal problem in neonates.[55] A neonatal piglet model for this inflammatory disorder was developed and used to investigate the role of platelet activating factor in its pathogenesis. Rodent models were also investigated; however, the neonatal piglet model is more relevant to humans due to more similar anatomy and physiology. Each piglet was anesthetized and a cuff-type electromagnetic flow probe was surgically placed around a branch of the cranial (superior) mesenteric artery. The location was selected to monitor the mesenteric blood flow for additional data to support the model. The animals were allowed to recover and the procedure for the development of the model occurred after stabilization of the readings from the monitor. The animals received intravenous injections of an endotoxin (lipopolysaccharide, 2 mg/kg). They were then allowed to breathe normal room air for 45 minutes, followed by a 45-minute period of breathing 10% oxygen, then another 45-minute period of breathing room air. The animals were then killed by lethal doses of pentobarbitone sodium and examined for gross and microscopic changes. This treatment caused a reduction of mesenteric artery blood flow in addition to the intestinal lesions consistent with necrotizing enterocolitis.

A change in immune functionality of the gastrointestinal system may occur due to allergy.[56] A rat model was developed to assist the study of gastrointestinal allergy. Allergic sensitivity to certain proteins was induced in rats by injecting proteins and adjuvants in various regimes. Sensitivity was also established in suckling rats by oral administration of the protein. A hypersensitive gastrointestinal reaction to challenge was demonstrated by electron microscopy, by light microscopy with the aid of conventional staining techniques, and also by a radionuclide procedure utilizing ^{51}Cr-labeled albumin.

GASTROINTESTINAL BLEEDING

Bleeding from the GI tract may indicate a variety of functional or pathologic problems. Detecting the presence of blood in feces is in most cases easier than finding the bleeding site. Occult blood tests may be performed on fecal samples.[57] A variety of methods can be used to detect occult bleeding, including the use of chemical tests, microscopic examination of feces for erythrocytes or hemoglobin crystals or its derivatives, spectroscopic analyses for hemoglobin or its derivatives, and ^{51}Cr-labeled erythrocytes. Fecal occult tests may produce false positives in dark feces that may be due to injected iron; in this case, simple testing is needed to rule out iron.[57,58]

CLINICAL CHEMISTRY ANALYSES

Simple blood sampling and analyses can provide insights into functional problems with the GI tract.[59] Electrolyte and fluid imbalance may be due to emesis, diarrhea, or a variety of mechanisms for maintaining electrolyte and fluid homeostasis. Chloride secretion from the pancreas varies inversely to the bicarbonate concentration that varies directly with flow rate. Hypocalcemia may also accompany severe pancreatic toxicity.

Glucose homeostasis is controlled by the liver and changes in that organ may produce imbalances. Hormones and other chemicals also have additional control of glucose levels, and include insulin (which is highly variable), glucagons, growth hormone, adrenaline, and cortisol. Urinary levels of glucose may also be determined to detect functional imbalances of glucose metabolism. Electrolyte metabolism may be altered during carbohydrate metabolism disturbances.

The measurement of enzymes is important for assessing gastrointestinal function, but many tests are specialized and are not common, especially in standard toxicology tests. Plasma P amylase is a specific assay for pancreatitis. Lipases are secreted by the pancreas. Alkaline phosphatase can change with gastrointestinal conditions such as intestinal obstruction or infarction, parasitic infection, obstruction of the biliary system, contraction of the sphincter of Oddi by specific drug, withdrawal of food, and age-related changes. Alkaline phosphatase is also secreted by bone, liver, and placenta. Since the liver can affect gastrointestinal functionality, liver function testing should also be performed.[60]

PAIN

Pain due to gastrointestinal disorders may arise from numerous sources including esophagitis, gastroesophageal reflux, restriction of the esophagus, tumors, infections and inflammation, constipation, irritable bowel syndrome, gall stones, pancreatitis, and metabolic and hormone disorders. Determination of the degree and location of pain in laboratory animals is difficult to reproduce due to communication barriers. To determine whether a specific chemical causes pain in the GI tract, one might look for gross (as a result of an endoscopy or at necropsy) or histopathological effects only as indications of possible pain.

REFERENCES

1. National Digestive Diseases Information Clearinghouse (NDDCH): Digestive disease statistics. http://www.digestive.niddk.nih.gov/statistics/statistics.htm (accessed 1/18/2006).
2. Daniel, E., Collins, S., Fox, J., and Huizinga, J. (1989): Pharmacology of drugs acting on gastrointestinal motility, in Rauner, B., Ed., *Handbook of Physiology*, American Physiological Society, Bethesda, chap. 19.
3. Schultz, S.G. (1989): The gastrointestinal system, in Schultz, S.G. and Wood, J.D., Eds., *Handbook of Physiology*, Vol. 1, Part 2, American Physiological Society, Washington, D.C., p. 818.
4. Christensen, J. (1983): The oesophagus, in Christensen, J. and Wingate, D., Eds., *A Guide to Gastrointestinal Motility*, Wright PSG, Boston, p. 75.
5. Smout, A. and Akkermans, L. (1992): Normal and disturbed motility of the gastrointestinal tract, *Diagnosis*, 1023: 216.
6. Bateson, M. and Bouchier, I. (1981): Oesophagus, in *Clinical Investigation of Gastrointestinal Function*, 2nd ed., Blackwell Scientific, Boston, p. 24.
7. Goyal, R.K. and Paterson, W.G. (1989): Esophageal motility, in Schultz, S.G. and Wood, J.D., Eds., *Handbook of Physiology*, Section 6, The Gastrointestinal System, Vol. 1, Part 2, American Physiological Society, Washington, D.C., chap. 22.
8. Richter, J., Sinar, D., Cordova, C., and Castell, D. (1982): Verapamil: a potent inhibitor of esophageal contractions in the baboon, *Gastroenterology*, 82: 882.
9. Winship, D., Poindexter, R., Thayer, W., and Spiro, H. (1965): Esophageal motility in the monkey, *Gastroenterology*, 48: 231.

10. Davenport, H. (1982): Gastric motility and emptying, in *Physiology of the Digestive Tract*, 5th ed., Chicago, Year Book Medical Publishers, p. 52.

11. You, C. and Chey, W. (1987): Functional disorders in gastric emptying, in Cohen, S. and Soloway, R., Eds., *Functional Disorders of the Gastrointestinal Tract*, Churchill Livingstone, New York, chap. 2.

12. Itoh, T., Higuchi, T., Gardner, C., and Caldwell, L. (1986): Effect of particle size and food on gastric residence time of non-disintegrating solids in beagle dogs. *J. Pharm. Pharmacol*, 38: 801.

13. Moran, T., Ameglio, P., Schwartz, G., Peyton, H., and McHugh, P. (1993): Endogenous cholecystolinin in the control of gastric emptying of liquid nutrient loads in rhesus monkeys, *Am. J. Physiol.*, 265: R371.

14. Chang, F., Lee, S., Yeh, G., and Wang, P. (1996): Influence of blood glucose levels on rat liquid gastric emptying, *Dig. Dis. Sci.*, 41: 528.

15. Anika, M.S., (1982): Effects of cholecystokinin and careulein on gastric emptying, *Eur. J. Pharmacol.*, 85: 195.

16. Morgan, K., Muir, T., and Szurszewski, J. (1981): Electrical basis for contraction and relaxation in canine fundal smooth muscle, *Physiol. Soc.*, 311: 475.

17. Summers, R., Kent, T., and Osborne, J. (1970): Effects of drugs, ileal obstruction, and irradiation on rat gastrointestinal propulsion, *Gastroenterology*, 59: 731.

18. Summers, R. and Kent, T. (1970): Effects of altered propulsion on rat small intestinal flora, *Gastroenterology*, 59: 740.

19. Christensen, J., Stiles, M., Rick, G., and Sutherland, J. (1984): Comparative anatomy of the myenteric plexus, *Gastroenterology*, 86: 706.

20. Christensen, J. (1989): Colonic motility, in Schultz, S.G. and Wood, J.D., Eds., *Handbook of Physiology*, Section 6, The Gastrointestinal System, Vol. 1, Part 2, American Physiological Society, Washington, D.C., p. 939.

21. Rostad, H. (1973): Colonic motility in the cat. I. Extraluminal strain gage technique: influence of anesthesia and temperature, *Acta Physiol. Scand.*, 89: 79.

22. Wienbeck, M. and Christensen, J. (1971): Effects of some drugs on electrical activity of the isolated colon of the cat, *Gastroenterology*, 61: 470.

23. Flores, J.O. (2001): Gastric acid determination, in Longe, J.L., Ed., *The Gale Encyclopedia of Medicine*, 2nd ed., Gale Group, Farmington Hills, MI.

24. Chey, W.D. and Chey, W.Y. (2003): Evaluation of secretion and absorption functions of the gastrointestinal tract, in Yamada, T., Ed., *Gastroenterology*, 4th ed., Lippincott Williams & Wilkins, New York, p. 3075.

25. Youngberg, C., Wlodyga, J., Schmaltz, S., and Dressman, J. (1985): Radiotelemetric determination of gastrointestinal pH in four healthy beagles, *Am. J. Vet. Res.*, 46: 1516.

26. Lui, C., Amidon, G., Berardi, R., Fleisher, B., Youngberg, C., and Dressman, J. (1986): Comparison of gastrointestinal pH in dogs and humans, *J. Pharm. Sci.*, 75: 271.

27. Wolfe, M. and McGuigan, J. (1982): Release of gastric inhibitory peptide following a peptone meal in the dog, *Gastroenterology*, 83: 864.

28. Friis-Hansen, L., Sundler, F., Li, Y., Gillespie, P., Saunders, T., Greenson, J., Owyang, C., Rehfeld, J., and Samuelson, L. (1998): Impaired gastric acid secretion in gastrin-deficient mice, *Am. J. Physiol.*, 274: G561.

29. Davenport, H. (1982): Secretion of bile, in *Physiology of the Digestive Tract*, 5th. ed., Year Book Medical Publishers, Chicago, p. 155.

30. Davenport, H. (1982): Pancreatic secretion, in *Physiology of the Digestive Tract*, 5th ed., Year Book Medical Publishers, Chicago, p. 143.
31. Faichney, A., Chey, W., Kim, Y., Lee, K., Kim, M., and Chang, T. (1981): Effect of sodium oleate on plasma secretion concentration and pancreatic secretion in dog, *Gastroenterology*, 81: 458.
32. Davenport, H. (1982): Chemical messengers of the digestive tract, in *Physiology of the Digestive Tract*, 5th ed., Year Book Medical Publishers, Chicago, p. 21.
33. Vaccaro, M.I., Tiscornia, O.M., Calvo, E.L., Cresta, M.A., and Celener, D. (1992): Effect of ethanol intake on pancreatic exocrine secretion in mice, *Scand. J. Gastroenterol.*, 27: 783.
34. Favus, M.J. (1985): Factors that influence absoption and secretion of calcium in the small intestine and colon, *Am. J. Physiol.*, 248: G147.
35. Zweibaum, A., Laburthe, M., Grasset, E., and Louvard, D. (1991): Use of cultured cell lines in studies of intestinal cell differentiation and function, in Rauner, B., Ed., *Handbook of Physiology*, American Physiological Society, Bethesda, MD, chap. 7, p. 223.
36. Scott, R.B., Eidt, P.B., and Shaffer, E.A. (1985): Regulation of fasting canine duodenal bile acid delivery by sphincter of Oddi and gallbladder, *Am. J. Physiol.*, 249: G622.
37. Chen, J.W.C., Thomas, A., Woods, C.M., Schloithe, A.C., Toouli, J., and Saccone, G.T.P. (2000): Sphincter of Oddi dysfunction produces acute pancreatitis in the possum, *Gut*, 47: 539.
38. Ayres, P.H., Medinsky, M.A., Muggenburg, B.A., and Bond, J.A. (1985): Alteration of gastrointestinal transit time in the rat after bile duct cannulation surgery, in Medinsky, M.A. and Muggenburg, B.A., Eds., *Inhalation Toxicology Research Institute Annual Report 1984–1985*, Lovelace Biomedical and Environmental Research Institute, Albuquerque, NM, p. 341.
39. Calabrese, E.J. (1984): Gastrointestinal and dermal absorption: interspecies differences, *Drug Metabol. Rev.*, 15: 1013.
40. DeSesso, J.M. (1991): Identification of critical biological parameters affecting gastrointestinal absorption, GRA&I, Issue 20.
41. Bateson, M. and Bouchier, I. (1981): Absorption, in *Clinical Investigation of Gastrointestinal Function*, 2nd ed., Blackwell Scientific Publications, Boston, p. 53.
42. Romano, T. and Dobbins, J. (1989): Evaluation of the patient with suspected malabsorption, *Malabsorption Nutr. Status Supp.*, 18: 467.
43. Ghoos, Y., Vantrappen, G., Rutgeerts, P., and Schurmans, P. (1981): A mixed triglyceride breath test for intraluminal fat digestive activity, *Digestion*, 22: 239.
44. Schwabe, A.D. and Hepner, G.W. (1979): Breath tests for detection of fat malabsorption, *Gastroenterology*, 76: 216.
45. Newcomer, A., Hofmann, A., DiMagino, E., Thomas, P., and Carlson, G. (1979): A sensitive and specific test for fat malabsorption, *Gastroenterology*, 76: 6.
46. Watkins, J., Schoeller, D., Klein, P., Ott, D., Newcomer, A., and Hofmann, A. (1977): ^{13}C-trioctanoin: a nonradioactive breath test to detect fat malabsorption, *J. Lab. Clin. Med.*, 90: 422.
47. Goon, D. and Klaassen, C. (1989): Dosage-dependent absorption of cadium in the rat intestine measured *in situ*, *Toxicol. Appl. Pharmacol.*, 100: 41.

48. Verma, M., Ganguly, N.K., Majumdar, S., and Walia, B.N.S. (1995): Cr-labelled ethylenediaminetetraacetic acid and D-xylose absorption in *Escherichia coli* enterotoxin-induced diarrhoea in mice, *Scand. J. Gastroenterol.*, 30: 886.

49. Bateson, M. and Bouchier, I. (1981): Small intestine, in *Clinical Investigation of Gastrointestinal Function*, 2nd ed., Blackwell Scientific Publications, Boston, p., 82.

50. Bienenstock, J. and Befus, A. (1985): The gastrointestinal tract as an immune organ, in *Gastrointestinal Immunity for the Clinician*, Shorter, R. and Kirsner, J., Eds., Grune & Stratton, New York, chap. 1.

51. Hanauer, S. and Kraft, S., (1985): Intestinal immunology, in Berk, J., Ed., *Gastroenterology*, 4th ed., W.B. Saunders, Philadelphia, p. 1607.

52. Wershil, B. and Galli, S. (1991): Gastrointestinal mast cells: new approaches for analyzing their function *in vivo*, *Gastroentero. Clin. N. Am.*, 20: 613.

53. MacDonald, T.T. (2003): A mouse model of intestinal fibrosis? *Gastroenterology*, 125: 1889.

54. Lawrance, I., Wu, F., Leite, A., Willis, J., West, G., Fiocchi, C., and Chakravarti, S. (2003): A murine model of chronic inflammation-induced intestinal fibrosis down-regulated by antisense NF-kB, *Gastroenterology*, 125: 1750.

55. Ewer, A., Al-Salti, W., Coney, A., Marshall, J., Ramani, P., and Booth, I. (2004): Role of platelet activating factor in a neonatal piglet model of necrotising enterocolitis, *Gut*, 53: 207.

56. Freier, S. (1982): Gastrointestinal allergy in the experimental animal: use of radioiodinated serum albumin in the assessment of new drugs: final report for October 15, 1977–November 30, 1979. GRA&I, Issue 5.

57. Bateson, M. and Bouchier, I. (1981): Gastrointestinal bleeding, in *Clinical Investigation of Gastrointestinal Function*, 2nd ed., Boston, Blackwell Scientific Publications, p. 16.

58. Lifton, L. and Kreiser, J. (1982): False-positive stool occult blood tests caused by iron preparations: controlled study and review of literature, *Gastroenterology*, 83: 860.

59. Evans, G.O. (1996) Assessment of gastrointestinal toxicity and pancreatic toxicity, in *Animal Clinical Chemistry: A Primer for Toxicologists*, Taylor & Francis, London, p. 137.

60. Bateson, M. and Bouchier, I. (1981): Liver biochemistry, in *Clinical Investigation of Gastrointestinal Function*, 2nd ed., Blackwell Scientific Publications, Boston, p. 153.

3 Safety Pharmacology and the GI Tract

Henry I. Jacoby

CONTENTS

INTRODUCTION

Long before safety pharmacology became a familiar term, pharmacologists and toxicologists evaluated developmental compounds for side and/or adverse effects on multiple organ systems in animal models. They did this mainly to evaluate compounds early in the development process that exhibited unwanted effects at doses equal to or greater than those showing efficacy. These studies were felt to be important in obtaining as much information as possible about serious toxicological potential and also about those properties that produced unwanted and sometimes annoying effects that seriously impacted patient compliance. This is especially true with drugs for chronic therapy where even minor side effects can affect compliance. These studies have various names: ancillary, general, or developmental pharmacology, and may have been performed in discovery or development departments of pharmaceutical companies.

Only within the last 10 to 15 years have attempts been made to codify the numbers and types of studies required for regulatory approval.

DEFINITION OF SAFETY PHARMACOLOGY

The origins of safety pharmacology are grounded upon observations that organ functions (like organ structures) can be toxicological targets in humans exposed to novel therapeutic agents, and that drug effects on organ functions (unlike organ structures) are not readily detected by standard toxicological testing.[1] Non-clinical safety assessment programs are usually designed to meet the needs of early clinical studies and guidelines on non-clinical safety[2] of the International Conference on Harmonization (ICH) or local regulatory agencies.

In addition to the repeated dose toxicity studies in one rodent and one non-rodent species, genotoxicity and safety pharmacology evaluations are critical to the full evaluation of drug safety and usually are conducted prior to the start of the Phase I clinical studies. Due to their relevance for human safety, the conduct of preclinical safety and pharmacokinetic studies before the start of clinical studies and granting of marketing authorization has become a critical, mandatory, and fairly standardized field regulated by national and international health authorities.[3]

However, there is no consistent official definition of *safety pharmacology*. Kinter et al.[4] define it as the systematic approach of investigating a candidate drug for activity to stimulate, potentiate, or inhibit the activity of physiological or pharmacological responses or interaction with another drug, whether *in vitro* or *in vivo*. Safety pharmacology studies are designed to assess the potential adverse effects of a compound on the physiologic functions of one or more organs or organ systems, in either intact or acutely prepared models that are of proven relevance to humans, whether healthy or sick.

Adverse effects of a compound on body function can be consequences of either primary or secondary pharmacological properties. Safety pharmacology, therefore, must cover pharmacologic properties at dose levels that must be relevant to clinical use and not excessive. In addition, safety pharmacology should focus on effects that are difficult to detect within toxicity studies. Definition of safety margins may also be important and it may be important to assess the therapeutic index, i.e., the margin between the primary and secondary actions of a drug.

Basic Considerations

Administration route and frequency — The intended human route should be employed if possible. Usually, a single administration is sufficient.

Dose levels — Generally, three doses are chosen. The low dose is equal to or slightly higher than the dose that produces the primary pharmacological action. The intermediate and high doses are chosen in order to establish a possible dose–response relationship.

Species, sex — For each test an appropriate animal species is chosen according to background data related to the pharmacological effects, to its (the species) acceptance as a predictor of pharmacological drug effects, and to the recognition by regulatory authorities that the species is acceptable for pharmacodynamic studies. Use of rats and dogs is recommended because these species are most commonly used in toxicological evaluations, and pharmacokinetic and toxicokinetic data for these species are often available.

Experimental design — The number of animals per group is chosen on the basis of the variability of measured parameters in order to test the absence or presence of examined effects using appropriate statistical tests.

The U.S. Food & Drug Administration (FDA) and other governmental regulatory agencies drafted guidelines for safety pharmacology that have been issued.[2] As of summer 2005, the *S7A Safety Pharmacology Studies for Human Pharmaceuticals Guidelines* provide suggestions and recommendations. It should be emphasized that as of mid-2005, no official viewpoint specifies the necessity of studies on most organ systems or how they are to be performed. Present requirements are basically limited to adverse effects on the cardiovascular system, specifically potential effects on arrhythmias. No specific testing for safety related to the gastrointestinal system is recommended at present. Alternative approaches may be used if such approaches satisfy the requirements of the applicable statutes and regulations.

Safety Pharmacology Core Battery

Central nervous system — Effects of the test substance on the central nervous system should be assessed appropriately. Motor activity, behavioral changes, coordination, sensory and motor reflex responses, and body temperature should be evaluated. For example, a functional observation battery,[5] modified Irwin's,[6] or other appropriate test[7] can be used.

Cardiovascular system — Effects of the test substance on the cardiovascular system should be assessed appropriately. Blood pressure, heart rate, and an electrocardiogram should be evaluated. *In vivo, in vitro* and/or *ex vivo* evaluations including methods for determining repolarization and conductance abnormalities should also be considered.

Respiratory system — Effects of the test substance on the respiratory system should be assessed appropriately. Respiratory rate and other measures of respiratory function (e.g., tidal volume[8] or hemoglobin oxygen saturation) should be evaluated. Clinical observation of animals is generally not adequate to assess respiratory function and thus these parameters should be quantified by using appropriate methodologies.

Follow-up and supplemental safety pharmacology studies — Adverse effects may be suspected based on the pharmacological properties or chemical class of the test substance. Concerns may arise from the safety pharmacology core battery, clinical trials, pharmacovigilance, experimental *in vitro* or *in vivo* studies, or literature reports. When such potential adverse effects raise concern for human safety, they should be explored in follow-up or supplemental safety pharmacology studies as appropriate.

FOLLOW-UP STUDIES FOR SAFETY PHARMACOLOGY CORE BATTERY

Central nervous system — Behavioral pharmacology, learning and memory, ligand-specific binding, neurochemistry, visual, auditory, and/or electrophysiology examinations.

Cardiovascular system — Cardiac output, ventricular contractility, vascular resistance, and effects of endogenous and/or exogenous substances on cardiovascular responses.

Respiratory system — Airway resistance, compliance, pulmonary arterial pressure, blood gases, and blood pH.

SUPPLEMENTAL SAFETY PHARMACOLOGY STUDIES

Supplemental studies are meant to evaluate potential adverse pharmacodynamic effects on organ system functions not addressed by the core battery or repeated dose toxicity studies when there is a cause for concern.

Renal–urinary system — Effects of the test substance on renal parameters should be assessed. For example, urinary volume, specific gravity, osmolality, pH, fluid/electrolyte balance, proteins, cytology, and blood chemistry determinations such as blood urea nitrogen, creatinine, and plasma proteins can be used.

Autonomic nervous system — Effects of the test substance on the autonomic nervous system should be assessed. For example, binding to receptors relevant for the autonomic nervous system, functional responses to agonists or antagonists *in vivo* or *in vitro*, direct stimulation of autonomic nerves and measurement of cardiovascular responses, baroreflex testing, and heart rate variability can be used.

Gastrointestinal system — Effects of the test substance on the gastrointestinal system should be assessed. For example, gastric secretion, gastrointestinal injury potential, bile secretion, transit time, and ileal contraction *in vitro*.

Other organ systems — Effects of the test substance on organ systems not investigated elsewhere should be assessed when there is reason for concern. For example, dependency potential or skeletal muscle, immune, and endocrine functions can be investigated.

Data from general pharmacology studies (U.S., Japan, European Union) or safety pharmacology studies in the assessment of a marketing application have been accepted worldwide. The Japanese Ministry of Health and Welfare issued its *Guideline for General Pharmacology* in 1991. The guideline states that general pharmacology studies should include those designed to identify unexpected effects on organ system function and to broaden pharmacological characterization (pharmacological profiling). However, there has been no internationally accepted definition of the terms *primary pharmacodynamics*, *secondary pharmacodynamics*, or *safety pharmacology*.

The need for international harmonization of the nomenclature and the development of an international guidance for *safety pharmacology* has been recognized. The *safety pharmacology studies* term first appeared in ICH's M3 *Timing of Nonclinical Safety Studies for the Conduct of Human Clinical Trials for Pharmaceuticals*[2] and S6 *Preclinical Safety Evaluation Of Biotechnology-Derived Pharmaceuticals*[9] as studies that should be conducted to support use of therapeutics in humans. Details of the safety pharmacology studies including their definitions and objectives were left for future discussion.

GENERAL PRINCIPLES FROM DRAFT GUIDELINE

The specific studies that should be conducted and their designs will vary based on the individual properties and intended uses of the individual pharmaceuticals. General principles for safety using scientifically valid methods should be used, and when there are internationally recognized methods that are applicable to pharmaceuticals, these methods are preferable. The objectives of safety pharmacology studies are to:

1. Identify undesirable pharmacodynamic properties of a substance that may have relevance to its human safety.
2. Evaluate adverse pharmacodynamic and/or pathophysiological effects of a substance observed in toxicology and/or clinical studies.
3. Investigate the mechanisms of the adverse pharmacodynamic effects observed and/or suspected.

Regardless of the route of administration, exposure to the parent substance and its major metabolites should be similar to or greater than that achieved in humans when such information is available. Assessment of effects by more than one route may be appropriate if the test substance is intended for clinical use by more than one route of administration (e.g., oral and parenteral) or where significant qualitative and quantitative differences in systemic or local exposure are observed or anticipated.

Generally, any parent compound and its major metabolites that achieve or are expected to achieve systemic exposure in humans should be evaluated in safety pharmacology studies. Evaluation of major metabolites is often accomplished through studies of the parent compound in animals. If the major human metabolites are found to be absent or present only at relatively low concentrations in animals, assessment of the effects of such metabolites on safety pharmacology endpoints should be considered. If metabolites from humans are known to substantially contribute to the pharmacological actions of the therapeutic agent, it could be important to test such active metabolites. When *in vivo* studies on the parent compound have not adequately assessed metabolites, the tests of metabolites can be used in *in vitro* systems based on practical considerations. *In vitro* or *in vivo* testing of individual isomers should also be considered when a product contains an isomeric mixture.

The following are some situations in which safety pharmacology may not be required:

1. Locally applied agents (e.g., dermal or ocular): if the pharmacology of the test substance is well characterized, and where systemic exposure or distribution to other organs or tissues is demonstrated to be low.
2. Cytotoxic agents for treatment of end-state cancer patients: safety pharmacology studies prior to the first administration in humans may not be needed. However, for cytotoxic agents with novel mechanisms of action, there may be value in conducting safety pharmacology studies.
3. Biotechnology-derived products that achieve highly specific receptor targeting are often sufficient to evaluate safety pharmacology endpoints as a part of toxicology and/or pharmacodynamic studies; therefore, safety pharmacology studies can be reduced or eliminated for these products.
4. Biotechnology-derived products that represent a novel therapeutic class and/or products that do not achieve highly specific receptor targeting: a more extensive evaluation by safety pharmacology studies should be considered.
5. A new salt having similar pharmacokinetics and pharmacodynamics.

A pharmacology committee was established in November 2004 at the Center for Drug Evaluation and Research (CDER) to develop regulatory guidance for use by sponsors and applicants, to apply current scientific knowledge to emerging technical problems, and to aid in the review process. The Safety Pharmacology Subcommittee was initially formed as an *ad hoc* committee to ascertain the need for a formal guidance document covering the safety pharmacology studies that should be conducted for pharmaceuticals intended for human use. The PTCC Safety Pharmacology Subcommittee has been constituted as a permanent subcommittee of the PTCC to provide CDER divisions with consultations and recommendations on safety pharmacology issues and studies. Establishment of this committee should increase the consistency of safety pharmacology requirements among CDER drug product review divisions. The committee's functions are to review, consult, and provide written recommendations on safety pharmacology issues and studies to CDER divisions.

Gastrointestinal Safety Studies

Effects on the gastrointestinal tract are not considered to be of primary importance based on a hierarchy of organ systems. Vital organs or systems, the functions of which are acutely critical for life (e.g., the cardiovascular, respiratory, and central nervous systems), are considered the most important ones to assess in safety pharmacology studies. Other organ systems (e.g., the renal and gastrointestinal systems) whose functions can be transiently disrupted by adverse pharmacodynamic effects without causing irreversible harm are of less immediate investigative concern. The guidelines suggest evaluation of gastric secretion, gastrointestinal mucosal injury potential, bile secretion, and transit time.

The investigator has discretion on which testing shall be used, depending on the class of pharmacological agent being developed.[10] The gastrointestinal tract extracts nutrients, electrolytes, minerals, and water, and is prone to injury as a result of oral drug administration. Clinical assessment of the GI tract is often limited to measurements of transit time and observations of vomiting or diarrhea, despite the existence of methods and techniques capable of assessing specific changes in GI function at the membrane, cell, and whole animal levels.

In some specific cases, membrane studies, measurement of the uptake of solutes, and electrolyte transport assessing the affects of compounds on transepithelial GI transport and flux may be required, but are not considered essential prior to the initial human trials. Such methods lend themselves to permeability, immunohistochemistry, morphology, and molecular biology techniques. In anesthetized animals, ligated segments of the intestine can be infused with test compounds, providing information about absorptive and secretory processes important for the treatment of diarrhea. Finally, advances in the field of imaging combined with endoscopy have resulted in a wireless capsule that allows inspection of GI tract anatomy and pathology without surgical intervention.

The tests recommended for gastrointestinal safety include: ulcerogenic effect (rat), gastric acid secretion (rat), gastric emptying (rat), fecal output models (mice or rats), emetic effect (ferret), intestinal transit (mice or rats), biliary secretion (rat), and pancreatic secretion (rat). This chapter will not consider *in vitro* organ bath systems because they do not appear to offer useful additional information.

General Recommendation for GI Safety Study Design

Acceptance by local animal use committee — All methods used should be approved by the appropriate animal care committee.
Protocol — Detailed protocols should be written and used for all safety pharmacology studies. All parameters should be spelled out.
Dose range testing — A dose range starting at the "therapeutic" dose and increasing at multiples of two to five for at least three doses.
Choice of test animal — If possible, an animal similar (species, sex, and source) to that in which efficacy has been shown should be used.

Test material — The test material should be similar to that shown to be active (same batch, if possible). Care should be taken to use the same vehicle, salt, and method of preparation.

Time course — The duration of the study should be based on information derived from efficacy studies.

Good laboratory practice (GLP) — If required, the necessary SOPs and protocols should conform to GLP and have all necessary approvals and audits.

ANIMAL MODELS FOR EVALUATION OF SAFETY PHARMACOLOGY

This section describes animal models available and accepted for evaluation of safety pharmacology on the gastrointestinal tract. Most of these methods are straightforward and do not require extensive equipment or surgical skills. They have been chosen on the basis of reported usage in the literature and personal experience.

DRUG-INDUCED GASTROINTESTINAL MUCOSAL LESIONS (ULCEROGENICITY)

Esophagus

Erosion of the mucosa of the esophagus has not been a common problem with orally administered drugs because the time the drug is in contact with the esophageal mucosa is usually limited. Most tablet or capsule formulations are coated and involve little contact with the mucosa. With a liquid preparation, unless the compound has corrosive activity, clearance of the formulation is usually rapid. However, in some circumstances, transport through the esophagus is delayed due to pathophysiology or disintegration of the formulation in the esophagus in the lumen, causing the releasing of a potentially damaging substance. Problems can also occur if the patient is supine and transport along the esophagus is delayed.

Suspect Classes of Compounds and Mechanisms

A potential problem with bisphosphonates has been observed and special recommendations as to when and how the tablet or capsule should be administered are required. Initial instructions were to take the formulation prior to breakfast and remain in an upright position for 30 minutes. Bisphosphonates appear to produce specific mucosal pathology of the esophageal mucosa. Other drugs may be corrosive or have other specific effects on esophageal mucosa upon prolonged exposure.

Animal Models Available

Acute dosing in rats with a solution or suspension of test agent is not a suitable model. Esophageal ulcerogenicity is rarely evaluated in animal studies because test compounds are usually delivered directly into the stomach via gavage. A test using anesthetized dogs has been described.[11] An endotracheal tube (internal diameter, 5.0 mm) is passed into the esophagus, with the cuff inflated directly caudal to the larynx. A rubber catheter is then passed through the tube, extending caudally just past the end of the tube. An infusion pump delivers the test liquid through the catheter over a 30-minute period. The cranial portion of the dog is elevated so that the liquid will flow aborally.

The infusions are generally administered for 5 consecutive days and the dogs are euthanized on the fifth day for gross and histopathologic examinations of the esophagus. For delivery of compounds in tablet form, a clear tube can be passed into the cranial third of the esophagus. The tablet tied to a premeasured length of silk suture is then introduced into the esophagus through the tube by using endoscopic retrieval forceps. The tablets are left in place for 1 hour and the dogs are then euthanized and examined. These techniques allowed for accurate and reliable testing in dogs of the esophageal irritancy of compounds in either the liquid or tablet form.

Endoscopy may also be useful for evaluation of acute dosing with a capsule or tablet formulation administered to a dog followed by esophageal and gastric endoscopy. A dog model to examine the possible mechanism for the esophageal adverse events has been published and showed that under low pH conditions, alendronate sodium can cause esophageal irritation.[12] No esophageal irritation occurred at pH 3.5 or higher where the drug exists primarily as the sodium salt. The animal studies also showed that alendronate sodium could exacerbate preexisting esophageal damage. Exposure of the esophageal mucosa for a prolonged period to alendronate sodium tablet can also cause mild esophageal irritation. These findings suggest that the esophageal irritation in patients taking bisphosphonates can be from prolonged contact with the tablet, reflux of acidic gastric contents, and exacerbation of preexisting esophageal damage.

Why Test?

Alendronate does not cause predictable esophageal, gastric, or duodenal mucosal damage when used as directed.[13] However, post-marketing surveys and endoscopic studies suggest that its use may be associated with significant predictable esophageal mucosal pathology. Because treatment of osteoporosis may be needed in as many as 30% of all postmenopausal women, and considering that alendronate could be used in all postmenopausal women as prevention, the definition of potential mucosal toxicity is crucial.

Stomach

One of the primary sites for the occurrence of adverse effects of a drug is the gastric mucosa. Although it was long known that drugs could produce gastric upset, and in some cases lesions and ulcerations leading to bleeding, there were no animal models for prediction of acute effects on mucosal integrity other than observations of lesions on necropsy after chronic treatment.

Classes of Compounds with Potential Liability and Possible Mechanisms

Any class of compound may produce gastric damage. The propensity to injure the gastric mucosa, which under normal conditions is resistant to acid conditions and the presence of proteolytic enzymes, is usually dependent on the ability of a compound to modify the protective barrier. This allows the acid and enzymes to contact mucosal cells lacking the protective coating of mucus. Drugs that are organic acids, have detergent actions, or affect the levels of protective prostaglandins are all suspect.

Borsch and Schmidt[14] published a survey of the damaging effects of acetylsalicylic acid, nonsteroidal anti-inflammatory drugs (NSAIDS), and corticosteroids on the gastroduodenal mucosa. They showed that these effects could be quantified in humans by blood loss studies, histology, and endoscopy. They pointed out the pathophysiology of these lesions and stressed the cytoprotective role of endogenous prostaglandins. This and other epidemiologic data strongly support an association between frequent and heavy intake of acetylsalicylic acid and other related compounds with gastrointestinal bleeding and gastric ulcer, whereas the association with duodenal ulcers is far less clearly established.

The ulcerogenic potency of corticosteroids, at least in the small or medium dose range, probably has been overstated in the past. Intensive ulcer therapy making use of H_2 receptor antagonists and proton pump inhibitors often allows healing of small ulcers with diameters up to 1 cm despite continued treatment with low dose corticosteroids or NSAIDs, whereas continuation of these drugs is associated with very poor healing in ulcers larger than 1 cm.

Aspirin and the then new class of NSAIDs were found to produce significant and predictable lesions after single doses in fasted rats only in the mid 1960s.[15] Other agents such as alcohol and steroids were shown to have similar effects. It was not until 1971 when Vane and his associates[16] showed that the mechanisms of action of aspirin and NSAIDS were due to inhibition of prostaglandin formation and that these were essential to the integrity of the upper gastrointestinal mucosa.[17] Cyclooxygenase (COX) leads to the formation of prostaglandins (PGs) that cause inflammation, swelling, pain, and fever.[18] By inhibiting this key enzyme in PG synthesis, aspirin-like drugs also prevented the production of physiologically important PGs that protect the stomach mucosa from damage by hydrochloric acid, maintain kidney function, and aggregate platelets when required.

This conclusion provided a unifying explanation for the therapeutic actions and shared side effects of the aspirin-like drugs. More recently with the discovery of a second COX gene, it became clear that there are two isoforms of the COX enzyme. The constitutive isoform, COX-1, supports the beneficial homeostatic functions, whereas the inducible isoform, COX-2, becomes up-regulated by inflammatory mediators and its products cause many of the symptoms of inflammatory diseases such as rheumatoid and osteoarthritis. Compounds that had selective COX-2 inhibitory activity were found to have potent analgesic and anti-inflammatory action but with less propensity to produce gastrointestinal mucosal damage.

Oral administration of indomethacin and other NSAIDS produced hemorrhagic gastric lesions in both normal and arthritic rats, although the severity of lesions was significantly greater in the latter group. In contrast, neither rofecoxib nor celecoxib caused any gastric damage in normal rats, but both drugs provoked hemorrhagic gastric lesions in arthritic rats. The expression of COX-2 mRNA and immunopositive cells was observed in the gastric mucosa of arthritic but not normal rats. The gastric mucosal prostaglandin (PGE_2) content was significantly elevated in arthritic rats in a rofecoxib-sensitive manner.[19]

Since COX-2 inhibitors produce gastric lesions in arthritic rats, similar to the nonselective COX inhibitors, it may be important to test potential anti-inflammatory agents in both normal and arthritic rats to evaluate the true gastric mucosal toxicity. COX-2 is up-regulated in the stomachs of arthritic rats, and PGs produced by COX-2 play a role in maintaining the integrity of the gastric mucosa. Dose-dependent administration of celecoxib and rofecoxib as COX-2 inhibitors and non-COX-1 inhibitors, respectively, did not produce toxic injuries on healthy gastrointestinal mucosa, thus providing a broad therapeutic spectrum.[20] On the other hand, when administered in the presence of altered gastrointestinal mucosa, they worsened and complicated gastric ulcers and also induced necrosis in the small intestine, thereby restricting clinical use.

The chronic use of NSAIDs, whether COX-1 or -2 inhibitors, is under attack due to an apparent increase in cardiac-related deaths in patients on high doses. It is not clear whether the use of COX-2 inhibitors in patients susceptible to gastrointestinal pathology is a risk worth taking.

Pathogenesis of gastric damage induced by NSAIDs involves multiple elements, such as deficiency of prostaglandins (PG), gastric hypermotility, neutrophil activation, and luminal acid.[21] PG deficiency may be critical in the increase of mucosal susceptibility to injury, and neutrophil activation alone is not ulcerogenic in the gastric mucosa, nor does it potentiate the ulcerogenic effects of other elements. Luminal acid is a prerequisite for later extension of damage to severe lesions.

Ethanol is a well known gastric mucosal irritant. Ethanol (80% v/v P.O.) given repeatedly to rats induces subchronic gastritis.[22] It can also produce gastric lesions after a single dose. Subchronic gastritis potentiated gastric ulcer formation, such as that produced by acetic acid. The induction of gastritis resulted in an activation of TNF-α expression followed by apoptosis in the gastric mucosa. This could lead to an increase in the severity of ulcerative damage in the stomach. It may be useful to test therapeutic agents likely to be given to humans with gastritis in mice with subchronic gastritis.

Models Available

Testing is usually simple and consists of oral dosing in 18- to 24-hour fasted rats and sacrificing after 3 to 5 hours. The stomachs are removed and filled with either saline or formalin. The mucosa is inspected, usually under low magnification, for the presence or absence of hemorrhagic spots, lesions, and ulcerations. Numerous attempts have been made to use scores and automated methods to provide quantitative data. However, in general, most investigators are interested in whether their compound produces a significant degree of mucosal damage and how this dose relates to the dose producing a therapeutic effect.

Multiple factors influence the rat model and its usefulness in predicting activity in humans.[23] The most important factor in using this model is to ensure a fasting period with a sufficient duration so that the stomach is devoid of food or ingested feces. Presence of material in the gastric content will interfere with observation of gross lesions and hemorrhagic spots and may provide enough buffering to raise the pH of the stomach above 4.

Why Test?

This test should be done for all clinical candidates that are to be administered orally. Gastric irritation is such a common side effect that this information should be available prior to the first human trials.

Small Intestine

The small intestine is also a common site for NSAID toxicity. Although NSAID strictures and perforations are relatively rare in humans, two thirds of regular NSAID users may be prone to small bowel enteropathy. With the use of a capsule camera, it is now possible to visualize the whole small intestine in a human. This will allow clinical trials to include evaluation for the potential of small intestinal pathology. Previously only limited visualization with flexible endoscopes could be achieved.

Classes of Compounds with Potential Liability and Possible Mechanisms

NSAID enteropathy is a step-wise process involving direct mucosal toxicity, mitochondrial damage, breakdown of intercellular integrity, enterohepatic recirculation, and neutrophil activation by luminal contents including bacteria.[24,25] Unlike upper gastrointestinal toxicity, cyclooxygenase-mediated mechanisms are probably less important. No temporal relationship was noted between prostaglandin inhibition and the formation of lesions in the small intestine, since the lesions became macroscopically apparent and developed at a time when cyclooxygenase inhibition was already declining.

Aspirin caused a prolonged inhibition of small intestine cyclooxygenase activity, yet failed to cause significant intestinal damage.[26,27] Thus, inhibition of prostaglandin synthesis alone may not be sufficient to initiate the processes that ultimately result in intestinal lesions. The prostaglandin-independent processes affected by indomethacin that lead to intestinal damage are as yet unknown. The use of animal models is unraveling new mechanisms for determining mucosal toxicity beyond the cyclooxygenase model.

Since one 5-HT$_3$ antagonist, alosetron, has been found to produce ischemic lesions in the small intestine, similar compounds may have to be evaluated prior to clinical trials.

Models Available

The fed rat is the usual model for evaluation of small intestinal lesions, at least those due to NSAIDs. The drug is administered with *ad lib* access to food and water. The rat is observed for 2 to 3 days. Indomethacin and other NSAIDs will produce significant lesions and even perforations in the small intestine.[28] Fed rats were 8 times more susceptible to intestinal damage than fasted rats, whereas fasted rats were 13 times more susceptible to gastric damage than fed rats.

The only model useful for specific evaluation of potential damage to small intestinal and colonic mucosa was published by Fara.[29] He used an *in situ* rabbit colon or intestine model as a sensitive and reproducible test to evaluate the topical effect of up to three substances applied to the colonic mucosa and found that doxycycline hyclate tablets and propranolol hydrochloride tablets produced macroscopic and histologic damage. Potassium released from Slow-K (potassium chloride) and Micro-K Extencaps caused more irritation than controlled-release GITS KCl (gastrointestinal therapeutic system KCl) Slow-K. This model may be useful in evaluating sustained or enteric-coated formulations for potential lesion-producing activity, and may be the only suitable way of evaluating potential problems with formulated products that are too large to be dosed to most laboratory animals.

Why Test?

All compounds believed to have anti-inflammatory activity or have effects on cyclooxygenase should be tested. Because of problems in humans (ischemic colitis) with at least one serotonin$_3$ antagonist, alosetron, this type of compound should also be evaluated. The initial enthusiasm for the use of 5HT$_3$ antagonists has been somewhat blunted by the withdrawal of alosetron because of ischemic colitis, but it remains to be seen whether this adverse event will be noted with other 5HT$_3$ antagonists.[30,31]

Alosetron is a potent and selective serotonin antagonist that recently became the first FDA-approved agent for diarrhea-predominant irritable bowel syndrome. Since approval, significant side effects including severe constipation, fecal impaction, and ischemic colitis have been noted with its use. Clinical, endoscopic, and pathologic features of the focal colitis strongly suggested ischemia and were observed in patients who should not have received the compound. Symptoms correlated temporally with alosetron use and abated with discontinuation of the drug.[32] Unfortunately, there are no test models known that will predict this type of small bowel enteropathy.

DRUG EFFECTS ON GASTRIC ACID SECRETION

Although guidelines suggest that experimental drugs should be evaluated for effects on gastric acid secretion, such testing does not appear to be needed for most classes of compounds.

Classes of Compounds with Potential Liability and Possible Mechanisms

Compounds that appear to be similar to known gastric antisecretory agents, muscarinic agonists and antagonists, and histamine agonists and antagonists should be tested to evaluate potential effects on acid secretion.

Models Available

Several models are available for evaluation in intact unanesthetized animals — the only appropriate approach. The pylorus-ligated rat has been the test most often used for evaluation of antisecretory activity. Drugs can be administered by any route, using an appropriate pretreatment time. Oral administration should occur at least 30 minutes prior to ligation so that the drug may have time to distribute to the small intestine. Topical activity can be evaluated by dosing after ligation. The test should be done in rats of the same source as therapeutic testing. Males or females may be used, although there has been some indication of gender differences.

The rat is anesthetized with a short-lasting volatile or intravenous anesthetic. Anesthetics having anticholinergic or α_2 agonist activity should not be used since they will inhibit secretion.[33,34] After a midline incision, a cotton ligature is placed snugly around the distal antrum (pylorus). The location and tightness of the ligation are important. The test duration is usually 3 hours, although other times have been used. The rat is euthanized, the stomach carefully removed, and the contents emptied into a calibrated centrifuge tube and centrifuged to obtain a clear supernatant. The volume is determined and an aliquot taken and titrated to pH 7.4. Results are noted as volume, titratable acidity, and total acid output.[35] The pH of the original sample should also be determined prior to dilution. Drugs may affect volume, concentration H^+, and the product of the two, total acid output (TAO). In many cases, the mechanism by which the compound inhibits secretion may be determined by which parameter is inhibited.

Ligation of the pylorus has been shown to stimulate acid secretion, so this model is not appropriate to evaluate compounds that may have gastric acid stimulatory activity. For this, a model in which gastric acid secretion is not stimulated is needed. The rat gastric fistula model, either chronic[36] or acute[37] preparation, is appropriate. For an acute gastric fistula preparation, a flanged plastic tube is inserted into the gastric lumen under anesthesia. The rat is allowed to recover from surgery and gastric juice is collected for 1 to 3 hours. Gastric acid secretion is about 50% of maximum so that both inhibitory and stimulatory effects may be observed. If another species is required, the chronic gastric fistula dog may be used.[37] The dog does not secrete acid in the fasted state. Thus it is the most sensitive for evaluation of compounds with potential acid secretory stimulatory activities. If antisecretory activity must be evaluated in dogs, the compound in question must be tested against gastric acid stimulated by gastrin, histamine, and other acid secretory agents.

Why Test?

Unless tests of gastric acid secretion are suggested for safety pharmacology purposes, they add little to information needed prior to clinical testing. If a series of compounds is similar to those having known effects, this type of test may be either postponed or eliminated.

EFFECTS OF DRUGS ON GASTROINTESTINAL PROPULSIVE MOTILITY

Gastric Emptying

Although gastric emptying testing is not specifically required by guidelines, data on the effects of experimental compounds on gastric emptying is important.

Classes of Compounds with Potential Liability and Possible Mechanisms

Drugs affecting gastric emptying may cause a variety of objectionable side effects that can be evaluated early in the discovery process. Compounds affecting the autonomic nervous system (agonists or antagonists), drugs having serotonergic (agonist or antagonist) activities, and a wide variety of compounds may have profound effects on gastric emptying. Drugs influencing emptying can also result in significant effects on pharmacokinetics, either increasing or decreasing blood levels achieved after oral administration. Drugs augmenting gastric emptying may also be useful in the treatment of patients with gastroparesis.

Models Available

The charcoal meal test is usually specified for evaluation of gastrointestinal propulsive motility. Unfortunately, it is not a good model for evaluation of gastric emptying, and can only provide an indirect indication of effects on gastric emptying. There are many specific test models to evaluate effects on solid or liquid emptying. When deciding what test to use, it is important to remember that drug activity may differ depending on whether solid or liquid meals are used.

Liquid meals — Emptying of a non-nutrient liquid solution of a non-absorbable dye (phenol red or carmine red) in conscious rats is a common method. Gastric emptying is measured at different time points after administration of a semi-viscous liquid (methylcellulose) containing a non-absorbable dye as the marker. The volume of gastric emptying is calculated from the amount of dye remaining in the stomach, taking into consideration the volume of gastric secretions. Depending on the duration of the test, this method may be optimized for evaluation of agents augmenting (10 to 20 minutes) or inhibiting gastric emptying (30 to 90 minutes). It may also be performed in chronically cannulated rats fitted with stainless steel gastric cannulas.[38]

Rosalmeida et al. conducted a typical study.[39] Phenol red dissolved in water was administered in small volumes to fasted rats. After test agent administration, the rats were gavaged (1.5 ml) with a test meal (phenol red in 5% glucose solution, 0.5 mg/ml) and sacrificed 10, 20, or 30 minutes later. The volume of gastric contents was determined by analysis of the dye remaining in the stomach, then compared to volumes from vehicle-treated animals. Sildenafil delayed gastric emptying of a liquid meal. Phenol red has also been used in mice (0.15 ml/mouse).[40]

Feldman and Putcha[41] studied the activities of atropine sulfate, trihexyphenidyl HCl, benztropine mesylate, diphenhydramine HCl, and ethopropazine HCl on gastric emptying and intestinal transit of a phenol red solution in rats.

Inhibition of gastric emptying and intestinal transit were only observed after single and multiple oral doses of diphenhydramine and ethopropazine.

Glucose solution and other liquid meals — The emptying of a glucose meal or other meal containing a thickening agent or plain water may be quantitated by comparison of gastric weight after a set period. Although results may be affected by secretion into the gastric lumen, the method provides a rough estimate of emptying of a liquid load.[50]

Charcoal meal — Lotti et al.[42] described a simple test in mice used to evaluate CCK antagonists based upon visual determination of the gastric emptying of a charcoal meal. CCK-8, but not various other peptide and nonpeptide agents, effectively inhibited gastric emptying in this test system.

Drug absorption — The absorption of a compound known not to be absorbed from the stomach but having consistent duodenal absorption characteristics has been used to quantify gastric emptying of a liquid meal.[43] The usual compound used is acetaminophen because it is not absorbed through the gastric mucosa and blood levels are observed only after the compound reaches the duodenum. An oral dose (100 mg/kg) was administered and blood samples were collected before and up to 12 hours after administration. Plasma assays were performed using a high performance liquid chromatography method with ultraviolet detection. The calculated population pharmacokinetic parameters Ka, Kel (first order absorption and elimination constants) and Vd/F (apparent volume of distribution) provided information on the effects of drugs on transport of acetaminophen into the duodenum compared to vehicle controls.

Radioisotopes — Emptying of liquid nutrient meals tagged with radioisotopes has been used as a model in animals and is a common method in humans. The method is useful for defining regulation of gastric emptying of nutrient liquid meals in mice. In larger animals, a γ-camera may be used to quantify radioactive material remaining in the stomach. Solutions of non-absorbable radioisotopes such as radiolabeled chromium have been used for estimating gastric emptying. In one study, results were compared to emptying of a charcoal meal. Gastrointestinal propulsive motility was assessed in rats 15 minutes after intragastric instillation of a test meal containing charcoal (10%) and $Na^{251}CrO_4$ (0.5 μCi/ml).[44] Gastric emptying was determined by measuring the amount of radiolabeled chromium contained in the small intestine as a percentage of the initial amount received. Gastrointestinal transit was evaluated by calculating the geometric center of distribution of the radiolabeled marker.

Solids: beads or pellets — The use of beads or non-dissolving tablets to evaluate the effects of drugs on gastric emptying has been established as a method for discovery of agents with gastroprokinetic activity.[45] Jacoby and Brodie[46] published a study using 1-mm Amberlite pellets in rats and small enteric-coated barium tablets tracked by fluoroscopy in rhesus monkeys to evaluate gastric emptying produced by metoclopramide. Other variations of the use of small pellets (polystyrene, plastic, glass) have been used to evaluate drug effects on gastric emptying.[47,48] Twenty-four-hour fasted rats are dosed with the test compound via the appropriate route and at the appropriate dose. A set number of pellets is administered by an appropriate size gavage tube and after 10 to 60 minutes the rat is euthanized and the stomach carefully removed. The number of beads remaining in the stomach is counted and compared to counts from a group of rats receiving the vehicle control. The experiment can be designed to detect agents increasing gastric emptying (shorter duration) or those inhibiting gastric emptying (longer duration). Some information as to intestinal propulsion can be obtained by counting pellets in segments of the small intestine. The study may also be done in rats with delayed gastric emptying due to streptotozin-induced diabetes.

Asai, Vickers, and Power[49] studied the effect of clonidine on gastric motility by examining gastric emptying of indigestible solids. Clonidine or saline was injected intraperitoneally, and ten steel balls (1.0 mm in diameter) were inserted into the stomach. Gastric emptying was examined at 3 hours. Clonidine delayed gastric emptying of the balls. Yohimbine, but not naloxone, significantly antagonized the inhibitory effect of clonidine.

Solids: chow meal — The use of a meal of ground rat or mouse chow may be useful in the estimation of gastric emptying of a semi-liquid meal. Differences in gastric weight between treated and control animals provide a rough index of emptying. Animals are deprived of food for 18 to 24 hours and allowed free access to preweighed solid chow for a set period (1 to 3 hours). The food is then removed and gastric emptying can be determined over several hours by measuring the wet weight of the stomach. For a more accurate estimate, the ground meal can be labeled with a radioisotope that binds to the meal or ground-up liver from an animal fed a radioisotope such as technetium can be used.

Why Test?

Slowing gastric emptying can affect absorption of an agent and may be responsible for drug interactions by interference with the absorption of concomitantly taken medication. Inhibition of gastric emptying in rats may also predict other adverse effects such as gastroparesis. Augmentation of gastric emptying may also affect the pharmacokinetics of co-administered agents and may indicate a useful pharmacological action.

Small Intestinal Propulsion

Classes of Compounds with Potential Liability and Possible Mechanisms

Opioids and a number of other classes of agents have significant effects on small bowel propulsive motility. The charcoal meal test will usually pick up both stimulants and inhibitors of propulsion and is one of the tests recommended in the guidelines.

Animal Models Available

Charcoal meal — This test is most commonly used to determine effects on propulsive motility. It can be performed in the fasted rats or mice. Charcoal meal has long been used as a measure of small intestinal propulsive motility since

Macht and Barba-Gose published the method in 1931.[51] It is recommended in most guidelines. The test agent is given by the appropriate route and a small volume (depending on the size of the test animal) of non-activated charcoal suspended in 1 to 2% carboxy or hydroxypropyl cellulose is administered orally. The test animal is euthanized at an appropriate time (1 to 3 hours) and the stomach and small intestine are removed. The distance of the furthest sign of charcoal in the intestine is noted and compared to the total length of the small intestine (pylorus to ileocecal valve).

The inhibitory effect of repetitiously administered loperamide, a peripheral μ-opioid receptor agonist and well recognized antidiarrheal agent, on mouse gastrointestinal transit was compared with that of morphine in order to examine the development of tolerance to μ-opioid receptor agonist-induced constipation (antitransit effect).[52] When administered subcutaneously 15 minutes before the oral injection of charcoal meal, loperamide (0.1 to 30 mg/kg) and morphine (1 to 8 mg/kg) dose-dependently and significantly inhibited gastrointestinal transit of charcoal with ID_{50} values of 1.6 mg/kg and 3.6 mg/kg, respectively.

Other tests using radionuclides have also been used but require special laboratories for handling radioactive materials and do not provide significantly more information.

Why Test?

Drugs affecting small intestinal propulsive motility may possess either inhibitory or stimulatory activity on small intestinal propulsive motility. These tests are good predictors for evaluating the possibility that a test compound has constipating or laxative activity.

Colonic Propulsive Motility

The purpose for testing the effects of compounds on colonic motility is primarily to predict the potential for producing constipation or diarrhea. Several simple tests have shown good correlation to clinical effects. They may also provide information as to mechanism and duration of action.

Classes of Compounds with Potential Liability and Possible Mechanisms

All compounds in development should be tested for effects on intestinal propulsive motility. These tests provide a simple method for determining constipation or diarrhea as a potential adverse effect for many classes of compounds, and may provide information indicating a better or worse profile in a series of compounds or show that one compound performs better than reference compounds. A large number of mechanisms including opioids, anticholinergics, and serotonin agonists and antagonists may manifest themselves through effects on intestinal propulsion.

Animal Models Available

Fecal pellet output — Monitoring the output of fecal pellets by mice or rats is one of the simplest tests available for evaluation of potential effects on intestinal propulsive motility. It can be useful for predicting constipation or diarrhea in mice or rats, although other species may be used. The test agent is administered by the appropriate route to rats or mice that are provided with access to food and water. Results may be monitored by counting fecal pellets and noting composition (solid, semisolid, not formed) or by weighing fecal output (wet or dry weight). Care must be taken to prevent loss of fecal pellets through the cage floor.

Drugs increasing colonic propulsion and excretion either by affecting motility or increasing fluid content (inhibition of absorption or increasing secretion) can be easily detected.[53] Serotonin and a serotonin$_3$ receptor agonist, 2-methyl-5-HT, dose-dependently increased fecal pellet output in conscious rats. The selective 5-HT$_3$ receptor antagonists (GK-128, granisetron, ramosetron, azasetron, and ondansetron) depressed the increase in fecal pellet output caused by 2-methyl-5-HT. Granisetron and ramosetron dose-dependently reduced the spontaneous excretion of fecal pellets.

Croci and Bianchetti[54] showed the effects of several α_{2A}-adrenoceptor antagonists on fecal output and water content in rats. The rat colon appears to be under tonic inhibitory control of prejunctional α_2-adrenergic receptors, whose blockage by specific antagonists induces fecal excretion. The α_{2A}-receptor subtype appears to be the most likely candidate for controlling fecal excretion through inhibition of acetylcholine release.

Fecal pellet output has also been used to evaluate potential antidiarrheal activity. Oral doses of castor oil increase both the fecal output (dry or wet weight) and the frequency of diarrhea in mice. Bismuth subsalicylate significantly prevented the enhancement of charcoal meal transport induced by castor oil in both mice and rats.[55] Increased fecal output (dry or wet weight) and increased frequency of diarrhea in mice were significantly reduced by bismuth subsalicylate in a dose-related fashion. Blockade of castor oil diarrhea was also used to discover the first synthetic antidiarrheal agents by Awouters et al.[56]

The time course of castor oil-induced diarrhea in fasted rats was quantified by weighing stools every 15 minutes for 8 hours after the challenge and then after 24 hours. Diarrhea began within 1 hour as a series of rapidly occurring evacuations over 20 to 40 minutes. Pretreatment with small doses of loperamide caused a significant reduction. Riviere et al.[57] used prostaglandin E$_2$ to produce diarrhea in mice. When given by intraperitoneal administration, PGE$_2$ induced a dose- and time-dependent diarrhea. Fecal output measurement provides a convenient method for investigation of mechanism of action of antidiarrheal agents.

Glass bead expulsion — The expulsion of glass beads inserted into the distal colons of rats or mice has been utilized as assay to investigate potential effects on colonic propulsive motility. This test is relatively specific for effects on propulsion and can detect most agents producing constipation in humans. It has been used to screen for antidiarrheal agents. In rats, it may also be useful for evaluation of agents increasing or decreasing colonic propulsive motility. However, in mice, it is only suitable for agents inhibiting propulsion.

The test is simple and consists of inserting a glass bead (~2 to 4 mm) through the anus into the distal colon. It can detect compounds that exert significant constipating activity or may be used as a primary screen for irritable bowel syndrome. A single 3-mm glass bead is inserted 2 cm into the distal colon of each mouse using a glass rod, one end of which was fire-polished so as to be rendered atraumatic. After bead insertion, the mice are placed in individual plastic cages lined with white paper to aid visualization of bead expulsion. The time required for expulsion of the glass bead is determined to the nearest 0.1 minute for each mouse. Mice that did not expel the beads within 0.5 to 1 hour are necropsied to confirm the presence of the bead in the lumen of the large intestine. Mice for which bead localization could not be confirmed were not included in the results.

Drugs interfering with expulsion may work by local effects in the distal colon blocking afferents, inhibiting smooth muscle propulsive motility directly or indirectly through receptor-mediated effects on the nervous network in the colon or through CNS-mediated effects. The rat provides a better model for detection of agents that increase propulsive motility since expulsion by rats is much slower than by mice. This test may be useful to evaluate laxatives such as $5HT_4$ agonists that have direct effects on propulsive motility.

Studies using glass beads have been used to evaluate mechanisms of action. Since drugs may be administered ICV in mice, the beads have also been used to investigate the site of action when compared to peripherally administered compounds,[58–60] and also to study the effect of peptides and opioids,[61,62] urocortins,[63] radio waves,[64] and nociceptin.[65]

Yamada and Onoda[66] studied the colonic prokinetic activity of oral T-1815 and compared it with that of yohimbine and naloxone in mice by designing an experiment in which colonic propulsive motility is inhibited by clonidine (3 to 30 μg/kg s.c.) or loperamide (0.3 to 3.0 mg/kg s.c.). Yohimbine (0.3 to 10 mg/kg) and T-1815 (0.1 to 10 mg/kg) showed a dose-dependent reduction of the delay in evacuation induced by clonidine, but naloxone had no effect. The loperamide-induced retardation of colonic propulsion was reduced by naloxone (0.3 to 10 mg/kg) and T-1815 (0.1 to 10 mg/kg) in a dose-dependent manner, but yohimbine had no effect. In normal animals, yohimbine and naloxone had no significant effect on evacuation, while a slight acceleration was observed with T-1815 at 10 mg/kg.

Why Test?

Diarrhea and constipation are two of the most commonly observed side effects of therapeutic agents. The tests available are excellent at predicting the possibilities in clinical studies and may be useful for choosing a lead compound in early developmental studies. All compounds should be tested with one or more of these methods prior to the first clinical trial.

Drug-Induced Emesis

Nausea and vomiting are the most frequent adverse effects observed in clinical trials. Although emetic activity may be classified as a CNS-related side effect, emesis produces significant disturbance of gastrointestinal functions and may produce problems in short- and long-term safety evaluations in dogs or monkeys.

Classes of Compounds with Potential Liability and Possible Mechanisms

All compounds related to known emetogenic agents should be tested. A wide variety of clinically useful compounds are associated with nausea and vomiting. This testing may provide information as to improvement of side effect profiles compared to positive controls. Among classes of compounds that have known emetogenic activities are cytotoxics, dopamine agonists, and antidepressants.

Animal Models Available

Since most rodents are not capable of vomiting, initial studies in rats, mice, and guinea pigs do not provide information concerning emetogenic activity. The dog has been the standard model for testing; however, dog use may be a problem in early drug development due to expense and supply. King[67] reviewed animal models including nonhuman primates, dogs, cats, and ferrets. The categories of pharmacologic compounds include those that act on identified membrane receptors (e.g., cholinergic agonists, catecholamines, and neuroactive peptides) and those that act on unidentified receptors (e.g., cardiac glycosides and veratrum alkaloids, among others). Emphasis is placed on emetic dose–response relations and threshold ED_{50} and ED_{100} values calculated from these relations as indices of species sensitivity to emetic stimuli. For the more noxious emetics, the cytotoxins, and radiation, the latency to the first emetic episode and duration of emesis were also compared across species.

Several alternatives to the use of dogs have been suggested. One, the house musk shrew, has been used; however, it was not found to be sensitive to many well known emetic agents such as morphine. In fact, opioids had anti-emetic activity.[68] There are few references to the use of this animal and its validity in testing has not been proven.

The ferret has been shown to be an excellent model for screening anti-emetics and is used extensively in the development of anti-emetics useful against chemotherapy and radiation-induced emesis. The use of ferrets to evaluate emetogenic or anti-emetic activity is documented[69] and there appears to be good correlation between emetogenic activity in ferrets and in humans.

The pathophysiology of the emetic reflex and the clinical management of emesis are very complicated. Animal models of chemotherapy- and radiotherapy-induced emesis successfully predicted the clinical efficacy of the 5-HT_3 receptor antagonists for the control of acute emesis.[70] Further studies in animals have provided valuable information relating to the pathophysiology of emesis and the mechanisms of action of 5-HT_3 receptor antagonists. These agents inhibit emesis by blocking the action of 5-HT at 5-HT_3 receptors on the vagus nerve in the gastrointestinal tract and in the hindbrain vomiting system.

Serotonin is believed to be released from enterochromaffin cells following cytotoxic therapy or radiation. The mechanism by which 5-HT is released from enterochromaffin cells is unknown. Although various mechanisms have been proposed, none has provided convincing supportive evidence. Emetics may produce acute or delayed vomiting. This is specifically true for cytotoxic agents similar to cisplatin. Ferrets, when given a dose of cisplatin and observed for 3 days, show a pattern of emesis similar to that seen in humans with two distinct phases: acute and delayed emesis. Ondansetron and other 5-HT$_3$ compounds are effective in reducing the emetic response over days 1 through 3. When a higher dose of cisplatin is used, emesis usually occurs in less than 2 hours. This can also be blocked by serotonin antagonists.

The typical emesis study is done using descented and castrated male ferrets that are individually housed in stainless steel cages and provided ~75 g of ferret diet each day and water *ad lib*. Dosing may be done in either overnight fasted or fed ferrets. After oral dosing, the ferrets are observed for signs of lip licking, malaise, retching, vomiting, and drooling for an appropriate time period. Ferrets have also been used occasionally for safety evaluation studies.[71]

Why Test?

Although not required in guidelines for inclusion of safety pharmacology, drug-induced emesis testing of all clinical candidates should be conducted prior to Phase I studies. The test is relatively inexpensive and does not require a great deal of test compound.

Liver and Gallbladder

Classes of Compound with Potential Liability and Possible Mechanisms

Any experimental compound may affect bile secretion and gallbladder function. However, only those compounds with known structural or pharmacologic similarities to substances that exhibit activities on these functions need be tested.

Models Available

Effect on bile flow — Studies on bile flow are usually not included in safety pharmacology testing but are performed during acute, short-term, or long-term safety evaluations. In some limited instances, data on effects on bile (content, volume) are required. Since rats do not have gallbladders, they are not appropriate species for the study of bile storage. Short-term studies of effects on bile formation and transport to the small intestine may be done in rats. Drug excretion and bile content can be studied using acute or chronic bile duct cannulation to directly collect bile. If these studies continue more than a few hours, some mechanism for returning bile to the small intestine must be used because catheterization of the common bile duct prevents recycling through the entero-porto-hepato-biliary circulation. Steady-state conditions can be ensured by constant infusion of bile or bile acids into the stomach or duodenum. Urine and feces can also be collected to allow quantitative excretion of the compound(s) of interest.

Enderlin and Honohan[72] published a method for long-term collection of bile using an externalized cannula brought through an intrascapular incision. The cannula was protected by a 30-cm, 16-gauge stainless steel tube attached to the skin through the incision. The rats were housed in cages at a level higher than the collection vials to aid in drainage of bile. A hole in each vial cap permitted the cannula to turn freely as a rat moved about the cage. This method allowed bile to be collected conveniently over long periods with minimal restraint of the animals.

In order to provide a steady state condition, Chipman and Cropper[73] describe a re-entrant cannula with a sampling arm that is inserted into the bile duct to allow intermittent collections of bile from unanesthetized minimally restrained rats for 30 days or more. The flow rate of bile (5.38 cm^3/hour/kg) was higher than that previously reported when using simple or re-entrant cannulas. This higher flow rate may be a result of allowing a minimum of 10 days post-operative recovery period before starting collection of bile and avoiding anesthesia and other stresses at the time of collection. Other methods may be found in References 74 through 78.

Why Test?

The usual reason for collecting bile is to evaluate and quantify drug excretion in the bile. However, bile collection may be used also to test the effects of compounds on bile flow if effects are suspected. A rabbit or dog model must be used to evaluate activity directly on the gallbladder.

Effects of Drugs on Exocrine Section of Pancreas

Classes of Compound with Potential Liability and Possible Mechanisms

Many classes of drugs may affect the volume and content of pancreatic fluid. The measurement of insulin and/or glucagon levels is usually a function of longer-term safety evaluations and is not usually considered a gastrointestinal safety study. Although such testing is not usually performed, in some cases the information gained can be helpful in designing clinical trials and in preventing potential adverse effects.

Animal Models Available

Several methods for collection of pancreatic juice are available. Again it is important that fluid and enzyme losses be replaced during experiments that last more than a day. A surgical procedure allows injection into the stomach and the duodenum by separate catheters, collection of the pancreatic juice during the experiments, recirculation of the pancreatic juice into the duodenum between experiments, and normal circulation of bile in rats.[79] The methods of Colwell[80] and Roze[81] may also be used for collection of pancreatic juice in unanesthetized rats.

Why Test?

Compounds suspected of having effects on volume and content of pancreatic juice should be tested.

REFERENCES

1. Bass, A., Kinter, L., and Williams, P., Origins, practices and future of safety pharmacology. *J. Pharmacol. Toxicol. Meth.*, 49, 145, 2004.
2. International Conference on Harmonization, *M3 Timing of Nonclinical Safety Studies for the Conduct of Human Clinical Trials for Pharmaceuticals* (FDA, 1997).
3. Guzmán, A., Safety pharmacology, pharmacokinetics and toxicology: an obstacle race in the development of a pharmaceutical compound. *Meth. Findings Exp. Chem. Pharmacol.*, 25, Suppl. A, 2003.
4. Kinter, L.B. et al., Research overview status of safety pharmacology in the pharmaceutical industry, 1993. *Drug Develop. Res.*, 32, 208, 1994.
5. Mattsson, J.L., Spencer, P.J., and Albee, R.R., A performance standard for clinical and functional observational battery examinations of rats. *J. Amer. Col. Toxicol.*, 15, 239, 1996.
6. Irwin, S., Comprehensive observational assessment: a systematic, quantitative procedure for assessing the behavioural and physiologic state of the mouse. *Psychopharmacologia* (Berlin), 13, 222, 1968.
7. Haggerty, G.C., Strategies for and experience with neurotoxicity testing of new pharmaceuticals. *J. Amer. Col. Toxicol.*, 10, 677, 1991.
8. Murphy, D.J., Safety pharmacology of the respiratory system: techniques and study design. *Drug Develop. Res.*, 32, 237, 1994.
9. International Conference on Harmonization, *S6 Preclinical Safety Evaluation of Biotechnology-Derived Pharmaceuticals* (FDA, 1997).
10. Harrison, A.P. et al., Gastrointestinal tract models and techniques for use in safety pharmacology. *J. Pharmacol. Toxicol. Meth.*, 49, 187, 2004.
11. Smith, S. et al., Novel techniques for testing of esophageal irritancy of liquids and tablets in dogs. *Contemp. Top. Lab. Anim. Sci.*, 37, 66, 1998.
12. Peter, C.P., Handt, L.K., and Smith, S.M.. Esophageal irritation due to alendronate sodium tablets: possible mechanisms. *Dig. Dis. Sci.*, 43, 1998, 1998.
13. Lowe, C.E. et al., Upper gastrointestinal toxicity of alendronate. *Am. J. Gastroenterol.*, 95, 634. 2000.
14. Borsch, G. and Schmidt, G., What's new in steroid and nonsteroid drug effects on gastroduodenal mucosa? *Pathol. Res. Pract.*, 180, 437, 1985.
15. Robert, A. and Nezamis, J.E., Histopathology of steroid-induced ulcers: an experimental study in the rat. *Arch. Pathol.*, 77, 407, 1964.
16. Vane, J.R., Inhibition of prostaglandin synthesis as a mechanism of action for aspirin-like drugs. *Nat. New Biol.*, 231, 232, 1971.
17. Vane, J.R. and Botting, R.M., The mechanism of action of aspirin. *Thromb. Res.* 15, 255, 2003.
18. Whittle, B.J., Temporal relationship between cyclooxygenase inhibition, as measured by prostacyclin biosynthesis, and the gastrointestinal damage induced by indomethacin in the rat. *Gastroenterology*, 80, 94, 1981.

19. Kato, S. et al., Ulcerogenic influence of selective cyclooxygenase-2 inhibitors in the rat stomach with adjuvant-induced arthritis. *J. Pharmacol. Exp. Ther.*, 303, 503, 2002.
20. Laudanno, O.M. et al., Gastrointestinal damage induced by celecoxib and rofecoxib in rats. *Acta Gastroenterol. Latinoam.*, 30, 27, 2000.
21. Takeuchi, K. et al., Analysis of pathogenic elements involved in gastric lesions induced by non-steroidal anti-inflammatory drugs in rats. *J. Gastroenterol. Hepatol.* 12, 36. 1997.
22. Liu, E.S. and Cho, C.H., Relationship between ethanol-induced gastritis and gastric ulcer formation in rats. *Digestion*, 62, 232, 2000.
23. Suwa, T. et al., Comparative studies on the gastrointestinal lesions caused by several nonsteroidal anti-inflammatory agents in rats. *Agents Actions*, 21, 167, 1987.
24. Fortun, P.J. and Hawkey, C.J., Nonsteroidal anti-inflammatory drugs and the small intestine. *Curr. Opin. Gastroenterol.*, 21, 169, 2005.
25. Szabo, S., Mechanisms of mucosal injury in the stomach and duodenum: time-sequence analysis of morphologic, functional, biochemical and histochemical studies. *Scand. J. Gastroenterol. Suppl.* 127, 2. 1987.
26. Brodie, D.A., Tate, C.L., and Hooke, K.F., Aspirin: intestinal damage in rats. *Science*, 9, 183, 1970.
27. Mariani, L., Factors influencing the indomethacin-induced intestinal lesions in the rat. *Eur. J. Toxicol. Environ. Hyg.,* 8, 335, 1975.
28. Brodie, D.A. et al., Indomethacin-induced intestinal lesions in the rat. *Toxicol. Appl. Pharmacol.*, 17, 615, 1970.
29. Fara, J.W. et al., Assessment and validation of animal models to evaluate topical effects of substances on gastrointestinal mucosa. *Pharm. Res.* 5, 165, 1988.
30. Spiller, R., Serotonergic modulating drugs for functional gastrointestinal diseases. *Br. J. Clin. Pharmacol.*, 54, 11, 2002.
31. Friedel, D., Thomas, R., and Fisher, R.S., Ischemic colitis during treatment with alosetron. *Gastroenterology*, 120, 557, 2001.
32. Kamm, M.A., The complexity of drug development for irritable bowel syndrome. *Aliment. Pharmacol. Ther.*, 16, 343, 2002.
33. Mullner, K. et al., Involvement of central K(ATP) channels in the gastric antisecretory action of 2-adrenoceptor agonists and beta-endorphin in rats. *Eur. J. Pharmacol.,* 435, 225, 2002.
34. Kunchandy, J., Khanna. S., and Kulkarni, S.K., Effect of 2 agonists clonidine, guanfacine and B-HT 920 on gastric acid secretion and ulcers in rats. *Arch. Int. Pharmacodyn. Ther.*, 275, 123, 1985.
35. Brodie, D.A. and Knapp, P.G., The mechanism of the inhibition of gastric secretion produced by esophageal ligation in the pylorus-ligated rat. *Gastroenterology,* 50, 787, 1966.
36. Komarov, S.A., Bralow, S.P., and Boyd, E., A permanent rat gastric fistula. *Proc. Soc. Exp. Biol. Med.*, 112, 451, 1963.
37. Jacoby, H.I. et al., Antisecretory actions of aminophylline in the rat and dog. *Digestion*, 19, 237, 1979.
38. Setler, P.E. and Smith, G.P., Gastric emptying in rats with chronic gastric fistulas. *Am. J. Dig. Dis.*, 14, 137, 1969.

39. de Rosalmeida, M.C. et al., Sildenafil, a phosphodiesterase-5 inhibitor, delays gastric emptying and gastrointestinal transit of liquid in awake rats. *Dig. Dis. Sci.*, 48, 2064, 2003.

40. Miyasaka, K. et al., Enhanced gastric emptying of a liquid gastric load in mice lacking cholecystokinin-B receptor: a study of CCK-A, B, and AB receptor gene knockout mice. *J. Gastroenterol.*, 39, 319, 2004.

41. Feldman, S. and Putcha, L., Effect of anti-Parkinsonism drugs on gastric emptying and intestinal transit in the rat. *Pharmacology*, 15, 503, 1977.

42. Lotti, V.J. et al., A new simple mouse model for the *in vivo* evaluation of cholecystokinin (CCK) antagonists: comparative potencies and durations of action of nonpeptide antagonists. *Life Sci.*, 39, 1631, 1986.

43. Gandia, P. et al., Influence of simulated weightlessness on the pharmacokinetics of acetaminophen administered by the oral route: a study in the rat. *Fundam. Clin. Pharmacol.*, 18, 57, 2004.

44. Pu, H.F. et al., Effects of juice from *Morinda citrifolia* (Noni) on gastric emptying in male rats. *Chin. J. Physiol.*, 47, 169, 2004.

45. Brodie, D.A., A comparison of anticholinergic drugs on gastric secretion, gastric emptying, and pupil diameter in the rat. *Gastroenterology*, 50, 45, 1966.

46. Jacoby, H.I. and Brodie, D.A., Gastrointestinal actions of metoclopramide: an experimental study. *Gastroenterology*, 52, 676, 1967.

47. Tabosa, A. et al., A comparative study of the effects of electroacupuncture and moxibustion in the gastrointestinal motility of the rat. *Dig. Dis. Sci.*, 49, 602, 2004.

48. Yamano, M. et al., Effects of gastroprokinetic agents on gastroparesis in streptozotocin-induced diabetic rats. *Naun. Schmied. Arch. Pharmacol.*, 356, 145, 1997.

49. Asai, T., Vickers, M.D., and Power, I., Clonidine inhibits gastric motility in the rat. *Europ. J. Anaesth.*, 14, 316, 1997.

50. Matsuda, H. et al., Inhibitory mechanism of costunolide, a sesquiterpene lactone isolated from *Laurus nobilis*, on blood ethanol elevation in rats: involvement of inhibition of gastric emptying and increase in gastric juice secretion. *Alcohol Alcoholism*, 37, 121, 2002.

51. Macht, D.I., and Barba-Gose, J., Two new methods for pharmacological comparison of insoluble purgatives. *J. Am. Pharm. Assoc.* 20, 558, 1931.

52. Tan-No, K. et al., Development of tolerance to the inhibitory effect of loperamide on gastrointestinal transit in mice. *Eur. J. Pharm. Sci.*, 20, 357, 2003.

53. Ito, C. et al., Effect of GK-128 [2-[(2-methylimidazol-1-yl)methyl]-benzo[f]thiochromen-1-one monohydrochloride hemihydrate], a selective 5-hydroxytryptamine$_3$ receptor antagonist, on colonic function in rats. *J. Pharmacol. Exp. Ther.*, 280, 67, 1997.

54. Croci, T. and Bianchetti, A., Stimulation of faecal excretion in rats by 2-adrenergic antagonists. *J. Pharm. Pharmacol.*, 44, 358, 1992.

55. Goldenberg, M.M., Honkomp, L.J., and Castellion, A.W., The antidiarrheal action of bismuth subsalicylate in the mouse and the rat. *Am. J. Dig. Dis.*, 20, 955, 1975.

56. Awouters, F. et al., Loperamide antagonism of castor oil-induced diarrhea in rats: a quantitative study. *Arch. Int. Pharmacodyn. Ther.*, 217, 29, 1975.

57. Riviere, P.J. et al., Prostaglandin E2-induced diarrhea in mice: importance of colonic secretion. *Pharmacol. Exp. Ther.*, 256, 547, 1991.

58. Jacoby, H.I. and Lopez, I.A., Method for the evaluation of colonic propulsive motility in the mouse after ICV administered compounds. *Dig. Dis. Sci.* 29, 551, 1984.

59. Raffa, R.B., Mathiasen, J.R, and Jacoby, H.I., Colonic bead expulsion time in normal and mu-opioid receptor deficient (CXBK) mice following central (ICV) administration of μ- and -opioid agonists. *Life Sci.*, 41, 2229, 1987.

60. Jacoby, H.I., Bonfilio, A.C. and Raffa, R.B., Central and peripheral administration of serotonin produces opposite effects on mouse colonic propulsive motility. *Neurosci. Lett.*, 122, 122, 1991.

61. Raffa, R.B. and Jacoby, H.I., Effect of the Phe-D-Met-Arg-Phe-NH$_2$-related peptides on mouse colonic propulsive motility: a structure-activity relationship study. *J. Pharm. Exp. Ther.* 254, 809, 1990.

62. Negri, L. et al., Effects of antisense oligonucleotides on brain delta-opioid receptor density and on SNC80-induced locomotor stimulation and colonic transit inhibition in rats. *Br. J. Pharmacol.*, 128, 1554, 1999.

63. Martínez, V. et al., Central CRF, urocortins and stress increase colonic transit via CRF$_1$ receptors while activation of CRF$_2$ receptors delays gastric transit in mice. *J. Physiol.*, 556, 221, 2004.

64. Radzievsky, A.A. et al., Single millimeter wave treatment does not impair gastrointestinal transit in mice. *Life Sci.*, 71, 1763, 2002.

65. Osinski, M.A., Bass, P. and Gaumnitz, E.A., Peripheral and central actions of orphanin FQ (nociceptin) on murine colon. *Am. J. Physiol. Gastrointest. Liver. Physiol.* 276, G125, 1999.

66. Yamada, K. and Onoda, Y., Comparison of the effects of T-1815, yohimbine and naloxone on mouse colonic propulsion. *J. Smooth Muscle Res.* 29, 47, 1993.

67. King, G.L., Animal models in the study of vomiting. *Can. J. Physiol. Pharmacol.*, 68, 260, 1990.

68. Selve, N. et al., Absence of emetic effects of morphine and loperamide in *Suncus murinus. Eur. J. Pharmacol.* 2, 256, 1994.

69. Marty, M., Chemotherapy-induced nausea and vomiting: from experimentation to experience. *Bull. Cancer*, 83 ,1014, 1996.

70. Naylor, R.J. and Rudd, J.A., Mechanisms of chemotherapy/radiotherapy-induced emesis in animal models. *Oncology*, 53, Suppl. 1, 8, 1996.

71. Kinsella, T.J. et al., Preclinical study of the systemic toxicity and pharmacokinetics of 5-iodo-2-deoxypyrimidinone-2'-deoxyribose as a radiosensitizing prodrug in two, non-rodent animal species: implications for phase I study design. *Clin. Cancer. Res.*, 6, 3670, 2000.

72. Enderlin, F.E. and Honohan, T., Long term bile collection in the rat. *Lab. Anim. Sci.*, 27, 490, 1977.

73. Chipman, J.K. and Cropper, N.C., A technique for chronic intermittent bile collection from the rat. *Res. Vet. Sci.*, 22, 366, 1977.

74. Gallo-Torres, H.E., Methodology for the determination of bioavailability of labeled residues. *J. Toxicol. Environ. Health,* 2, 827, 1977.

75. Balabaud, C. et al., Bile collection in free moving rats. *Lab. Anim. Sci.* 31, 273, 1981.

76. Tomlinson, P.W., Jeffery, D.J., and Filer, C.W., A novel technique for assessment of biliary secretion and enterohepatic circulation in the unrestrained conscious rat. *Xenobiotica*, 11, 863, 1981.

77. Rath, L. and Hutchison, M., A new method of bile duct cannulation allowing bile collection and re-infusion in the conscious rat. *Lab. Anim.*, 23, 163, 1989.

78. Heitmeyer, S.A. and Powers, J.F., Improved method for bile collection in unrestrained conscious rats. *Lab. Anim. Sci.*, 42, 312, 1992.

79. Cavarzan, A. et al., Action of intragastric ethanol on the pancreatic secretion of conscious rats. *Digestion,* 13, 145, 1975.

80. Colwell, A.R. Jr., Collection of pancreatic juice from rats and consequences of its continued loss. *Am. J. Physiol.,* 164, 812, 1951.

81. Roze, C., Ling, N. and Florencio, H., Inhibition of gastric and pancreatic secretions by cerebroventricular injections of gastrin-releasing peptide and bombesin in rats. *Regul. Pept.,* 3, 105, 1982.

4 Gastrointestinal Tract Development and Its Importance in Toxicology

Joseph V. Rodricks, Allison A. Yates, and Claire L. Kruger

CONTENTS

SUMMARY

This chapter presents current knowledge regarding the development of the human gastrointestinal tract, including dietary, neuroendocrine, and immunological influences on gastrointestinal (GI) tract development and the course of bacterial colonization of the gut. Two aspects of gut development related to assessment of exposures to foreign chemicals or to dietary ingredients are considered: first, such chemicals or dietary constituents may alter normal GI tract development either by direct effects, by adversely affecting one or more of the regulatory influences over gut development, or by altering the normal course of bacterial colonization. Second, absorption of chemicals or dietary ingredients and the effects of microbial enzymes on them may be different in the immature tract compared to the mature tract; thus, the immature may be more or less susceptible to foreign substances than the mature.

GI TRACT DEVELOPMENT IN HUMANS

EMBRYONIC DEVELOPMENT

In early human embryonic development, most of the components of the gastrointestinal (GI) tract arise from the endoderm germ cell layer during the second and third weeks of gestation. During the fourth week, a tube forms the primitive gut and develops into three portions known as the foregut, midgut, and hindgut that extend the length of the embryo. The oral cavity forms from the buccopharyngeal membrane arising from the mesoderm layer. The open tube contains amniotic fluid at this stage as well as later stages when it is swallowed.

The earliest differentiated organ is the liver, formed from the liver bud of the open GI tube. The midgut is a herniated umbilicus external to the abdomen during this stage of development. An important step in early development is the rotation of this midgut to allow the GI tract to be in the appropriate position to develop mesentery derived from the mesoderm layer (see Figure 4.1). During the time that the midgut is herniated, the small intestine coils, the cecum forms, and by week 8 of gestation the descending colon is apparent (Hamilton, 2000).

Early in development, the GI tract differentiates to form identifiable structures along its length — the esophagus, stomach, duodenum, jejunum, and the small and large intestines. Continued growth of the GI tract results in bending of the tract and organ movement from the tube-like form to localizing in permanent anatomical positions (see Figure 4.1) (Hill, 2005).

During embryonic development the primitive gut is first formed, and then through a sequence of cellular proliferation during weeks 5 and 6, the lumen is occluded due to this cell growth during weeks 6 and 7, and then re-established by week 9, first in the esophagus, then the stomach–duodenum, then the small intestine, and finally in the colon by week 10. This gradient in sequencing from proximal to distal sites occurs both in structural development and in subsequent secretory development.

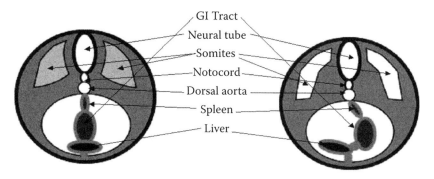

FIGURE 4.1 Rotation of midgut to initiate curvature of primitive anatomical units. (Source: adapted from Hill, 2005.)

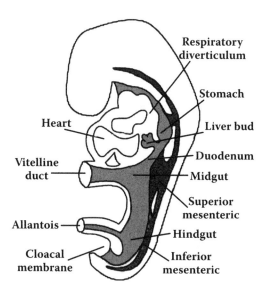

FIGURE 4.2 Origins of major components of GI tract and its blood supply. (Source: adapted from Hill, 2005.)

The blood supply to the GI tract derives from the common dorsal mesentery, arising from the mesoderm layer (see Figure 4.2). The midgut and hindgut are supplied by the superior mesenteric and inferior mesenteric arteries. The portal vessel is derived from the vitelline circulation, also from the mesoderm (Hill, 2005). The pancreas arises from the hepatic diverticulum and the duodenum, and as it differentiates it establishes both the α and β cells responsible for endocrine and exocrine function. During week 5, the spleen arises from the mesoderm, with the cells responsible for hematopoiesis derived from the yolk sac wall.

By the end of the first 8 weeks, the intestinal loops return to the abdominal cavity and the appendix appears as the fetal development period begins. During late embryonic and early fetal development — approximately the first trimester — cell differentiation occurs at a rapid pace. Undifferentiated stem cells are present throughout the GI tract by week 5, giving rise in the small intestine and colon first to committed stem cells and then developing into four distinct lines of cells:

1. Paneth's cells (secretory cells) found in the bases of crypts of Lieberkühn that contribute to mucosal barrier function by the apical release of granules containing a variety of antimicrobial products, including peptides termed cryptdins (crypt defensins)
2. Goblet cells responsible for mucus production
3. Enteroendocrine cells that appear by week 8 and are responsible in the duodenum for synthesis and release of hormones such as secretin and cholecystokinin (CCK) in response to nutrients and neural factors present in the upper GI tract
4. Columnar absorptive cells that become the major mucosal cells involved in absorption and local metabolism of nutrients as well as toxic contaminants

During week 11 crypt formation begins, with villi formation completed by week 13. Paneth's cell defensins are considered early markers of crypt ontogeny (Ayabe et al., 2000; Babyatsky and Poldosky, 2003; Ouellette and Bevin, 2001).

Fetal Development

Digestion, absorption of nutrients, and elimination of waste products are the primary functions of the GI tract; digestion and absorption of nutrients require developed digestive enzymes and transport systems and functioning smooth muscle and enteric nervous systems (Doughty, 2004). As demonstrated by the timing of the development of a number of GI systems, structural development occurs prior to the maturation of secretory function and normal motility throughout most of fetal life (Doughty, 2004).

Structure

As secretory cells differentiate and primitive structures form, muscle and neural cells develop into organized tissue as well. During week 5, circular smooth muscle is detected in the esophagus, where neuroblasts are found dispersed among the muscle cells. By week 6, the rotation of the primitive gut results in linking the left and right vagi nerves to the anterior and posterior areas of the stomach. By week 8, enervation of the small intestine is initiated as synaptic protein and glial supporting tissue penetrate the outer layers of the developing circular musculature in the intestines; by week 9, the longitudinal muscle layer (inner layer within the mesenchyme) is formed along with the myenteric plexus, a network of nerve fibers between the outer longitudinal and middle circular muscle layers (Babyatsky and Podolsky, 2003; Hill, 2005).

The enteric nervous system initiated during week 7 in the stomach can be detected in the rectum by week 13, another example of the longitudinal gradient of development from a proximal to a distal direction. By the end of week 13, the submucous plexus is formed between the middle circular muscle layer and the submucosa, and mature ganglion cells are detected in the esophagus. Functionally, fetal swallowing is initiated during week 11. During week 14, the anatomical components of the stomach are distinguishable (curvatures, corpus, antrum, and pylorus). By the end of the second trimester around week 26, the structural features of the GI tract are well developed (Babyatsky and Podolsky, 2003; Erdman and Pollack, 2001; Hamilton, 2000).

Functional Development

As the fetal period begins, cells responsible for secretory function become apparent. Within the primordial stomach, rudimentary glands develop mucous neck cells, then parietal and chief cells by week 8, with mRNA for muc1, 4, 5B, and 6 detected in epithelial mucin in the stomach at that time. By the second trimester, the spleen is generating both red and white blood cells, thus initiating a mechanism for developing oxygen transport as well as leukocytes to the gut.

Secretory Function

By week 10, a fully differentiated spectrum of endocrine cell types is present in the stomach and duodenum. Sucrase–isomaltase, maltase, and trehalase enzymes are present in the small intestine at 60 to 70% of adult levels. Active transport of glucose is not demonstrated until week 20. Substance P and neurokinin A can be detected in the stomach also at week 10. During week 11, gastric lipase appears, and dipeptidases are detected in the small intestine microvilli. By week 12, intestinal lactase is measurable and pancreatic muc5B appears. Within the developing pancreas, secretory acini (responsible for pancreatic enzyme production and secretion) and islets of Langerhans (responsible for insulin, glucagon, and somatostatin production, among other hormones) appear also in week 12.

Intrinsic factor- and histamine-containing cells are evident in the stomach by week 14, followed by the attainment of adult levels of gastric lipase by week 16. Because pancreatic lipase, which is first detected during week 16, is not fully functional at adult levels until late into the first year of life (see Table 4.1), gastric lipase becomes the primary determinant of lipolytic activity in premature and newborn infants. Protein digestion at this gestational age is also developing; while microvilli dipeptidases were first detected during week 11 (as was gastric lipase), by week 16 they too are at adult levels. Leucine aminopeptidase activity in the *distal* small intestine is high at this gestational age (one of the few examples of a distal-to-proximal direction in development).

While detected during week 10 of gestation, proximal to distal gradients for activity of lactase and other glucosidases are evident by week 17. As the second trimester continues, ductal and acinar cells in the developing pancreas are

TABLE 4.1

Comparison of Functionality at Birth vs. Maturity

Structure/Function	At Birth	When Fully Mature (Adult Level)
Esophagus		
Striated muscle in mid-esophagus	Same as adult	At birth
LES pressure		3–6 wks of age
Swallowing	Poorly coordinated; rate = 450 ml/d in presence of mean amniotic fluid volume of 850 ml	
Neuronal density	Decreased to adult level	
Vagus nerves innervate striated muscle		Maturation of ennervation complete by 2 yrs of age
Stomach/Duodenum		
Rate of DNA synthesis	Markedly higher than adult level, leading to significant mucosal growth	
Gastrin G cells	Appear in gastric antrum	
Gastrin	High levels in neonatal plasma may act to increase crypt and villus density and parietal and ECL cells	
Histamine response	Immature	1 yr of age
Somatostatin D cells	Appear in gastric mucosa	
Gastric lipase activity		3 mos of age
Parietal cells secrete HCl	HCl <50% of adult values; pH ≈ 4–5	1 yr of age, pH ≈ 1–2
Pepsinogen secreted by chief cells	<50% of adult values	Mature chief cells; pepsinogen at adult level by 1 yr
Intrinsic factor		Increases rapidly to adult value by day 10
Motility	Not fully developed	
Enterochromaffin-like cells	Accelerate 1–3 wks of age	
Small Intestine/Colon		
Bacterial colonization	None	Within a few days of birth
Microvilli	Lengthening	
Disaccharidases		At birth
Glucose transporters		At birth
Fructose transporter	Not present until after birth	
Enterokinase	20% of adult level	
Brush border and cytosolic peptidases		At birth
Amino acid transporters		At birth
Pinocytosis	Higher rates in infant than in adult	
Bile acid reabsorption	Passive in infant	By weaning

TABLE 4.1 (CONTINUED)
Comparison of Functionality at Birth vs. Maturity

Structure/Function	At Birth	When Fully Mature (Adult Level)
Micelle formation	Poor due to low level of bile acids, pancreatic lipase	
Passive and carrier-mediated absorption	Increased at birth above adult levels	
Heavy metal (Cu, Fe, Zn, Pb) absorption	Efficiency > than in adults	Returns to normal at weaning
Lactoferrin receptors	Present for milk at birth	
Contractile activity and motility	Near adult levels	
Fat-soluble vitamin absorption	Poor	Matures with weaning, normal fat absorption
Folate absorption	Less	
Vitamin B$_{12}$ absorption	Not well absorbed in proximal ileum	
Pancreatic lipase	10% of adult level	By weaning

Sources: From Babyatsky, M.W. and Podolsky, D.K. 2003, in *Textbook of Gastroenterology*, 4th Ed., Philadelphia: Lippincott Williams Wilkins; Philipps, A.F. and Sherman, M.P. 2003, in *Rudolph's Pediatrics*, 21st Ed., New York: McGraw Hill; and Pacha, J. 2000. *Physiol. Rev.* 80: 1633.

undergoing rapid cell mitosis during week 19, and Peyer's patches (aggregates of lymph nodules) emerge during week 20 in the small intestine. By week 22 bile secretion is demonstrated, and by week 24 increased lactase activity is present, indicating that induction by maternal lactose is not necessary.

By the end of the second trimester (around week 26), six amino acid transporters for neutral and charged amino acids are found in muscosal cells, and fetal macromolecular transport across the mucosal cell can be demonstrated — an important activity that aids in the digestion of proteins and lipophilic compounds present in amniotic fluid.

Early in the third trimester, trypsin activity is measurable in the small intestine, reflecting developing pancreatic function and the presence of active enterokinase. By week 30, enterokinase activity is at about 6% of adult levels. By week 32, pancreatic lipase activity is at 50% of the level at birth (although still low compared to adult levels). Lactase activity surges throughout the third trimester, while other disaccharidases reach adult levels prenatally (Babyatsky and Podolsky, 2003).

Muscular Function and Motility

While muscle cells and nerve cells are visible in the early gut by week 9, the muscularis mucosa is present throughout the small intestine to the colon by week 20, and neuronal density within the esophagus peaks by week 20 as well, resulting in swallowing rates of 13 ml/day at this gestational age, with sucking behavior apparent. Contraction pressure within the intestines is at about 60% at week 25 compared to the level reached at term, indicating early ability to move intestinal contents along the developing gut. By the end of the second trimester (week 26), contraction is noted after electrical stimulation, indicating more coordinated activity. Motility measured at week 28 is about 20 to 25% that seen in a term infant.

During the third trimester, given that structural development is somewhat complete, improved function is noted. By week 32 the lower esophageal sphincter is functional, allowing more coordinated swallowing patterns to develop, although mature patterns of contractile activity and motility are not seen until near term, and coordinated contraction of smooth muscle in the colon and function of the internal and external anal sphincters (perhaps due to the proximal–distal gradient in development) are poorly developed before birth. Random peristaltic activity can be detected by the 26th week but effective peristalsis is usually not present until week 33, with nutritive sucking and coordinated swallowing not developing until week 34 (Doughty, 2004).

Postnatal Development

Many physiologists separate postnatal development into three time periods: birth and the first few days after birth (when colostrum is available), the suckling period, and the weaning period (Pacha, 2000). The weaning period marks the beginning of notable changes in digestive and transport functions that result in maturation of the GI system (Walthall et al., 2005). Macromolecules given as tracers late *in utero*, either introduced into amniotic fluid or the intestinal lumen, are absorbed into mucosal cells in humans and a number of other species including monkeys, guinea pigs, and rats, thus demonstrating a high rate of pinocytosis that is highly active in the first 10 days after birth and decreases substantially with weaning (Babyatsky and Podolsky, 2003), providing a mechanism by which intact proteins are absorbed. This can be demonstrated in premature infants as well during the first few months of life. It has been suggested that the lack of a fully protective barrier during the first months of life may play a significant role in subsequent sensitivity to dietary and environmental proteins (Babyatsky and Poldolsky, 2003).

Birth

Humans have been classified as precocial animals in that prior to birth, essential functions such as sight, hearing, hair, etc. are in place to allow for normal growth and development. This is in contrast to other animals such as rodents that have altricial characteristics: they become fully functioning during postnatal development rather than prenatally. Thus, functional maturation in humans occurs *in utero*, allowing viability in spite of prematurity prior to birth and even earlier for many functional attributes such as absorption, swallowing, etc. Thus, animal models used to evaluate potential human toxicity during pre- and postnatal periods must be chosen carefully to appropriately represent human age-dependent functional development.

Structure

At term, the small intestine is typically 250 to 300 cm (approximately one-half the length of the adult small bowel) and the large intestine and colon together are typically 30 to 40 cm in length (approximately one-fifth normal adult length) (Doughty, 2004). Thus the neonatal colon, mirroring the cephalocaudal pattern of development, is comparatively less functional than the small intestine. Solute and electrolyte absorption and bile reabsorption are not yet at mature stages.

Function

At birth, while normal levels of many enzymes are present in humans so that digestion and subsequent absorption of nutrients can occur, a few important functions are not fully mature (see Table 4.1). A comparatively high rate of macromolecular transport important to protein and lipid digestion occurs due to pinocytosis during the first 2 weeks of life. This allows mucosal enzymes to assist in digestion of proteins and lipids when pancreatic proteolytic enzymes are not yet available in adequate amounts. These are assisted by higher than normal levels of lysosomal proteases in enterocytes (e.g., cathepsins) that allow protein digestion.

In the early postnatal period, unhydrolyzed triglycerides are found in feces, a result of only passive bile acid reabsorption that continues until weaning. Bile acid concentrations are initially too low to allow for micelle formation, which requires pancreatic lipase as well as bile acids. During the first 4 to 6 weeks of life, intraluminal bile acids increase and absorptive mechanisms develop, leading to improved but not mature lipid absorption (Babyatsky and Podolsky, 2003).

Fewer chief cells are present in the neonatal stomach compared to the levels found in an adult stomach, with generally low levels of pepsin produced. The number of chief cells increases with age as the stomach increases in size and thickness. The mass of parietal cells (per unit area) at birth is two to three times greater than that of the adult stomach, but with thinner walls than found in that of an adult (Walthall et al., 2005). Acid output increases, as does pepsin production, resulting in improved digestion of proteins.

Innate resistance to environmental and pathogenic microorganisms in the neonate is provided by Paneth's cells; considerable quantities of these cells are present in the small intestine, in all probability keeping bacterial levels low compared to levels present in the colon. Paneth's cells produce and secrete antimicrobial peptides known as defensins. Gram-negative and Gram-positive bacteria and their bacterial products have been shown to stimulate their secretion (Bourlioux et al., 2003; Porter et al., 2002).

In terms of muscle function, mature patterns of contractile activity and motility are not found until near term in humans, with coordinated contraction of colonic smooth muscle and anal sphincters responses poorly developed (Babyatsky and Podolsky, 2003). Sympathetic stimulation of the autonomic nerves reduces secretion and motility, while parasympathetic stimulation has been shown to increase peristalsis and secretion; these functions are immature at birth (Doughty, 2004).

Suckling Period

By 1 month of age, pepsin activity is only at 18% of adult levels, and since the pH for maximum enzymatic activity of pepsin is ≈2, while it may be present, it is not functioning at an optimal level due to the relatively high gastric pH, which is about 4.0 to 4.5 (Adkins and Lonnerdal, 2003). At the same time, the pancreas is still developing, with pancreatic function not attaining the adult stage until much later in infancy. Pancreatic enzymes such as trypsinogen that require intestinal enterokinase for cleavage to active forms are low at birth as well, limiting the luminal digestion of proteins; at birth, enterokinase activity is about 25% of that at 1 year of age (Atkins and Lonnerdal, 2003). It has been hypothesized that proteins in human milk may not be hydrolyzed in the small intestine, thus enabling them to exert a host-defense function beyond providing essential amino acids (Adkins and Lonnerdal, 2003).

ROLE OF NUTRIENTS AND DIETARY COMPONENTS IN NORMAL DEVELOPMENT

The nutrient needs of the developing GI tract are uniquely met by both the nutrients present in the lumen derived from amniotic fluid and gut secretions during the fetal period or milk and gut secretions postnatally, as well as those provided by arterial blood flow. The comparatively high rate of mucosal cell turnover within the GI tract is functionally of great importance, allowing a means to protect an individual from adverse effects of constant exposure to potentially injurious substances present in the lumen, particularly in the colon, where mutagens and carcinogenic substances may be present.

Nutrients thus presented to the developing GI tract can act to regulate growth, functional patency, and cellular differentiation in three ways: by exerting direct effects on mucosal cells before joining the systemic circulation; by stimulating hormonal production due to presence in the GI tract or post-absorption; and by affecting motor activity. Exposure to nutrient and other trophic factors in the diet has been shown to directly enhance villus height and crypt depth in the small intestine to a greater extent than in the ileal region. This has been shown to be a direct effect on the intestinal section itself, as transposition of ileal and jejunal intestinal loops results in increased villus size in the ileal segment (Babyatsky and Podolsky, 2003; Erdman and Pollack, 2001; Perin et al., 1997; Sanderson, 1999; Thiesen et al., 2000).

The presence of protein and fat in the duodenum and proximal small intestine results in the secretion of CCK from specialized I cells in the duodenum. CCK is thought to play key roles in stimulating pancreatic secretion, gallbladder contraction, and slowing down gastric motility, thus optimizing protein and fat digestion, which in neonates is still immature (Sidhu et al., 2000).

Exposures during critical periods of fetal and postnatal development are thought to have lasting or lifelong effects on subsequent structures or functions of organs (Hertzman, 1995) as well as impacting risk of chronic disease in later life (Barker, 2002). Relating perinatal exposure to long-term effects must take into account that factors that raise disease risk or promote good health accumulate gradually over the course of life both independently and in patterned ways (Ben-Shlomo and Kuh, 2002), so that connecting early exposure or lack thereof to later health consequences, both positive and negative (life-course epidemiology), is not yet a well researched model for establishing disease causation.

Fetal under-nutrition has been linked with increased risk of disease in later life, specifically coronary heart disease, type 2 diabetes, stroke, and hypertension (Barker, 2004). Nutrient supply, including oxygen, has been shown to have more influence on fetal growth than genes (Harding, 2001). Smaller babies have fewer cells than would be proportionally expected in key organs such as the kidney and GI tract (Barker, 2004); this has been proposed as possibly a selective reduction resulting from diverting blood flow from the trunk to protect the brain. Along this line, it has been hypothesized that the tissue resistance seen to insulin in type 2 diabetes in adults may be a continuation of the fetal response noted in which glucose concentrations are maintained in the blood to provide adequate glucose to the brain at the expense of glucose transport into muscle, resulting in lower levels of muscle growth (Phillips, 1996).

DEVELOPMENT OF IMMUNOLOGICAL FUNCTION

DEVELOPMENT OF GASTROINTESTINAL MICROBIOTA

After birth, the GI tract exists in symbiosis with a large number and variety of bacteria that contribute to the health of an individual. Gut microorganisms contribute to diverse mammalian processes. *In toto*, the gut microflora acts as an effective barrier against opportunistic and pathogenic microorganisms. Other advantageous effects include modulation of the immune system, development of intestinal microvilli, production of short chain fatty acids (SCFAs) upon which the colonic mucosa is dependent for energy, fermentation of non-digestible dietary fiber, and anaerobic metabolism of peptides and proteins, resulting in recovery of metabolic energy for the host and removal of carcinogens and toxins (Nicholson et al., 2005; Cummings et al., 2004; Dai and Walker, 1999).

At birth, the intestinal tract of the human infant is sterile. During vaginal birth, the infant is colonized by bacteria from its mother (vaginal microflora, feces) and, to a lesser extent, from the environment; diet plays an important role in the further development of the microbiota (Boehm et al., 2005; Dai and Walker, 1999; Hammerman et al., 2004; Mackie et al., 1999).

The GI microflora of vaginally delivered infants is quite different from that of infants delivered via cesarean section; C-section infants often have a microflora dominated by environmental or hospital isolates. Following birth, the mother delivers additional microbial strains to the infant during suckling, kissing, and caressing (Mackie et al., 1999). Other factors that influence the constituents of the infant gut microflora include birth environment (home or hospital), hygiene measures in place at the time of birth, developmental stage at birth (term or preterm), use of antimicrobials, and diet (breast fed or formula fed) (Heavey and Rowland, 1999; Orrhage and Nord, 1999). Over several years, the microflora of a child will change until it becomes identical to that of an adult (Stark and Lee, 1982).

The first components of the infant microflora (during the first 1 to 2 days) are Streptococci and enterobacteria (Conway, 1997). Enterococci have also been identified in infant feces during the first days of life (Stark and Lee, 1982; Balmer et al., 1989; Lundequist et al., 1985). The physiochemical environment of the infant gut changes during the first week of life; facultatively anaerobic bacteria begin to predominate as oxygen in the gut is utilized and depleted. Anaerobes including Bifidobacteria and Bacteroides begin to appear; these strains are found as early as day 2 in the breast-fed infant's microflora, although peak counts are reached closer to day 7 (consistent with the depletion of oxygen). Other anaerobic bacteria that appear during this change include *Clostridium* spp., *Eubacterium* spp., and Lactobacilli (Stark and Lee, 1982; Lundequist et al., 1985; Balmer and Wharton, 1989).

The earliest studies of infant microflora found a difference between those who were breast-fed and those who ingested formula. Breast-fed infants have a microflora dominated by Bifidobacteria that easily out-compete other genera and whose presence is thought to depend on the occurrence of certain glycoproteins in human breast milk (Cummings et al., 2004). In contrast, formula-fed infants have a more complex flora that resembles the adult gut in that Bacteroides, Clostridia, Bifidobacteria, Lactobacilli, Gram-positive cocci, coliforms, and other groups are all represented in fairly equal proportions (Cummings et al., 2004).

Formula-fed infants have also been found to have higher fecal levels of potentially harmful bacterial metabolic by-products (Edwards and Parrett, 2002). Results from individual studies, however, are variable. Some investigators found no differences between the microflora of formula-fed and breast-fed infants (Kleessen et al., 1995; Lundequist et al., 1985). Some studies found that choice of feeding had no effect on levels of Bifidobacteria (Balmer and Wharton, 1989; Kleessen et al., 1995; Stark and Lee, 1982).

In summary, studies in term infants have shown that the normal microflora of infants is variable and that these variations may be due to differences in an infant's environment, composition of formula, and limitations of the different bacteriological identification schemes utilized in studies of microflora (Heavey and Rowland, 1999; Orrhage and Nord, 1999; Conway, 1997; Wold and Adlerberth, 2000; Fanaro et al., 2003).

In preterm infants in an intensive care setting, an abnormal pattern of bowel colonization develops when compared with patterns of healthy full-term infants. A critical factor in preterm infant flora development is the delay in appearance of Bifidobacteria; they first appear in the stools of very low birth weight infants at a mean age of approximately 10 days and become predominant around 20 days. This is in contrast to full-term breast-fed infants in whom bifiobacterial flora appear as early as 2 to 4 days of age (Hammerman et al., 2004; Dai and Walker, 1999). In contrast to the more complex and diverse patterns of colonization seen in healthy term neonates, a delay in establishing normal intestinal microflora and the resulting abnormal pattern of colonization may predispose to overgrowth of potentially pathogenic species. This can create a reservoir of antibiotic-resistant bacteria, with the potential of contributing to the pathogenesis of one of the most common gastrointestinal medical or surgical emergencies occurring in neonates: necrotizing enterocolitis (NEC) (Hammerman et al., 2004; Dai and Walker, 1999).

NON-IMMUNOLOGICAL PHYSICAL BARRIERS

The first step in producing systemic invasive infections is adherence of bacterial cells to the surface of the intestine (Dai et al., 2000). The normal intestinal tract is a dynamic environment wherein fluids and solids are constantly moved by peristalsis; the failure of a bacterium to adhere to the surface of this environment will result in its eventual elimination. Many bacteria utilize specific receptors on their membranes or cell walls to interact with intestinal epithelial cells, thus binding them to the surface of the intestine; these interactions are often mediated through lectins (Mouricout, 1997). In addition, many bacterial toxins require epithelial cell receptors in order to bind to and therefore affect the intestine (Popoff, 1998).

Prevention of bacterial adhesion to the intestine is therefore a critical step in preventing pathogen colonization. The use of probiotic strains of bacteria has proven effective in reducing the adherence of pathogens to the intestinal epithelium. Probiotic treatments seek to establish strains of bacteria (including *Bifidobacteria* spp. and *Lactobacillus* spp.) as components of normal microflora; these probiotic strains are non-pathogenic, non-invasive, and able to out-compete pathogens for receptor sites on intestinal cells, thus preventing attachment (Duffy, 2000).

To cause systemic infection, colonizing bacteria must also translocate across the intact intestinal barrier. Bacterial translocation (e.g., the passage of viable bacteria from the lumen of the gastrointestinal tract to extraintestinal internal locations such as the lymph nodes, liver, spleen, kidney, and bloodstream) is a major concern in the progression of infections caused by enteropathogenic bacteria (Dai et al., 2000). Bacteria colonize the gut by adhering to a glycoprotein or glycolipid receptor in the microvillus membrane. Several studies suggest that the glycosylation in the microvillus membrane is under developmental regulation. In adult animals, glycosylation results in complete carbohydrate side chains on microvillus membrane glycoproteins and glycolipids. In contrast, the newborn animal intestine has immature glycosylation that provides differences in the availability of terminal glycoconjugates. This may account for enhanced pathogenicity and pathogen toxin binding (Dai and Walker, 1999). Studies of human neonatal intestine suggest that pathologic colonization of bacteria may occur because of immaturity in glycosylation of the mucosal surface molecules (Chu et al., 1989).

The intestinal mucosa provides a natural physical cellular barrier, limiting potentially harmful microorganisms present in the intestinal lumen from colonizing enterocytes, as described earlier. The gastrointestinal tract of the preterm neonate is physiologically immature in its development at the time of birth, rendering it more susceptible to bacterial translocation than that of the adult. Many species of pathogenic bacteria are able to alter the permeability of the intestine and invade deep tissue; these include, among others, *Salmonella* spp., *Listeria monocytogenes*, *Yersinia* spp., and *Shigella* spp. Infection of the intestinal epithelium often leads to diarrhea; when the diarrhea fails to resolve the infection, bacteria may move into deeper tissue and eventually cause systemic infections and related symptoms (Pucciareli et al., 1997).

However, anaerobic lactic acid bacteria (*Lactobacillus acidophilus*, Bifidobacteria) have a protective role against the translocation of other bacteria. This is mediated by the production via fermentation of SCFAs that produce an acid environment unfavorable for many pathogens as well as production of antimicrobial bacteriocins. Bacteriocins are proteins or protein complexes with bactericidal activities directed against species that are closely related to the producer bacterium (Hammerman et al., 2004; Dai and Walker, 1999). Several studies have investigated the enteric flora of infants with NEC and found a decline in the concentration of anaerobic species and increased colonization with Gram-negative bacteria (Hammerman et al., 2004).

GUT-ASSOCIATED LYMPHOID TISSUE (IMMUNOLOGICAL) BARRIER (GALT)

The intestine is one of the human body's most critical immune organs. The gut-associated lymphoid tissue (GALT) is the largest mass of lymphoid tissue in the human body. One quarter of the intestinal lumen surface is composed of lymphoid tissue and more than 70% of all immune cells are located in the intestine (Gaskins, 1997). The intestinal immune response is mediated through the follicles and Peyer's patches and then distributed into the mucosa, epithelium, and secretory sites. Immunoglobulin A (IgA) production is abundant in the intestine; secreted IgA is resistant to proteolysis in the lumen of the intestine and does not activate complement or inflammatory responses. Because IgA secreted by the GALT is a component of the common mucosal immune system, immune responses mediated by GALT-derived IgA can affect immune responses at other mucosal surfaces including the respiratory tract, salivary glands, and mammary glands (Isolauri et al., 2001). Thus the GALT provides important immunological stimulation and programming for the systemic immune system.

Very little antigen exposure occurs *in utero*. Therefore, at birth the immune system is naïve from an immunological standpoint. During early postnatal life, exposure to antigens is a prerequisite for promoting the expansion of the immune organs (Kelly and Coutts, 2000).

Studies in germ-free animals exposed to dietary antigens but not bacterial antigens revealed only a rudimentary immune system (Kelly and Coutts, 2000). In the neonate, therefore, generation of appropriate immune responses and development of immune regulatory networks are dependent on the development and presence of normal intestinal flora and exposure to dietary antigens.

The microflora of the intestine can have significant effects on the GALT. Studies examining the absence of a normal microflora demonstrated increased antigen transport across the gut mucosa (Isolauri et al., 2001). Additionally, intestinal colonization by nonpathogenic bacteria is an important antigenic stimulus for the maturation of the GALT; as the gut microflora is established, the capacity of the GALT to produce IgA-secreting cells increases.

The stimulatory effect of the microflora on the secretory IgA system and on B cell function in general is well established (Gaskins, 1997). For example, bacterial colonization of the mouse intestine during early post-natal growth plays a critical role in the development of antibody-secreting cells in the small intestine. Bacterial colonization is also thought to explain the characteristic increase in IgA-positive plasma cells in the lamina propria at weaning. A study that made use of the severe combined immunodeficient mouse model provides strong evidence that antigenic components of the microflora are critical to the earliest natural IgA responses in that animal species (Gaskins, 1997). The consistent demonstration that oral ingestion of probiotic Lactobacilli can stimulate multiple components of the secretory IgA system is often used as support for the notion that direct feeding of microbial probiotics can modulate host immunity in humans and animals (Gaskins, 1997).

Oral tolerance (e.g., the ability to consume antigenic materials without eliciting a massive immune response) is a critical step in the maturation of an infant's immune system. The GALT must continually protect against invasive organisms and harmful antigens while remaining silent when confronted with normal antigens present in food. Microbial probiotics have been shown to be critical to the development and maintenance of oral tolerance (Kalliomaki and Isolauri, 2003). The microflora is known to modulate a number of cytokines and other immune signaling molecules, so the fact that oral tolerance is mediated by T cells, IL-10, and TGF- suggests that it can be impacted by the type of bacteria present in the gut (Tlaskalova Hogenova et al., 2004).

Additionally, the timing of any such probiotic treatment is critical: in studies with germ-free mice, the application of Bifidobacteria (a demonstrated probiotic) during the neonatal period resulted in oral tolerance, while treatment at any subsequent age did not (Sudo et al., 1997). This observation is supported by the work of Gronlund and colleagues who evaluated the effect of microflora modulation on the development of humoral immunity; they concluded that the type of bacteria present in the gut microflora and the times at which they are present may affect the abundance of IgA- and IgM-secreting immune cells in the intestine (Gronlund et al., 2000).

The GALT also plays a major role in food allergy. Formula protein allergy is one of the first forms of food allergy in infants and may occur as early as the first week of life (Vanderhoof and Young, 2003). The effects of early allergic reactions are often observed in the GI tract (diarrhea, discomfort) but can also be manifested as respiratory or cutaneous reactions as an infant ages. Probiotics have been shown to lessen the effects of existing allergies to food. In one study, 31 infants with atopic eczema induced by consumption of cow's milk showed decreases in symptoms when treated with a probiotic Lactobacillus strain (Majamaa and Isolauri, 1997). The exact mechanism by which probiotics mitigate the effects of allergy-inducing antigens has not been fully elucidated. However, it has been suggested that the ability of these organisms to adhere to the GI tract via specific receptors can modulate the induction of an immune response. In addition, stimulation of additional mucin secretion may play a role in this phenomenon (Vanderhoof and Young, 2003).

The immune response to microorganisms relies on both innate mechanisms and acquired components of immunity that require memory of previous exposure. The innate immune system must discriminate between potential pathogens and commensal bacteria with the use of a restricted number of preformed receptors (Bourlioux et al., 2003). Strains of bacteria interact with the cells lining the GI tract. As these bacteria lyse or shed molecules, receptors monitor the composition of the lumen in an effort to determine what microbes are present. An example of these receptors is a class of molecules known as Toll-like receptors or TLRs (Kalliomaki and Isolauri, 2003). These receptors are able to recognize certain bacterial molecules including lipopolysaccharides, lipoteichoic acid, CpG dinucleotides, and others. TLRs can sense what types of bacteria are present in the gut and induce cytokine production or signal the immune system in the event that a pathogen is present. It has been suggested that the normal flora or probiotics may have a different set of microbe-associated molecular patterns (MAMPs) from foreign or pathogenic bacteria, and thus may send different signals to the immune system (Schiffrin and Blum, 2002; Tlaskalova-Hogenova et al., 2004). Probiotics may produce anti-inflammatory MAMPs, while the molecules released by pathogens may elicit an immune response. This signaling has been suggested to be critical in the maintenance of immunologic homeostasis in the gut (Blum and Schiffrin, 2003).

IMPLICATIONS FOR TOXICITY

Age-dependent changes in gastrointestinal structure and function contribute significantly to age-dependent changes in toxicity. The principal causes of those changes are related to factors affecting the pharmacokinetic profiles of foreign compounds, although increased vulnerability of the neonatal GI tract to the direct action of some toxicants can also alter systemic responses. There are, of course, numerous age-dependent changes other than those occurring in the GI tract that affect both the pharmacokinetic and pharmacodynamic profiles of foreign compounds. Thus, the cumulative effects of age on both qualitative and quantitative manifestations of toxicity cannot be discerned solely from consideration of the status of the GI tract.

It is certainly the case, for example, that age-related changes in the GI tract that may serve to increase or decrease the toxicities of some substances may sometimes be countered by other (systemic) factors that are also age-related. Extreme caution is thus warranted when conclusions are drawn about the possible consequences for the whole organism of alterations in toxicity due to age-dependent effects of gastrointestinal structure or function (Schumann et al., 1999).

Much of the information available about age-dependent changes in toxicity is necessarily based on experimental studies, and, as pointed out in Chapters 9 and 10, there are several cross-species differences in GI tract structure and function that complicate interpretation of both rodent and non-rodent findings for purposes of assessing risks to humans. This situation holds even for well developed models of mature animals and is compounded further when drawing inferences from findings in immature animals.

Because of the highly incomplete state of knowledge regarding risks of toxicity in immature humans and the similarly incomplete understanding of available animal models, much of the following is based on known age-dependent changes in the structure and function of the human GI tract that could affect toxicity; further development of experimental models is necessary to reveal the actual consequences of such changes. There are, however, notable examples of the influence of GI tract immaturity and these will be highlighted.

In addition to the effects of age-dependent alteration of GI tract structure and function on the toxic properties of foreign compounds, much concern focuses on the effects of such compounds on developmental processes, particularly on neurological development (NRC, 2001), but the possible consequences of *in utero* and neonatal exposures on the development of the GI tract (that may in part be related to neurodevelopmental toxicity) are also of interest. This topic will also be discussed in the following section.

ALTERATIONS IN PHARMACOKINETIC PROFILES

Absorption

Absorption and metabolism of foreign compounds can be age-related. Absorption from the GI tract depends upon many factors including the type of diet and the timing of exposure relative to food intake, the pH levels of both GI tract contents and the foreign compound, the rate of passage of contents through the tract, and the surface area available for absorption. Certain disease states may also influence absorption. All these factors are altered in neonates, infants, and even young children relative to their status in adults. Their cumulative effects on any single drug or chemical are not readily predictable.

Gastric pH is decreased in neonates relative to adults, and secretion of acid may not reach adult levels until early puberty (Rane, 1992). Interestingly, pH appears to be increased during the first few days of life, then declines (Weber et al. 1975). Although diet can alter gastric acidity, especially one high in milk and formula, pH generally remains low until puberty and early adulthood (Rane,

1992). The absorption of hydrophilic compounds, particularly those that can undergo ionization, is most significantly affected by intragastric pH, because these compounds do not readily traverse the lipid membrane matrix when ionized. The relatively low pH of the immature GI tract will tend to most significantly affect basic compounds, a higher proportion of which will exist in ionic form in the immature GI tract than in the mature tract. Thus, based on gastric acidity alone, basic compounds should be less readily absorbed in the young than in adults. Absorption of lipid soluble compounds is generally little affected by pH (Renwick, 2001).

GI transit times can alter absorption. Gastric transit time is generally longer in neonates and infants than in older children and adults, and is also delayed by diet, particularly one of high caloric density (Premji, 1998). These factors tend to increase the opportunities for absorption of foreign compounds in the immature.

To make matters more complex, chemicals are generally less readily absorbed from the stomach than from the small intestine. The relatively lower pH and larger and well perfused surface area of the latter increases opportunities for absorption (Renwick, 2001). Although small intestine perfusion in the immature is not clearly greater than that of the adult, mucosal surface area and permeability are increased; again, the opportunity for increased absorption in the young relative to the adult is supported by these functional differences (Schumann et al., 1999; Sreedharan and Mehta, 2005).

A range of enzymes involved in digestion and other biochemical functions including pepsin, lipase, α-amylase, β-glucuronidase, and UDP-glucuronyl transferase change in activity during the developmental period (see above). Some of these changes may affect absorption of foreign compounds. Lower levels of bile acids present in neonates may alter enterohepatic circulation of metabolites and otherwise affect absorption (de Belle et al., 1979; Watkins, et al., 1973).

Altered drug absorption secondary to diseases such as infantile diarrhea, gastroenteritis, malabsorption syndrome, and inflammatory bowel disease has been reported for several pharmaceuticals (Maples et al., 2006). Reduced capacity for gastric emptying with consequent increased absorption has been reported for infants with congenital heart disease (Cavell, 1981).

The combined effects of these many factors influencing the GI absorption of foreign chemicals are not readily predictable, but most tend to support increased absorption in neonates, infants, and perhaps young children relative to adults. Documentation of these differences through experimental studies has not been a highly active area of research, but several well established examples exist in the literature on pharmaceuticals and environmental toxicants.

Among the latter substances, lead stands out as perhaps the most thoroughly investigated. In both human and non-human primates, the age dependence of lead absorption rates is striking, with perhaps four to five times greater uptake in children after oral exposure than has been observed in adults (Mahaffey, et al., 2000). Much less clear is the age range over which absorption rates approach those of adults. Some studies suggest that by ages 6 to 11, absorption rates become comparable to those of adults (Gulson et al., 1997). The combination of increased

TABLE 4.2
Differences in GI Tract Absorption between Very Young and Adults

Chemical	Differences (Species)
Lead	5-fold (humans)
Cadmium	20-fold (guinea pigs)
	4-fold (humans)
Strontium	9-fold (rats)
Plutonium	85- to 100-fold (rats)
Radium	24-fold (rats)

Source: Calabrese, E.J. 1986. *Age and Susceptibility to Toxic Substances*. New York: John Wiley & Sons.

absorption and increased intake resulting from ingestion of a given environmental level of lead explains why infants and children are most at risk from lead exposure (CDC, 1991; Plunkett et al., 1992).

More limited data on other heavy metals — mercury, cadmium, and nickel in particular — generally show the same trend observed for lead (Mahaffey et al., 2000; Calabrese, 1986). Studies of absorption are sometimes confounded by the fact that exposure of young children and adults to the same environmental sources and concentrations results in greater intake per unit of body weight. It is not always possible to separate and quantify the relative effects of increased intake and increased GI tract absorption (Mahaffey et al., 2000). Data on this issue compiled by Calabrese (1986) are presented in Table 4.2.

The pediatric pharmacology literature contains numerous examples of both increased and decreased drug bioavailability in neonates, infants, and children. Penicillin G, ampicillin, and nafcillin, for example, all display increased bioavailability in neonates relative to older children and adults (Maples et al., 2006). Reduced bioavailability and delayed absorption of phenobarbital, phenytoin, and acetaminophen have been reported in children (Maples et al., 2006). Increased bioavailability of drugs increases the risk of adverse side effects, while delayed absorption and reduced bioavailability may render them relatively ineffective.

Metabolism

Although liver is the primary site of foreign chemical metabolism, the GI tract is also a relatively active site. Moreover, microflora present in the mammalian GI tract, most especially those of the large intestine, are involved in a range of effects in the host, some of which are related to the metabolism and toxicity of foreign chemicals. Indeed, some have postulated that gut microflora may be substantially more significant contributors to both beneficial and detrimental health effects than we now recognize (Nicholson, et al. 2005). These two sources of enzymatic activity are discussed in sequence below.

Age-associated changes in foreign compound metabolism are well documented. Both phase I and phase II metabolizing enzymes are expressed to different degrees in neonates and adults. Fetal enzyme activity is virtually absent, increases in the neonatal period, and becomes fully mature in childhood. Although this general trend holds, it appears that the different subsets of CYP enzymes become active at different rates (Leeder and Kearns, 1997).

Caffeine metabolism in adults depends almost entirely on CYP1A2 activity (Kalow and Tang, 1993). Fetal activity of CYP1A2 is, however, virtually absent, and does not achieve mature status until the first 3 to 8 months of life (Cazeneuve et al., 1994). Other CYP isozymes are active preterm and yield qualitatively and quantitatively different metabolic profiles. Theophylline metabolism is similarly affected (Kraus et al., 1993).

The CYP3A subfamily of enzymes is highly important in drug metabolism; three isoforms (CYP3A4, 3A5, 3A7) are known (Maples et al., 2006). Isoform 3A7 is highly expressed in fetal tissue and then declines throughout infancy (Schuetz et al., 1994). At the same time 3A4 increases in activity throughout the neonatal period, reaches peak levels in childhood, and then declines to adult levels at puberty (deWildt et al., 1999). Clearance patterns for midazolam, cyclosporine, and carbamazipine have been demonstrated to be consistent with the age-related changes in CYP3A enzyme activity (Maples et al., 2006; Korinthenberg et al., 1994).

These types of age-dependent changes are well-documented for certain CYP enzymes such that effects on pediatric drug use are reasonably predictable. Much less is known about other classes of chemicals, but the pharmaceutical literature can provide much guidance.

EFFECTS OF FOREIGN COMPOUNDS ON NEONATAL GI TRACT

Irritating and corrosive compounds are well established causes of acute injury to the upper regions of the GI tract including the oral cavity (Tyler, 1999). The problem is most serious in children, related both to the potential for higher intakes of chemicals per unit of GI tract surface area and greater susceptibility. Many forms of acute poisoning leading to GI tract injuries appear in the literature, some related to commercial products and some related to non-food plant products, the latter often tempting to young children. Common irritants and corrosive materials are the heavy metals and strong acids and bases. Plants that induce gastric injuries and produce vomiting, diarrhea, and abdominal pain include pokeweed, holly, castor, and various members of the Solanaceae family (Sreedharan and Mehta, 2005).

Increased vulnerabilities of infants and children are well documented in the case of various bacterial toxins that are causes of food- and water-borne illnesses, where less-than-fully-developed immune status compromises the response.

The developing GI tract is a target for a number of chemical toxicants, although it appears that most involve *in utero* exposures during critical periods of fetal development. Anorectal malformations have been observed in rats following *in utero* exposure to ethylene thiourea (Hirai and Kuwabara, 1990); similar malformations have been observed in mice following *in utero* exposure to all-trans retinoic acid (Hashimoto et al., 2002). It seems that *in utero* exposure during GI tract development is required to produce these effects and that the neonatal animal would not be susceptible; direct studies to support such a conjecture are not available. Whether the effect of *in utero* or neonatal exposures in neuro-development may indirectly compromise GI tract development does not seem to have been investigated.

REFERENCES

Adkins, Y. and Lonnerdal, B. 2003. Potential host-defense role of a human milk vitamin B_{12}-binding protein, haptocorrin, in the gastrointestinal tract of breastfed infants, as assessed with porcine haptocorrin *in vitro*. *Am. J. Clin. Nutr.* 77: 1234–1240.

Ayabe, T., Satchell, D.P., Wilson, C.L., Parks, W.C., Selsted, M.E., and Ouellette, A.J. 2000. Secretion of microbicidal a-defensins by intestinal Paneth cells in response to bacteria. *Nature Immunol.* 1: 113–118.

Babyatsky, M.W. and Podolsky, D.K. Growth and development of the gastrointestinal tract, in Yamada, T. et al., Eds., *Textbook of Gastroenterology*, 4th ed. Philadelphia: Lippincott Williams & Wilkins.

Balmer, S.E. and Wharton, B.A. 1989. Diet and faecal flora in the newborn: breast milk and infant formula. *Arch. Dis. Childhood* 64: 1672–1677.

Barker, D.J.P. 2004. The developmental origins of well-being. *Phil. Trans. R. Soc. Lond.* B. 359: 1359–1366.

Barker, D.J.P., Eriksson, J.G., Foresen, T., and Osmond, C. 2002. Fetal origins of adult disease: strength of effects and biological basis. *Int. J. Epidemiol.* 31: 1235–1239.

Ben-Shlomo, Y. and Kuh, D. 2002. A life course approach to chronic disease epidemiology: conceptual models, empirical challenges and interdisciplinary perspectives. *Int. J. Epidemiol.* 31: 285–293.

Blum, S. and Schiffrin, E.J. 2003. Intestinal microflora and homeostasis of the mucosal immune response: implications for probiotic bacteria? *Cur. Issues Intest. Microbiol.* 4: 53–60.

Boehm, G., Stahl, B., Jelinek, J., Knol, J., Miniello, V., and Moro, G.E. 2005. Prebiotic carbohydrates in human milk and formulas. *Acta Paediatr. Suppl.* 94: 18–21.

Bourlioux, P., Koletzko, B., Guarner, F., and Braesco, V. 2003. The intestine and its microflora are partners for the protection of the host: report on Danone Symposium, Paris, June 14, 2002. *Am. J. Clin. Nutr.* 78: 675–683.

Calabrese, E.J. 1986. *Age and Susceptibility to Toxic Substances*. New York: John Wiley & Sons.

Cavell, B. 1981. Gastric emptying in infants with congenital heart disease. *Acta Pediatr. Scand.* 70: 517–520.

Cazeneuve, C., Pons, G., and Rey, E. 1994. Biotransformation of caffeine in human liver microsomes from fetuses, neonates, infants, and adults. *Br. J. Clin. Pharmacol.* 37: 405–412.

Centers for Disease Control. 1991. *Preventing Lead Poisoning in Young Children.* Atlanta: U.S. Public Health Service.

Chu, S.H., Ely, I.G., and Walker, W.A. 1989. Age and cortisone alter host responsiveness to cholera toxin in the developing gut. *Am. J. Physiol.* 256: G220–G225.

Collins, M.D. and Gibson, G.R. 1999. Probiotics, prebiotics, and synbiotics: approaches for modulating the microbial ecology of the gut. *Am. J. Clin. Nutr.* 69 (Suppl.): 1052S–1057S.

Conway, P.L. 1997. Development of intestinal microbiota, in Mackie, R.I. et al., Eds., *Gastrointestinal Microbiology.* London: Chapman & Hall.

Cummings, J.H., Antoine, J.M., Azpiroz, F., Bourdet-Sicard, R., Brandtzaeg, P., Calder, P.C., Gibson, G.R., Guarner, F., Isolauri, E., Pannemans, D., Shortt, C., Tuijtelaars, S., and Watzl, B. 2004. Gut health and immunity. *Eur. J. Nutr.* 43 (Suppl. 2): 118–173.

Dai, D., Nanthkumar, N.N., Newburg, D.S., and Walker, W.A. 2000. Role of oligosaccharides and glycoconjugates in intestinal host defense. *J. Pediatr. Gastroentrol. Nutr.* 30: S23–S33.

Dai, D. and Walker, W.A. 1999. Protective nutrients and bacterial colonization in the immature human gut. *Adv. Pediatr.* 46: 353–382.

de Belle, R.C., Vaupshas, V., Vitullo, B.B., Haber, L.R., Schaffer, E., Mackie, G.G., Owen, H., Little, J.M., and Lester, R. 1979. Intestinal absorption of bile salts: immature development in the neonate. *J. Pediatr.* 94: 472–476.

deWildt, S.N., Kearns, G.L., Leeder, J.S., and van den Anker, J.N. 1999. Glucuronidation in humans: pharmacogenetic and developmental aspects. *Clin. Pharmacokinetics.* 36: 439–452.

Doughty, D. 2004. Structure and function of the gastrointestinal tract in infants and children. *J. Wound Ostomy Continence Nurs.* 31: 207–212.

Duffy, L.C. 2000. Interactions mediating bacterial translocation in the immature intestine. *J. Nutr.* 130: 432S–436S.

Edwards, C.A. and Parrett, A.M. 2002. Intestinal flora during the first months of life: new perspectives. *Br. J. Nutr.* 88 (Suppl. 1): S11–S18.

Erdman, T.S. and Pollack, P.F. 2001. Neonatal alimentary system, in *Ross Pediatrics, Clinical Education Series.* http://rosslearningcenter.com/library/NeonatalAlimentarySystem.pdf. Accessed August 30, 2005.

Fanaro, S., Chierici, R., Guerrini, P., and Vigi, V. 2003. Intestinal microflora in early infancy: composition and development. *Acta Paediatr. Suppl.* 441: 48–55.

Gaskins, H.R. 1997. Immunological aspects of host/microbiota interactions at the intestinal epithelium, in Mackie, R.I. et al., Eds., *Gastrointestinal Microbiology.* London: Chapman & Hall.

Gronlund, M.M., Arvilommi, H., Kero, P., Lehtonen, O.P., and Isolauri, E. 2000. Importance of intestinal colonization in the maturation of humoral immunity in early infancy: a prospective follow-up study of healthy infants aged 0–6 months. *Arch. Dis. Child. Fetal Neonatal Ed.* 83: F186–F192.

Gulson, B.L., Mahaffey, K.R., Vidal, M, Jameson, C.W., Law, A.J., Mizon, K.J., Smith, A.J., and Korsch, M.J. 1997. Dietary lead intakes for mother/child pairs and relevance to pharmacokinetic models. *Environ. Health. Perspect.* 105: 1334–1342

Hamilton, J.R. 2000. The pediatric patient: early development and the digestive system, in Walker, W.A. et al., Eds., *Pediatric Gastrointestinal Disease.* Hamilton, Ontario: B.C. Decker.

Hammerman, C., Bin-Nun, A., and Kaplan, M. 2004. Germ warfare: probiotics in defense of the premature gut. *Clin. Perinatol.* 31: 489–500.

Harding, J. 2001. The nutritional basis of the fetal origins of adult disease. *Int. J. Epidemiol.* 30: 15–23.

Hashimoto, R., Nagaya, M, Ishiguro, Y., Inouye, M., Aoyama, H., Futaki, S., and Murata, Y. 2002. Relationship of the fistulas to the rectum and genitourinary tract in mouse fetuses with high anorectal malformations induced by all-trans retinoic acid. *Pediatr. Surg. Int.* 18: 723–727.

Heavey, P.M. and Rowland, I.R. 1999. The gut microflora of the developing infant: microbiology and metabolism. *Microb. Ecol. Health Dis.* 11: 75–83.

Hertzman, C. 1995. The biological embedding of early experience and its effects on health in adulthood. *Ann. NY Acad. Sci.* 896: 85–95.

Hill, M. 2005. Gastrointestinal tract development. http://embryology.med.unsw.edu.au/ Notes/git.htm. August 30, 2005.

Isolauri, E., Sutas, Y., Kankaanpaa, P., Arvilommi, H., and Salminen, S. 2001. Probiotics: effects on immunity. *Am. J. Clin. Nutr.* 73 (Suppl.): 444S–450S.

Kalliomaki, M. and Isolauri, E. 2003. Role of intestinal flora in the development of allergy. *Curr. Opin. Allergy Clin. Immunol.* 3: 15–20.

Kalow, W. and Tang, B.K. 1993. The use of caffeine for enzyme assays: critical appraisal. *Clin. Pharmacol. Ther.* 53: 503–514.

Kelly, D. and Coutts, A.G.P. 2000. Early nutrition and the development of immune function in the neonate. *Proc. Nutr. Soc.* 59: 177–185.

Kleessen, B., Bunke, H., Tovar, K. Noack, J., and Sawatzki, G. 1995. Influence of two infant formulas and human milk on the development of the faecal flora in newborn infants. *Acta Pediatr.* 84: 1347–1356.

Korinthenberg, R., Haug, C., and Hannak, D. 1994. The metabolization of carbamazepine to CBZ-10,11-epoxide in children from the newborn age to adolescence. *Neuropediatrics.* 25: 214–216.

Kraus, D.M., Fischer, J.H., Reitz, S.J., Kecskes, S.A., Yeh, T.F., McCulloch, K.M., Tung, E.C., and Cwik, M.J. 1993. Alterations in theophylline metabolism during the first year of life. *Clin. Pharmacol. Ther.* 54: 351–359.

Hirai, Y. and Kuwabara, N. 1990. Transplacentally induced anorectal malformations in rats. *J. Pediatr. Surg.* 25: 812–816.

Leeder, J.S. and Kearns, G.L., 1997. Pharmacogenetics in pediatrics: implications for practice. *Pediatr. Clin. North Am.* 44: 55–77.

Lundequist, B., Nord, C.E., and Winberg, J. 1985. The composition of the faecal microflora in breastfed and bottle fed infants from birth to eight weeks. *Acta Paediatr. Scand.* 74: 45–51.

Mackie, R.I., Sghir, A., and Gaskins, H.R. 1999. Developmental microbial ecology of the neonatal gastrointestinal tract. *Am. J. Clin. Nutr.* 69 (Suppl.): 1035S–1045S.

Mahaffey, K.R., McKinney, J., and Reigart, J.R. 2000. Lead and compounds, in Lippmann, M., Ed., *Environmental Toxicants, 2nd Ed.* New York: Wiley Interscience, chap. 14.

Majamaa, H. and Isolauri, E. 1997. Probiotics: a novel approach in the management of food allergy. *J. Allergy Clin. Immunol.* 99: 179–185.

Maples, H.D., James, L.P., and Stowe, C.D. 2005. Special pharmacokinetic and pharmacodynamic considerations in children, in Burton, M.E. et al., Eds., *Applied Pharmacokinetics and Pharmacodynamics*, 4th ed., Philadelphia: Lippincott Williams & Wilkins.

Mouricout, M. 1997. Interactions between the enteric pathogen and the host. *Adv. Exp. Med. Biol.* 412: 109–123.

National Research Council. 2001. *Evaluating Chemical and Other Agent Exposures for Reproductive and Developmental Toxicity: Report of Subcommittee on Reproductive and Developmental Toxicology.* Washington, D.C.: National Academy Press.

Nicholson, J.K., Holmes, E., and Wilson, I.D. 2005. Gut microorganisms, mammalian metabolism and personalized health care. *Nat. Rev. Microbiol.* 3: 431–438.

Orrhage, K. and Nord, C.E. 1999. Factors controlling the bacterial colonization of the intestine in breastfed infants. *Acta Pediatr.* 88 (Suppl.): 47S–57S.

Ouellette, A.J. and Bevin, C.L. 2001. Paneth cell defensins and innate immunity of the small bowel. *Inflammatory Bowel Dis.* 7: 43–50.

Pacha, J. 2000. Development of intestinal transport function in mammals. *Physiol. Rev.* 80: 1633–1667.

Perin, N.M., Clandinin, M.T., and Thomson, A.B.R. 1997. Importance of milk and diet on the ontogeny and adaptation of the intestine. *J. Ped. Gastroenterol. Nutr.* 24: 419–425.

Philipps, A.F. and Sherman, M.P. 2003. Neonatal nutrition and gastrointestinal function, in Wonsiewicz, M.J. et al., Eds., *Rudolph's Pediatrics, 21st Ed.* New York: McGraw Hill.

Phillips, D.I. 1996. Insulin resistance a programmed response to fetal undernutrition. *Diabetologia* 39: 1119–1122.

Popoff, M.R. 1998. Interactions between bacterial toxins and intestinal cells. *Toxicon* 36: 665–685.

Porter, E.M., Bevins, C.L., Ghosh, D., and Ganz, T. 2002. The multifaceted Paneth cell. *Cell. Mol. Life Sci.* 9: 156–170.

Premji, S.S. 1998. Ontogeny of the gastrointestinal system and its impact on feedings in the pre-term infant. *Neonatal Netw.* 17: 17–24.

Pucciareli, M.G., Siebers, A., and Finlay, B.B. 1997. Bacterial pathogen translocation across the gastrointestinal barrier, in Mackie, R.I. et al., Eds., *Gastrointestinal Microbiology.* London: Chapman & Hall.

Rane, A. 1992. Drug disposition and action in infants and children, in Yaffe, S.J. and Aranda, J.V., Eds., *Pediatric Pharmacology: Therapeutic Principles in Practice, 2nd Ed.* Philadelphia: W.B. Saunders.

Renwick, A.G. 2001. Toxicokinetics: pharmacokinetics in toxicology, in Hayes, A.W., Ed., *Principles and Methods of Toxicology,* Philadelphia: Taylor & Francis.

Plunkett, L.M., Turnbull, D., and Rodricks, J.V. 1992. Differences between adults and children affecting exposure assessment, in Guzelian, P. et al., Eds., *Similarities and Differences between Children and Adults: Implications for Risk Assessment.* Washington, D.C.: ILSI Press, p. 79.

Sanderson, I.R. 1999. The physiocochemical environment of the neonatal intestine. *Am. J. Clin. Nutr.* 69 (Suppl.): 1028S–1034S.

Schuetz, J.D., Beach, D.L., and Guzelian, P.W. 1994. Selective expression of cytochrome P450 CYP3A mRNAs in embryonic and adult human liver. *Pharmacogenetics* 4: 11–20.

Schiffrin, E.J. and Blum, S. 2002. Interactions between the microbiota and the intestinal mucosa. *Eur. J. Clin. Nutr.* 56 (Suppl. 3): S60–S64.

Schumann, K., Elsenhans, B., and Richter, E. 1999. Gastrointestinal tract, in Marquardt, H. et al., Eds., *Toxicology.* San Diego: Academic Press.

Sidhu, S.S., Thompson, D.G., Warhurst, G., Case, R.M., and Benson, R.S.P. 2000. Fatty acid-induced cholecystokinin secretion and changes in intracellular Ca^{2+} in two enteroendocrine cell lines, STC-1 and GLUTag, *J. Physiol.* 528: 165–176.

Sreedharan, R. and Mehta, D.I. 2005. Gastrointestinal tract. *Pediatrics* 113: 1044–1050.

Stark, P.L. and Lee, A. 1982. Microbial ecology of the large bowel of breast-fed and formula-fed infants during the first year of life. *J. Med. Microbiol.* 15: 189–203.

Sudo, N., Sawamura, S.M., and Tanaka, K. 1997. The requirement of intestinal bacteria flora for the development of an IgE production system fully susceptible to oral tolerance induction. *J. Immunol.* 159: 1739–1745.

Thiesen, A. Wild, G., Keelan, M., Clandinin, M.T., McBurney, M., Van Aerde, J., and Thomson, A.B.R. 2000. Ontogeny of intestinal nutrient transport. *Can J. Physiol. Pharmacol.* 78: 513–527.

Tlaskalova-Hogenova, H., Stepankova, R., Hudcovic, T., Tuckova, L., Cukrowska, B., Lodinova-Zadnikova, R., Kozakova, H., Rossmann, P. Bartova, J., Sokol, D., Funda, D. P., Borovska, D., Rehakova, Z., Sinkora, J., Hofman, J., Drastich, P. and Kokesova, A. 2004. Commensal bacteria (normal microflora), mucosal immunity and chronic inflammatory and autoimmune diseases. *Immunol. Lett.* 93: 97–108.

Tyler, T. 1999. Peroral toxicity, in Ballantyne, B. et al., Eds., *General and Applied Toxicology, 2nd Ed.*, Vol. 1, New York: Grove's Dictionaries Inc.

Vanderhoof, J.A. and Young R.J. 2003. Role of probiotics in the management of patients with food allergy. *Ann. Allergy Asthma Immunol.* 90 (Suppl. 3): 99–103.

Walthall, K., Cappon, G.D., Hurtt, M.E., and Zoetis, T. 2005. Postnatal development of the gastrointestinal system: species comparison. *Birth Defects Res. B: Dev. Reprod. Toxicol.* 74: 132–156.

Watkins, J.B., Ingall, D., Szczepanik, P., Klein, P.D., and Lester, R. 1973. Bile salt metabolism in the newborn: measurement of pool size and synthesis by stable isotope technique. *New Engl. J. Med.* 288: 431–434.

Weber, W.W. and Cohen, S.N. 1975. Aging effects and drugs in man, in Gillette, J.R. and Mitchell, J.R., Eds., *Concepts in Biochemical Pharmacology*, vol. 3. New York: Springer.

Wold, A.D. and Adlerberth, I. 2000. Breast feeding and the intestinal microflora of the infant: implications for protection against infectious diseases. *Adv. Exp. Med. Biol.* 478: 77–93.

5 Gastrointestinal Tract as Major Route of Pharmaceutical Administration

Robert W. Kapp, Jr.

CONTENTS

INTRODUCTION

The primary functions of the gastrointestinal (GI) tract are the breakdown of foodstuffs and the absorption of nutrients and water. These functions occur through the methodical mixing of food with digestive enzymes to create chyme which is moved by peristaltic motion across the mucosal cells of the GI tract to be absorbed. The small intestine is particularly well suited for this function because of its musculature, secretive cells, and immense surface area. Almost 80% of the chyme entering the small intestine is absorbed before it enters the colon. Because the small intestine is effective at absorbing the essential elements for life, it is also a target for the entry of a host of additional entities such as chemicals, bacteria, and toxic substances.

The body is designed to strive to permit only essential materials into the system. While its defenses are certainly not foolproof, the mammalian digestive system includes a series of inherent barriers that attempt to prevent the absorbance of materials not recognized as essential substances. These barriers include cell membranes of the intestinal mucosa that provide physical barriers. Recent studies also reveal that intestinal cells that produce enzymes can also metabolize many substances that attempt to minimize toxicants that pass through cell walls. Another defense is an aqueous boundary layer sometimes referred to as the "unstirred water layer" adjacent to the lumen of the GI tract that acts as a diffusion barrier to a number of substances.

Immediately adjacent to the lumen is an acid microclimate that poses yet another barrier for substances attempting to gain entry into the circulatory system. If a substance does not disintegrate or dissolve, the amount that can be absorbed into the bloodstream significantly decreases. The stomach pH of 3 to 5 not only degrades many chemical structures, but destroys millions of bacteria that could be absorbed into the bloodstream. If a xenobiotic is absorbed in spite of these barriers, it is transported to the liver prior to entering the general circulation in a process referred to as the first pass effect. A xenobiotic substance can be metabolized extensively in the liver before reaching the general blood circulation. Hence, a foreign substance must overcome numerous hurdles prior to its entrance into the general circulatory system. Drugs are among the many xenobiotics that are actively and passively prevented from absorption.

In spite of the myriad hurdles drugs must overcome to gain entry into the body via ingestion, ingestion remains the primary mode of drug administration. It is well known that the peroral route for drug administration is preferred by patients since it is in most cases the least stressful and most convenient mode. Unfortunately, many drug formulations pose inherent solubility, absorption, distribution, and stability issues resulting from exposure to the GI tract. Several major problems are associated with drugs administered via oral ingestion: (1) too-rapid transit time across the ideal absorption site, (2) intense degradation of peptide-based drugs in the GI tract, and (3) poor permeability across the lumen wall (Harding, 2003). Drug companies are under considerable pressure to produce drugs for oral administration because they are frequently less expensive to manufacture, are preferred by clinicians and patients alike, and can be made into a variety of delivery formats including fast release tablets, slow release tablets, capsules, and enteric-coated preparations.

One critical prerequisite of both the successful manufacture and clinical use of chemicals for oral administration is finding those with the highest potential to be absorbed in the GI tract, distributed into the circulatory system, and not metabolized before they can reach their ultimate receptor sites. Numerous factors determine the degree of absorption of a compound across the GI tract membranes and into the circulatory system. Physicochemical properties include solubility, pKa, molecular size, hydrophobicity, hydrogen bonding capacity, particle size, complexation, and chemical stability. Physiological factors include membrane permeability, surface area of site of adsorption, available transporters, variations in metabolism along the tract, amounts and types of foodstuffs present, amount of water present, enterohepatic circulation engagement, intestinal and pancreatic secretions, transit time, and local pH (Burton et al., 2002).

The purpose of this chapter is to describe the issues concerning the GI tract as a route of drug administration and the associated processes of drug absorption, bioavailability, and distribution. Because any xenobiotic or drug must overcome so many barriers to gain effective entry, the drug companies strive to manufacture oral medications that are successfully absorbed and ultimately transported to receptor sites.

STRUCTURE AND FUNCTION OF GASTROINTESTINAL TRACT

The primary function of the GI tract is the absorption of nutrients and water from the surrounding environment for sustenance. The tract is a specialized structure present in multicellular organisms that essentially obtains nourishment by the ingestion of organic material. This process provides the body cells with nutrients required to maintain life functions. The cell walls of the GI tract are composed of numerous tissue types that serve to break down foodstuffs and fluids into absorbable components and also create an environment for absorption of these components into the circulatory system.

The GI tract is a 25- to 30-foot series of hollow organs connected to form a pathway that starts at the mouth and proceeds through the pharynx, esophagus, stomach, small intestine, large intestine, and rectum, and ends at the anus. Although positioned within the body, the contents of the lumen of the GI tract are considered external and must traverse cell membranes to gain entry into the circulatory system. The digestive system functions to modify the ingested luminal content so that it can be absorbed from the lumen or exterior to the blood and/or lymph circulatory system or interior of the body (Kapp, 2007).

The digestion system is organized into two divisions: (1) the GI tract or alimentary canal that includes the mouth, pharynx, esophagus, stomach, small intestine, large intestine, rectum, and anus; and (2) the accessory structures including teeth, tongue, salivary glands, pharynx, liver, gallbladder, and pancreas (Kapp, 2007). The major organs of the digestive tract are illustrated in Figure 5.1.

Each portion of the GI tract is highly specialized. In conjunction with the accessory digestive organs connected through a series of ducts including the salivary glands, pancreas, liver, and gallbladder, the foodstuffs are turned into a thick semi-liquid mass of partially digested food (chyme) that is eventually

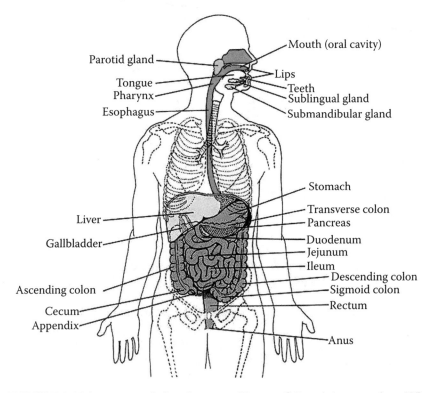

FIGURE 5.1 Major organs of digestive tract. (Tortora, G.J. and Anagnostakos, N.P., *Principles of Anatomy and Physiology*, 6th ed., 1990. Reprinted with permission of John Wiley & Sons.)

absorbed in the small intestine for transport into the circulatory and lymphatic systems. Table 5.1 summarizes the structures and primary functions of the various portions of the GI tract.

Each portion of the GI tract has a specialized function and varying conditions such as pH, transit time, and surface area. The oral cavity serves primarily as a place where foodstuffs or xenobiotics first enter the GI tract by tearing of food into smaller pieces through mastication. These substances rarely remain in the oral cavity long enough to be absorbed. However, some materials can be absorbed directly into the circulatory system via sublingual absorption. For example, nitroglycerin used to treat certain heart conditions is commonly administered in this fashion since the material can quickly get into the bloodstream and bypasses the first pass metabolism of the liver. This type of absorption, while important, is the exception rather than the rule for absorption in the GI tract.

As a substance is swallowed, it enters the esophagus en route to the stomach. The esophagus is thick and muscular and material quickly passes through this section with little to no absorption occurring in transit. The substance is delivered to the stomach which has a pH of 3 or lower and a capacity of about one liter. The highly acidic stomach contents not only destroy the bacteria that enter with the foreign materials, but activate pepsinogen in the break-down of proteins. The stomach fluid also contains mucus, which protects the stomach lining from the high acidity of the contents. The stomach mixes the contents into chyme for transport into the next part of the digestive tract.

From the stomach, the chyme passes into the duodenum of the small intestine where the pH varies from about 6 to 6.5 and the majority of the absorption into the circulatory system occurs. Numerous digestive or intestinal juices are added in the small intestine along with pancreatic and bile secretions that are critical to the digestive process. The surface area of the duodenum is extremely large, providing a vast area for absorption of food and xenobiotic substances. The cell wall of this portion of the small intestine has millions of finger-like projections called villi that can be found on projections called brush borders that are designed to provide a vast area for nutrient absorption. Each villus is embedded into the connective tissue of the wall of the small intestine and has an arteriole, a venule, a capillary network, and a lymphatic vessel (lacteal) that allows nutrients to pass through the capillary wall directly into the lymphatic and cardiovascular systems.

The jejunum and ileum lie beyond the duodenum. Although they comprise the longest part of the small intestine, they provide only a fraction of the absorptive surface. The jejunum possesses more absorptive surface area than the ileum, which possesses the least area. (Magee and Dalley, 1986). The pH becomes more basic as the distance from the stomach increases. The total time in transit through the entire small intestine is about 3 to 4 hours. The final section of the GI tract is the large intestine or colon. This section is the primary site of water and electrolyte resorption. The pH of the large intestine ranges from 5 to 7. The blood supply to the rectum is not transported to the liver for first pass metabolism. The colon is similar to the sublingual area in that anything absorbed there such as

TABLE 5.1
GI Tract Structures and Functions

Section of GI Tract	Function	Secretory Glands	Accessory Organs	pH	Transit Time	Membrane	Vascularization	Surface Area	First Pass Metabolism
Oral cavity	Mastication; begin liquefaction	Salivary glands	Teeth; tongue	~7	Brief	Thin	High	Limited	No
Esophagus	Conduit to stomach	Mucus secretion	Pharynx; larynx	5–6	Brief	Thick	Normal	Limited	NA
Stomach	Reservoir mixing	Gastric acid glands	None	<3	30–45 min	Normal	Normal	Moderate	Yes
Small intestine	Digestion and absorption	Intestinal juice; maltose; sucrase; lactase; amino-peptidase; dextrinase nuclease	Pancreas; liver; gallbladder	6–8	3–4 hr	Normal	High	Very large	Yes
Large intestine	Bacterial digestion; water resorption	Alkaline mucus	None	5–7	24–30 hr	Normal	Normal	Moderate	Yes

NA = not applicable.

Source: Adapted from Bourne, W.A.D., PHAR 7632, 7633, and 4634, College of Pharmacy, University of Oklahoma Health Sciences Center, Oklahoma City, 2001.

suppositories and enemas goes directly into systemic circulation. The transit time through the colon is quite long and can exceed 24 hours.

PHARMACOKINETICS

Pharmacokinetics broadly refers to the mathematics of movement of chemical substances through the body including the way in which the body's physiology affects the substances over time. The composition of the substance in question exerts an influence over the location of substance absorption, the specificity of where that substance may be transported, the degree of metabolism, and the rapidity of excretion. These four functions — absorption, distribution, metabolism, and excretion (ADME) — define the effectiveness of a pharmaceutical compound (Beers and Berkow, 2005) and all are critical to its success. The biological, physiological, and physicochemical factors that influence the transfer of drugs within the body also influence the rate and extent of ADME of those drugs. In many cases, pharmacological and toxicological actions are related to plasma concentrations of drugs. The study of pharmacokinetics allows a pharmacist to individualize therapy for a patient.

BIOAVAILABILITY

Bioavailability involves all the activities associated with the processes necessary for the entrance of an active xenobiotic substance (drug) into the body and its eventual arrival at a designated receptor site where it can have an effect. Hence, bioavailability is a pharmacokinetic term that describes the rate and extent to which a therapeutically active drug is absorbed from a drug matrix and becomes available at the receptor site of drug action (Shargel and Yu, 1999; Banakar and Makoid, 1997).

Oral absorptive mechanisms constitute a complex series of processes that are dependent upon a number of factors including chemical properties of the substance as well as physiological factors inherent within the lumen of the GI tract.

Interestingly, drug concentrations generally cannot be readily measured at a receptor site; therefore, most bioavailability studies involve the determination of drug concentration in the blood or urine. This is based upon the premise that a drug at a site of action is in equilibrium with drug in the circulatory system. It is therefore postulated that one can obtain an indirect measure of drug response by monitoring drug levels in the blood and/or urine. The bioavailability of a drug product affects the onset, intensity, and duration of therapeutic response and therefore can determine its therapeutic efficacy. Therefore, oral bioavailability can specifically be defined as the extent of original drug appearing in the blood after oral administration. F_{oral} is generally expressed by comparing the amount of drug in the circulatory system post-oral administration as compared to the amount of drug in the circulatory system post-intravenous administration. $f_{absorbed}$ is the fraction of the intact drug taken into the intestinal tissue. $f_{gut\ wall}$ is the fraction of drug that remains after intestinal metabolism and enters the portal vein. $F_{hepatic}$ is the fraction of drug that remains following first pass intestinal and hepatic metabolism (Pond and Tozer, 1985). One can express the mathematical relationship of the bioavailability of a drug in the following equation:

$$F_{oral} = f_{absorbed} \times f_{gut\ wall} \times f_{hepatic}$$

Thus, bioavailability can be equal to or (more often) less than the fraction of the substance absorbed, depending upon the degree of drug loss in the gut wall and through first pass metabolism. In most cases, the concern is the extent of absorption of drug, (that is, the fraction of the dose that actually reaches the bloodstream) because it represents the effective dose. In general, numerous factors can and do influence the bioavailability of a drug and many barriers can prevent a drug from reaching the ultimate receptor sites in order to be effective.

Christopher Lipinski's seminal manuscript (Lipinski et al., 1997) about the "rule of five" identifies a series of features commonly found in orally active drugs. The guidelines have been unofficially adopted by the pharmaceutical industry in an effort to predict which chemicals in early drug development may have the best possibilities of passive transcellular transport and permeability. The rule of five is so called because most of the parameters start with the number five or represent multiples of five. In general, an orally active drug has:

• Molecular weight below 500
• Low lipophilicity (expressed as cLogP less than 5)
• Not more than 5 hydrogen bond donors
• Not more than 10 hydrogen bond acceptors

Table 5.2 summarizes the most critical chemical factors affecting drug absorption. Table 5.3 summarizes the physical factors that affect drug absorption. Table 5.4 summarizes the most critical physiological factors affecting drug absorption. In addition to the factors listed in Tables 5.1 through 5.4, additional issues affecting drug–drug interactions are listed in Table 5.5.

ABSORPTION

Absorption is defined as the transfer of a substance from its site of entry to the circulatory or lymphatic system. The rate and efficiency of absorption of any substance administered orally are dependent upon numerous factors (Beers and Berkow, 2005). As a substance passes into the GI tract, it can be absorbed by one or more of several mechanisms. While no known mechanisms specifically transport only xenobiotics into the body, many existing nutrient absorption pathways in the GI tract are also used by foreign substances such as drugs to gain entry into the body. Generally, if a drug is an organic acid or base, it most likely will be absorbed via simple diffusion.

TABLE 5.2
Critical Chemical Factors Affecting Drug Absorption

Chemical Property of Drug	Variable	Effect
Particle size or molecular size	Degree of disintegration	Larger size results in less absorption
Hydrogen bonding	Degree of hydrogen bonding	Increases transit time and degree of absorption (Whitehead, 2005)
Partition coefficient	Pathway of absorption	Paracellular or transcellular route or not transported (Kulkami, 2002)
Hydrophilicity	Tight junctions between epithelial cells	Prevents drug from passing through cellular membrane tight junctions
Lipophilicity	Adipose tissue	Drug becomes trapped in adipose tissue
Ion trapping	Localization at non-receptor sites	Weak acid/or base drugs become trapped at sites such as kidney and cannot reach receptor site
Crystalline structure	Degree of hydration of active ingredient	Availability at membrane wall
Stability	Active ingredient intact long enough to be absorbed	Less stable drugs have decreased absorption
Low pH	Stomach	Degradation of active ingredients

By virtue of the structures of these substances, one can estimate that an organic acid exists primarily in lipid-soluble form in the stomach and in ionized form in the small intestines. Hence, an organic acid would be absorbed more readily in the acidic stomach than in the neutral small intestine. Organic bases, on the other hand, would be absorbed more readily in the more neutral pH of the small intestine rather than in the acidic stomach. However, since the pH is about neutral in the small intestine, both weak acids and weak bases are non-ionized and readily absorbed by passive diffusion. There are significant exceptions due to the large surface area of the small intestine, varying blood flow rates, and the law of mass action that maintains a gradient in the compartments.

In addition to the above passive transport mechanisms, a variety of active and facilitated mechanisms transport nutrients including monosaccharides, amino acids, and minerals into the mucosal epithelial cells. A xenobiotic transport mechanism called the multi-drug-resistant (mdr) protein or p-glycoprotein has been identified. This mechanism functions to move certain xenobiotics out of cells which, in turn, acts to decrease the net amount of GI absorption for some drugs and toxicants. The multi-resistant drug protein transport systems (mrps) have been shown to transport glucuronides and glutathione metabolites out of cells as well (Rozman and Klaassen, 2001). The iron transport mechanism also

TABLE 5.3
Critical Physical Factors Affecting Drug Absorption

Dosage Form	Variable	Effect
Solutions (e.g., syrups and elixirs)	Already in aqueous form	Readily absorbable
Suspensions	In aqueous form; suspended particles must be disintegrated	Less readily absorbable than solutions
Capsules	Most readily disintegratable form of solid dosage; drug inside capsule is easily dissolved	Less readily absorbable than suspensions
Uncoated tablets	Solids compressed into small pills; must be disintegrated before they can be dissolved	Less readily absorbable than capsules; must be disintegrated
Enteric-coated tablets	Tablet coatings are more difficult to disintegrate than uncoated tablets	Less readily absorbable than uncoated tablets; coating is designed not to disintegrate upon administration
Controlled-release capsules	Designed to slowly dissolve over time; absorption is sequential and constant	Less readily absorbable than enteric-coated tablets
Controlled-release tablets	Designed to dissolve over longer period for sequential and constant absorption	Less readily absorbable than controlled-release capsules

absorbs xenobiotics such as thallium while manganese and cobalt both utilize and also compete for access to the iron transport system. The calcium transport mechanism also absorbs lead. The pyrimidine transport system also absorbs 5-fluorouracil.

While these xenobiotics are actively transported into the mucosal epithelial cells of the GI tract, the majority of toxicants and drugs enter by simple passive diffusion. Low molecular weight lipid-insoluble compounds are absorbed through aqueous membrane pores at the tight junctions in membranes via passive diffusion. Another factor in the absorption of xenobiotics is that particulate drugs can be absorbed via vesicular transport — either by pinocytosis or phagocytosis.

As described in Tables 5.1 through 5.5, other factors that can markedly affect absorption include a drug's package design (tablet, capsule, controlled-release formulation, etc.); its physical and chemical properties; physiological characteristics of the patient; and disease states of the patient. Generally, however, the rate

TABLE 5.4
Critical Physiological Factors Affecting Drug Absorption

Physiological Properties	Variable	Effect
Intestinal contents	Amount of food or other chemicals already present with substance to be absorbed	Binding or complexation can affect amount of drug available for absorption (Galia, 1998)
Gastrointestinal microorganisms	Numbers and locations of microorganisms	Metabolism of active ingredients to inactive forms
Regional variations in pH of digestive fluids	Fluid volumes and secretion rates of intestinal enzymes	Changes in degradation rate and partition coefficients can increase or decrease absorption rates (Fallingborg, 1989)
Regional variations in absorptive capabilities of digestive tract	Duodenum is very absorptive; jejunum and ileum less absorptive	Certain areas of GI tract are more prone to enhance absorption than others
Intestinal motility	Transit can increase or decrease	The slower the transit rate, the more absorption can occur (Pang, 2003)
Gastric emptying	Gastric emptying rate can increase with stress, increased pH; can decrease with increased viscosity of GI tract content, exercise, ingestion of fatty acids or carbohydrates, decreased pH	The less time a substance remains in GI tract, the less absorption occurs (Pang, 2003)
Intestinal metabolism	Metabolism occurring in cell walls of GI tract	Increases first pass metabolism of liver which can deactivate or activate drug
Intestinal blood flow	Blood flow varies with stomach contents	Increased blood flow decreases transit time through gut and liver, lessening potential for first pass metabolism
Aqueous boundary layer or unstirred water layer	Water/mucus layer surrounding villi of small intestine	Substances must diffuse across this layer to gain access to mucosal cell membranes
Age, weight, sex	Each biological variable can affect absorption rates	Variable effects are noted in absorption rates with each variable
Pathology	Various disease states may affect rate of drug absorption	Variable effects noted in absorption rates with many disease states

TABLE 5.5
Drug–Drug Interactions

Item	Variable	Effect
pH	Acidic or basic — indirect effect	pH of one drug can change absorption of another by changing drug ionization state
Gastric motility	Change in rate of transit — indirect effect	One drug can speed or slow transit rate in GI tract which can affect absorption rate of second drug
Drug-induced malabsorption	Interference with mucosal function — indirect effect	One drug can change properties of intestinal mucosa which can affect absorption rate of second drug
Chelation	Complexing with another drug — direct effect	One drug can chemically bind with another, reducing absorption of both
Exchange resin binding	Adsorption of resin of one drug with active moiety of second drug — direct effect	One drug can bind with components of another, reducing absorption of both

of absorption is determined by the solubility of the active ingredient and the permeability of the cell wall to the solute. A drug product frequently consists of an active ingredient along with inactive ingredients such as diluents, disintegrants, stabilizers, and lubricants that are compressed in varying degrees to enhance absorption. If a drug is administered in solution, it is already in a form that is theoretically, at least, absorbable. Nevertheless, the solution must not degrade significantly in the presence of the acidic pH and enzymatic secretions of the GI tract.

If a drug is administered in a solid form such as a tablet or capsule, several additional steps in the process are necessary to facilitate absorption: (1) disintegration of the substance; (2) dissolution of the substance in proximity of the absorption site; and (3) transfer of the substance across the lumen of the GI tract into the circulatory or lymphatic system. Disintegration increases the surface area of the substance, which enhances the probability that the solid will dissolve into the solute. Surfactants, disintegrants, and lubricants are usually added during the manufacturing process to increase the solubility and dispersibility of the active ingredient. In the case of enteric-coated tablets, hydrophobic lubricants and extreme pressure may be applied during the manufacturing process to slow the dissolution process. This allows the active ingredient to be released over a longer period of time and is critical to time-release drugs. Dissolution is the rate of availability of the active ingredient for absorption or the time required for a given amount of drug to be released into solution from a solid dosage form. Dissolution time is usually measured *in vitro* under conditions that simulate those that occur *in vivo* in experiments in which the amount of drug in solution is determined as a function of time (Ritter et al., 2003).

Once a drug has entered the GI tract and is a liquid or a thoroughly dissolved solid, it must pass through several lipid cell membrane barriers prior to reaching the circulatory or lymphatic system. Immediately adjacent to the lumen cell wall is an aqueous boundary layer or "unstirred water layer" comprised of <5% mucus and 90% water (Carlstedt et al., 1985; Artursson, 1991). This layer acts as a diffusion barrier to drugs, toxicants, and chyme alike and represents yet another barrier to surmount in the absorption process. In addition to the unstirred water layer, another layer termed the acid microclimate exists at the surface of the luminal cell membrane. Once a substance traverses the unstirred water layer and the acid microlayer, it reaches the surface of the membrane of the lumen. The two main pathways for a substance to enter the membrane are the transcellular (through the cells) and the paracellular (between the cells). The next section describes each of these absorption mechanisms.

TRANSCELLULAR TRANSPORT

Substances entering the membrane via the transcellular route do so either passively or are actively transported. There are several types of transcellular transport processes including those that are completely passive, those that are active, and those that do not easily fit into either category in the conventional sense.

Passive Cellular Transport

This type of absorption expends no energy and is the most common route of absorption in the GI tract. Passive cellular transport is dependent upon the permeability of the membrane and the surface area available for absorption. Four types of passive cellular transport mechanisms are found in the GI tract: diffusion, filtration, osmosis, and facilitated diffusion.

Diffusion

This type of transport shows low chemical specificity and does not involve a carrier or the expenditure of energy. The process involves the absorption of a substance across a concentration from a membrane compartment of high concentration to a compartment of low concentration. Diffusion only occurs when there is a concentration gradient of a substance separated by a membrane. The physics of diffusion follows Fick's first law which describes the passive movement down a concentration gradient to equilibrate the substance in both compartments. Given enough time, the flow of substance will eventually result in homogeneity within the matrix, causing the net flow of substances to cease. Fick postulated that the flux of material across a given plane is proportional to the concentration gradient across the plane (Wilson, 2004). Mathematically this movement is described by the following equation:

$$F = -D \; (\partial C(x,t)/\partial x)$$

where F is the flux, D is the diffusion constant for the substance diffusing in the specific solvent, and $\partial C(x,t)/\partial x$ is the concentration gradient. The diffusion constant of a substance is also referred to as its diffusion coefficient and it is expressed in units of length^2/time (e.g., μm^2/hour). The negative sign [–] on the right side of the equation indicates that the substances flow in the direction of lower concentration.

This pathway is primarily for lipophilic substances. Fromm and Heirholzer (2000) have shown that different sections of the GI tract membrane have varying degrees of permeability because of thickness and fluidity of the basolateral membrane. Additional factors governing absorption with passive cellular transport include the available membrane surface area and transit time — both increasing proportionately with increasing values.

Filtration

This phenomenon occurs when water flows across membranes in large quantities due to hydrostatic pressure. Water flow tends to adhere to some substances with molecular weights of 150 to 300 and pulls the molecules through the same channels in the cell membrane. The movement and hydrostatic pressure of the water forces substances through the membrane in a way that is greater than that expected by random motion.

Osmosis

Osmosis is the passive movement of groups of water molecules through cell membranes. Water molecules — unlike other substances — tend to be drawn together by weak hydrogen bonds. This weak bonding makes the molecules stick to one another in an amorphous mass and their movement across the membrane is also referred to as bulk flow.

Facilitated Diffusion

Facilitated diffusion is a protein carrier-mediated process by which large substances can pass through cell walls. An example is glucose, which is not only too large to enter the membrane, but is also insoluble in lipids. The process involves binding of the substance to a specific carrier protein. The complex binds to a receptor site within the cell which transports the entire complex through the cell membrane and releases it on the other side. Since facilitated diffusion is a passive process, these substances only move down the concentration gradient.

ACTIVE CELLULAR TRANSPORT

The movements of many compounds across the mucosal epithelial membrane require active assistance and the expenditure of energy, generally because a substance has a large molecular weight, is insoluble, or is moving against a concentration gradient. Since these substances successfully traverse the

membrane, a system of transport mechanisms has been devised to explain the movements of numerous materials inside mucosal epithelial cells. This process is characterized by selectivity and requires energy expenditure by cells. The process of active transport moves molecules against their electrochemical gradient, a process that would not be possible if it were not coupled with the hydrolysis of adenosine triphosphate (ATP). This coupling can be either primary or secondary. In the primary active transport, transporters that move molecules against their electrical or chemical gradient chemically hydrolyze ATP. In the secondary active transport, transporters use energy derived from transport of another molecule in the direction of their gradient, to move other molecules in the direction against their gradient. This can be either in the same direction — symport — or in the opposite direction — antiport (Kimball, 2005).

Active transport processes have been identified for various ions, vitamins, sugars, and amino acids as well as some xenobiotic materials. The divalent metal ion transporter (dmt) assists with the absorption of metals while the nucleotide transporter (nt) and peptide transporter (pept) function in the transport of nucleotides and peptides, respectively. While these transporters seem to be quite different as they transport widely diverse substances, they are similar in many respects. The following characteristics are exhibited by most active transport systems:

1. The system is chemical-structural specific.
2. The system is carrier-mediated.
3. The system utilizes energy.
4. The system is competitive among other similarly structured chemicals that utilize the same transport system.
5. The system is transport-rate limiting either by saturation or competition and exhibits a transport maximum (T_m).
6. The system moves substances against concentration/energy gradients.

With few exceptions, actively transported substances are transported across the mucosal epithelial cell by forming a membrane-bound complex on the low concentration side of the membrane. The substance then crosses the membrane through specific channels by the expenditure of energy where it is released on the high concentration side of the membrane. The coupling of transport to the energy source may be direct or indirect (Rozman and Klaassen, 2001).

Direct Cellular Transport

Direct active transport or primary active transport is coupled directly to an exergonic reaction which is mostly hydrolysis of ATP. These transport proteins are termed ATPases or ATPase pumps. There are four types of transport ATPases.

P type ATPase — The P type is reversibly phosphorylated by ATP as part of the transport mechanism and includes, Na^+/K^+ ATPase of plasma membranes,

H^+ ATPase of GI tract epithelial cells, and Ca^{2+} ATPase of skeletal muscle cells and endoplasmic reticulum.

V type ATPase — The V type does not undergo phosphorylation. V type ATPases are involved with vesicle pumps that pump protons into organelles of the endosomal membranes.

F type ATPase — The F type is found only in bacteria, mitochondria, and chloroplasts. These ATPases are involved with proton transport in organisms that use the energy of ATP hydrolysis to drive ATP synthesis.

ABC type ATPase — The ABC type ATPases or ATP binding cassettes are transmembrane proteins that expose a ligand-binding domain at one surface and an ATP-binding domain at the other surface and are usually restricted to a single type of molecule. The bound ATP provides the energy to the ligand transfer. The human genome contains at least 48 ABC transporters including CFTR (cystic fibrosis transmembrane conductance regulator) and TAP (transporter associated with antigen processing) (Wright, 2005; Kimball, 2005).

Indirect Cellular Transport

Indirect or secondary active transport is characterized by the fact that the energy driving the system is that of two molecules — one going down its gradient drives the movement of the other substance against its gradient. Since the gradient is maintained by ATP hydrolysis, ATP is the indirect source of energy for this process. Generally, the driving ion in this scenario is Na^+ with its gradient established by the Na^+/K^+ ATPase. The two basic types of indirect active transport mechanisms are symport and antiport. (Kimball, 2005).

Symport

In this type of indirect active transport, the driving ion (usually Na^+) is forced through the membrane pump in the same direction as a second molecule or ion. An example of this is the Na^+/glucose transporter in which the transmembrane protein permits Na^+ ions and glucose to enter the cell together. The Na^+ ions flow down their concentration gradient while the glucose molecules are pumped against their concentration gradient. Eventually, the Na^+ is pumped back out of the cell by the Na^+/K^+ ATPase. This pump is used to actively transport glucose out of the GI tract and into the circulatory system.

Antiport

In this type of indirect active transport, the driving ion (also usually Na^+) diffuses through the pump in one direction and that transfer provides the energy for the active transport of another molecule in the opposite direction. An example of this type of pump is the H^+/K^+ ATPase that catalyzes the transport of H^+ out of gastric parietal cells (toward the lumen of the stomach) in exchange for a K^+ ion that enters the cells (away from the lumen of the stomach).

ENDOCYTOSIS

Endocytosis is the process by which a substance gains entry into a cell without passing through the cell membrane proper. The cell wall invaginates or changes shape in such a way that it encloses the substance, then the wall re-fuses, forming a vesicle that moves to the interior of the cell. This mechanism of absorption utilizes energy so it is considered a form of active transport. It is not believed that endocytosis is involved with the absorption of many drugs in a major way. The three distinct types of endocytosis are pinocytosis, phagocytosis, and receptor-mediated endocytosis (Beers and Berkow, 2005).

Pinocytosis

The cell invaginates, engulfing relatively small amounts of dissolved substances or liquids; hence the process is also referred to as "cellular drinking." The invagination and subsequent restructuring of the cell wall require energy (Bourne, 2001).

Phagocytosis

The cell changes shape by sending out projections around the substance. These projections are called pseudopodia or "false feet." The cell wall is attracted to the substance by a chemical (chemotaxis). The cell sends out projections in the membrane that make contact with the substance, achieving a non-specific receptor–ligand interaction. Subsequently, the membrane projections engulf the substance, eventually re-fusing the cell walls forming an intracellular vesicle. This type of endocytosis is limited to certain specialized cells such as neutrophils, macrophages, and amoebae so phagocytosis is not involved in the absorption of drugs per se (Bourne, 2001).

Receptor-Mediated Endocytosis

Specific receptors on the outer cell wall bind tightly to specific ligands on the outside of a cell. As that occurs, the cell sends out pseudopodia projections and engulfs the substance as described for phagocytosis. The difference is that the specific substances are very important to cell survival so the rate of absorption may be as much as 1000 times more efficient than pinocytosis. An example of this type of endocytosis is characterized by the uptake of iron. Iron, of course, is necessary for cell survival. It is transported in the blood complexed to a protein called transferrin. Interestingly, cell surfaces have receptors on their surfaces that specifically bind to transferrin. The iron complex is subsequently absorbed into the cell via endocytosis. Eventually, the iron is released for use by the cell. Since the receptor is specific, the cell can get the required amount of iron–transferrin complex even if the concentration is only a fraction of the content of the extracellular fluid. Cells can obtain cholesterol by the same receptor-mediated endocytosis (Kimball, 2005).

Exocytosis

Exocytosis is simply the reverse of endocytosis; the cell can release various substances such as secretions and toxins outside of the cell. Generally, membrane-bound (exocytic) vesicles move to the cell surface where they fuse with the cell wall. As they fuse, these vesicles turn inside out and empty their contents into the extracellular fluid. It is believed that the exocytic vesicles are created from endosomes that do not fuse with lysosomes or the endoplasmic reticulum or Golgi apparatus that take various cell products to the surface. These types of events occur in the pancreas in the process of the secretion of pancreatic enzymes. In addition, certain cells lining the intestinal lumen synthesize fat that is discharged by exocytosis into lacteals (Kimball, 2005).

PARACELLULAR TRANSPORT

The paracellular pathway involves the passive movement of substances through the intercellular spaces between epithelial cells. The controlling gateway of the paracellular pathway is the tight junction, which is an apically located cell–cell interaction of lumen epithelial cells. The tight junction permits the passage of ions while restricting the movement of large molecules. The porosity of the tight junction complex is dependent upon several factors including the molecular size of the substance, the net charge of the compound, intra- and extra-cellular calcium ion concentration, osmolarity, protein kinase inhibitors, and a complex network of proteins including claudin, occludin, and the junctional adhesion molecule (JAM).

Claudins constitute a group of about 20 tissue-specific tight junction proteins believed to be part of the structure containing two extracellular loops and varying amino acid residues and short intracellular tails (Fasano and Shea-Donohue, 2005; Furuse et al., 1998). Occludin is polypeptide that contains four transmembrane domains with two extracellular loops with internal amino and carboxy termini (Furuse et al., 1993; Fasano and Shea-Donohue, 2005). Junctional adhesion molecule is an immunoglobin identified as a component of the tight junction necessary to allow the transmigration of monocytes through the paracellular space (Martin-Padura et al., 1998; Coyne et al., 2002). A tight junction possesses a complex regulatory system that changes the network of tight junction proteins to the physiological needs of the organism. Tight junctions are estimated to be less than 0.1% of the total surface area of the intestinal tract. Further, the substances absorbed by this method are small hydrophilic molecules. It is believed that substances transported via the paracellular route are generally incompletely absorbed into the circulatory system. Hence the tight junctions are dynamic interactive structures that are critical in the physiology of absorption.

DISTRIBUTION

Distribution is the process by which an absorbed substance is reversibly transported through the circulatory or lymphatic system to various tissues throughout the body where it is able to react with various body tissues and/or endpoint receptors. Once a substance is absorbed into the circulatory system, it is almost immediately circulated throughout the entire body. While the blood and lymphatic systems transport the substances quickly, the substances are not absorbed evenly throughout the body. The rate of entry into the tissues and body compartments is influenced by many factors such as local pH, perfusion rates, tissue binding, blood flow to the tissue, tissue mass, partition characteristics of the tissue, and specific cell membrane permeability (Beers and Berkow, 2005).

APPARENT VOLUME OF DISTRIBUTION

The apparent volume of distribution (V_d) is the fluid volume required to contain the substance in the body at the same concentration equal to that in the plasma. This measure is a reference for the plasma concentration anticipated for a given amount of substance required to produce that concentration in the plasma. The following equation mathematically describes that relationship:

$$V_d = -\frac{Q}{C_p}$$

where Q is the amount of substance in the body at the same concentration as that present in the plasma which is represented by C_p. This equation, however, does not provide any information about the pattern of distribution since each substance is distributed within the body in a different way (Bourne, 2005).

PATTERNS OF DISTRIBUTION

Generally, drug distribution follows one of four basic patterns:

1. The substance remains bound within the vascular system such as those materials that tightly bind to plasma proteins.
2. The substance becomes uniformly distributed through the body water.
3. The substance is concentrated in one or more tissues that may or may not be the sites of action.
4. The substance is non-uniformly distributed throughout the body based upon membrane permeability and lipid solubility with the greatest concentrations often found in the kidney, liver and colon — a reflection of the substance being eliminated from the body.

Water-soluble substances usually remain in the blood and interstitial spaces. Acidic substances tend to bind to various blood protein components such as albumin. On the other hand, lipid-soluble substances tend to collect in adipose tissue and rather than rendering it inactive tend to extend the effect of the substance due to the storage depot effect. Some other substances are tightly bound to liver and kidney tissues. Equilibrium between blood and the target tissue is reached more rapidly in highly vascularized areas than in poorly perfused areas. At equilibrium, substance concentrations in tissues and in extracellular fluids are reflected by the plasma concentration (Bourne, 2005; Kimball, 2005).

BODY COMPARTMENTS

In general, absorbed substances are distributed primarily into the following major body compartments (Ritter et al., 2003):

1. Plasma ~5%
2. Intercellular fluid ~16%
3. Intracellular fluid ~35%
4. Transcellular fluid ~2%
5. Adipose tissue ~20%

Substances are transported via the circulatory system, partially unbound and partly bound as noted previously. Proteins such as albumin chemically freeze a substance; this renders it pharmacologically inactive while the unbound portion of the substance is considered the free fraction and is the pharmacologically active portion. Plasma protein binding significantly influences both the distribution and the relationship between the pharmacological activity and the substance concentration in the plasma. As the number of available binding sites approaches saturation at higher substance concentration levels, other substances may be displaced. This displacement activity is a critical function in chemical interactions.

RATE OF DISTRIBUTION

The rate of distribution is primarily a function of membrane permeability and blood perfusion. Membrane permeability is governed by the solubility of the substance (lipids can pass through the membrane quickly whereas water soluble compounds distribute less quickly). Substances that are ionizable in the blood will increase the rate of transfer across the membrane. The blood perfusion rate is the rate at which the blood is distributed throughout an organ. The perfusion rate varies widely from one organ to the next as indicated in Table 5.6.

The higher the flow of blood through an organ, the higher the concentration of a substance one can expect in that organ.

TABLE 5.6
Perfusion Rates (Highest to Lowest)

Organ	Perfusion Rate (ml/min/ml tissue)	Percent of Cardiac Output
Kidney	4.0	22
Thyroid	2.4	1
Adrenals	1.2	0.2
Liver	0.8	27
Heart	0.6	4
Brain	0.5	14
Fat	0.03	4
Muscle	0.025	15
Skin	0.024	6
Bone	0.02	5

Source: Adapted from Shargel, L. and Yu, A.B., *Applied Biopharmaceutics and Pharmacokinetics*, 4th ed., McGraw-Hill, New York, 1999.)

EXTENT OF DISTRIBUTION

The extent of distribution is affected by several factors including plasma protein binding because a drug usually remains in the circulatory system rather than transferring out into a tissue. Binding sites can be for acidic substances (albumins) or basic substances (α, β, and δ globulins) any of which can determine how tightly bound a substance may be to a plasma protein. The degree of interaction between the substance and the protein molecules in the circulatory system is determined partially by electrostatic interactions, van der Waals' forces, and hydrogen bonding. Very small changes in binding can release enough unbound substance into the plasma to make significant changes in the effect at the receptor site. Mathematically, the binding of a substance to a binding site is described by the following equation (Bourne, 2005):

$$D = [nP - rP] \overset{Ka}{\underset{Kd}{\leftrightarrow}} [DP]$$

where D is the concentration of free substance, nP is the total concentration of protein binding sites, and rP is the concentration of bound substance or bound protein with "r" substance molecules bound per protein molecule. Generally there can be one to four binding sites per each protein molecule.

Intracellular Binding

Substances may also bind to intracellular molecules which can be the pharmacological endpoint receptors for certain substances. The overall binding rate is influenced by tissue proteins, the affinity to lipids, or the binding to DNA.

METABOLISM

Metabolism or biotransformation generally refers to the process by which chemical changes occur to a substance following entry into the body. Enzymes located within specific tissues are responsible for changes in the structure of a substance and subsequently altering its pharmacologic properties. Biotransformation of a xenobiotic usually occurs within a matter of minutes or hours. The primary location for metabolic changes is the liver. Other locations include the lungs, kidneys, gastrointestinal epithelium, and skin. Some substances can be changed into less toxic substances or can be prevented from metabolizing into toxic derivatives altogether; hence the process can be an important defense mechanism. Unfortunately, the reverse is also possible: a substance can enter the body as a non-toxic entity and can be metabolized into a toxic derivative (Kapp, 2007, Rozman and Klaassen, 2001).

Phase I and Phase II Reactions

These metabolic reactions can be divided into two general types: phase I and phase II reactions. In phase I reactions, the structure of the toxicant is changed in a way that it is readied for additional changes during the next step in the process. Phase I reactions involve the formation of new or modified functional groups or cleavage and are non-synthetic reactions that can neutralize substances in three ways:

1. By making a structure hydrophilic
2. By dividing a substance into two or more less toxic substances
3. By transforming a substance into an activated form that can be further metabolized by other enzymes

The majority of phase I reactions are mediated by the cytochrome P-450 enzymes that oxidize lipophilic toxicants and add polar groups to the molecular structure. Next are the phase II reactions that involve conjugation with an endogenous compound and are considered synthetic reactions. (Coppoc, 2004). The seven major biochemical reactions occurring in phase II are:

- Glutathione conjugation
- Amino acid conjugation
- Methylation
- Acetylation

- Sulfation
- Glucuronidation
- Sulfoxidation

Each of these reactions metabolizes specific types of activated substances by adding a molecule to the structure that forms an inactive or significantly less active water-soluble metabolite.

First Pass Effects

The metabolic activity of the small intestine is referred to as the intestinal first pass effect. While the small intestine is primarily an absorptive organ, it also has the ability to metabolize drugs by many pathways involving preconjugation (phase I) and conjugation (phase II) reactions (Ilett 1990; Renwick and George, 1989). Many of the enzymes present in the liver are also found in the small intestine; however, the enzyme levels are considerably lower in the small intestine than in the liver (Lin et al., 1999). Certainly a factor that plays a critical role in the amount of substance absorbed is a phenomenon called the hepatic first pass effect. In this case, orally ingested substances are absorbed by the intestinal mucosal cells, enter the capillaries and veins of the GI tract as described in the previous sections, and are transported through the portal vein directly to the liver before entering the general circulation of the body.

The absorbed substance is exposed to the liver before it is allowed to pass through to the body. If the substance is lipophilic, non-polar, and has a low molecular weight, it is absorbed through the GI tract mucosal cells. Such substances are difficult to eliminate and can accumulate throughout the body to toxic levels. Many of these lipophilic substances are biotransformed into hydrophilic metabolites that do not easily enter the membranes of the potential target tissues. Endogenous materials such as bilirubin are also biotransformed into hydrophilic derivatives that are excreted into the bile and are ultimately eliminated in the feces.

Substances can also be biotransformed into derivatives that are more toxic than the parent compound. This activity is known as bioactivation and can be very toxic to an organism. This process is also called toxication and it has several pathways depending upon the chemical:

- Nucleophile formation
- Electrophile formation
- Free radical formation

In each of these scenarios, an electron-rich or electron-poor derivative that is very reactive is created and can cause significant toxicity to the organism (Gregus and Klaassen, 2001).

ELIMINATION

The elimination of chemical substances from the body involves the processes of metabolism as well as excretion and results in eliminating waste products of metabolism and other materials that are of no use to the organism. Hence, elimination is the sum of the processes of substance loss for the body. It is an essential process in all forms of life. Generally, chemical substances are eliminated from the body by two means: they are either metabolized to an alternative form or they are excreted via urine (Beers and Berkow, 2005). Both forms of elimination, however, often follow a first order process with the rates of excretion and metabolism dependent on the amount of unchanged drug in the body. Most substances are metabolized prior to being excreted by one or more of the reactions described in the metabolism section above.

Excretion is the removal of waste substances from body fluids. The main organs of excretion are the kidneys and accessory urinary organs through which urine is eliminated and the large intestine from which solid wastes are expelled. The skin and lungs also have excretory functions of eliminating water and salt (skin) and water and carbon dioxide (lungs). Other routes of excretion include bile, saliva, and milk. Substances are eliminated by several processes.

Polar substances are filtered from the blood in the kidneys and removed into urine. Non-polar substances, on the other hand, are generally reabsorbed from the kidney or distributed into adipose tissue. The liver metabolizes many substances that are non-polar, producing compounds that are more polar and more easily excreted. Enzymes in the liver form conjugates with substances or hydrolyze and oxidize them. The kinetics of a substance can be markedly altered by changes in metabolism or excretion. These processes considered together result in the elimination of a drug.

RENAL EXCRETION

Renal clearance is the total amount of a substance excreted over a specific time period. It depends upon all sources of renal excretion. The three processes involved in renal clearance are tubular secretion, glomerular filtration, and tubule resorption.

Substances and/or their biotransformed products are transported to the kidney tubules. Most substances enter the kidney tubule by tubule secretion. Tubular secretion is an active transport system consisting of two primary carriers — acidic for acidic substances and basic for basic substances. The tubules also permit small molecules and unbound chemicals to passively filter from the blood to the Bowman's capsule of the tubule. Large molecules and substances bound to plasma proteins such as albumin are not filtered and are not well excreted by this process, which is termed glomerular filtration. Lastly, some substances that enter the kidney tubule may be reabsorbed back into the blood stream. This is termed resorption and it is a passive diffusion process requiring no energy. Since water is resorbed back into the blood from the tubules to conserve body fluids, the process also transports some of these molecules; hence they are resorbed along with the water (Bourne, 2001).

Another factor that influences the excretion rate is urine pH. Generally drugs are weak acids and/or bases. Acidic substances are ionized more effectively in alkaline urine, whereas alkaline substances are more effectively ionized in acidic urine. Ionized substances are generally more soluble in water, which permits efficient dissolution in body fluids and ultimately better excretion.

BILIARY EXCRETION

Bile acids are synthesized from cholesterol in the liver and secreted into the small intestine where they facilitate the absorption of lipids and some fat-soluble vitamins. The majority of bile acids are reabsorbed from the intestine, returned to the liver via the portal venous circulation, and resecreted into bile in what is termed the enterohepatic cycle. Over 90% of the intestinal bile acids are reabsorbed so less than 10% are excreted in the feces. Substances and their metabolites that are excreted in bile are actively transported across the biliary membrane. In the intestine, bile is reclaimed through a combination of passive absorption in the jejunum, active transport in the distal ileum, and passive absorption in the colon (Hoffman, 1994).

Bile acids are actively transported in the terminal ileum by the well characterized ileal apical sodium bile acid cotransporter (ASBT or apical sodium-dependent bile acid transporter). This sodium transporter moves bile acids from the lumen of the small intestine across the membrane and into the portal circulation (Dawson et al., 2003; Jung et al., 2004).

Chemicals with molecular weights greater than 300 and those with both polar and lipophilic groups tend to be excreted in the bile. Conjugation with glucuronic acid is also generally excreted in the bile. In addition, substances secreted into the intestine undergo enterohepatic cycling upon hydrolyzation. Biliary excretion only eliminates substances that are not recycled in the enterohepatic cycle.

REFERENCES

Artursson, P. (1991). Cell cultures as models for drug absorption across the intestinal mucosa. *Crit. Rev. Therap. Drug Carrier Systems* 8: 305–330.

Banakar, U.V. and Makoid, M.C. (1997). *Pharmacokinetics in Drug Development: Practical Applications*. Technomic Publishing Company, Lancaster, PA.

Beers, M.H. and Berkow, R., Editors, *The Merck Online Manual of Diagnosis and Therapy*, 17th ed. http://www.merck.com/

Blanchette, J.B., Kavimandan, N., and Peppas, N.A. (2004). Principles of transmucosal delivery of therapeutic agents. *Biomed. Pharmacother.* 58: 142–151.

Bourne, W.A.D. (2001). Pharmacokinetics and Biopharmaceutics, PHAR 7632/7633 & 4634. College of Pharmacy, University of Oklahoma Health Sciences Center, Oklahoma City, OK. http://www.boomer.org/

Burton, P.S., Goodwin, J.T. Vidmar, T.J., and Amore, B.M. (2002). Predicting drug absorption: How nature made it a difficult problem. *Pharm. Exp. Therap.* 303: 889–895.

Carlstedt, I., Sheehan, J.K., Corfield, A.P., and Gallagher, J.T. (1985). Mucous glycoproteins: a gel of a problem. *Essays Biochem.* 20: 40–76.

Chiou, W.L. (2001). The rate and extent of oral availability versus the rate and extent of oral absorption: clarification and receommendation of terminology. *J. Pharmacokinetics Biopharm.* 28: 3–6.

Coppoc, G.L. (2004). Biotransformation. Purdue Research Foundation.

Coyne, C.B., Vanhook, M.K., Gambling, T.M., Carson, J.L., Boucher, R.C., and Johnson, L.G. (2002). Regulation of airway tight junctions by proinflammatory cytokines. *Mol. Biol. Cell* 13: 3218–3234.

Fallingborg, J., Christensen, L.A., Ingeman-Nielsen, M., Jacobsen, B.A., Abildgaard, K., and Rasmussen, H.H. (1989). *Aliment. Pharmacol. Therap.* 3: 605–613.

Fasano, A. and Shea-Donohue, T. (2005). Mechanisms of disease: role of intestinal barrier function in the pathogenesis of gastrointestinal autoimmune diseases. *Gastroenterol. Hepatol.* 2: 416–422.

Fromm, M. and Hierholzer, K. (2000). Epithelium, in *Physiology des Menschen*, Vol. 34, Schmidt, R.F. et al., Eds., Springer, Berlin, p. 719.

Furuse, M, Hirase, T., Itoh, M., Nagafuchi, A., Yonemura, S., Tsukita, S., and Tsukita, S. (1993). Occludin: a novel integral membrane protein localizing at tight junctions *J. Cell Biol.* 123: 1777–1788.

Furuse, M. Fujita, K. Hiiragi, T. Fujimoto, K., and Tsukita, S. (1998). Claudin-1 and -2: novel integral membrane proteins localizing at tight junctions. *J. Cell Biol.*, 141: 1539–1550.

Galia, E., Nicolaides, E., Horter, D., Lobenberg, R., Reppas, C., and Dressman, J.B. (1998). Evaluation of various dissolution media for predicting *in vivo* performance of class I and II drugs. *Pharm. Res.* 15: 698–705.

Gregus, Z. and Klaassen, C.D. (2001). Mechanisms of toxicity, in *Casarett & Doull's Toxicology: The Basic Science of Poisons*, 6th ed., Klaasen, C.D., Ed., McGraw-Hill, New York. pp. 35-81.

Harding, S.E. (2003). Mucoadhesive interactions. *Biochem. Soc. Trans.* 31: 1036–1041.

Hoffman, A.F. (1994). Intestinal absorption of bile acids and biliary constituents, in *Physiology of the Gastrointestinal Tract*, Johnson, L.R., Ed., Raven Press, New York, pp. 1845–1865.

Ilett, K.F., Tee, L.B.G., Reeves, P.T., and Minchin, R.F. (1990). Metabolism of drugs and other xenobiotics in the gut lumen wall. *Aliment. Pharmacol. Therap.* 46: 67–93.

Jung, D., Fantin, A.C., Scheurer, U., Fried, M., and Kullak-Ublick, G.A. (2004). Human ileal bile acid transporter gene ASBT (SLC10A2) is transactivated by the glucocorticoid receptor. *Gut* 53: 78–84.

Kapp, R.W. (2007). Gastrointestinal toxicology, in *Principles and Methods of Toxicology*, 5th ed., Taylor & Francis, Philadelphia, chap. 26.

Kimball, J.W. (2005). *Kimball's Biology Pages: Online Biology Textbook.* http://biology-pages.info

Kiuchi-Saishin, Y., Gotoh, S., Furuse, M., Rakasuga, A., Tano, Y., and Tsukita, S. (2002). *J. Am Soc. Nephrol.* 13: 875–886.

Kulkarni A., Han Y., and Hopfinger, A.J. (2002). Predicting Caco-2 cell permeation coefficients of organic molecules using membrane-interaction QSAR analysis. *J. Chem. Inf. Comput. Sci.* 42: 331–342.

Lin, J.H., Chiba, M., and Baillie, T.A. (1999). Is the role of the small intestine in first pass metabolism overemphasized? *Pharmacol. Rev.* 51: 135–158.

Lipinski, C.A., Lombardo, F., Dominy, B.W., and Feeney, P.J. (1997). Experimental and computational approaches to estimate solubility and permeability in drug discovery and development settings. *Adv. Drug Delivery Rev.* 23: 3–25.

Magee, D.F. and Dalley, A.F. (1986). *Digestion and the Structure and Function of the Gut*, Vol. 8, Continuing Education Series, Karger, Basel.

Martin-Padura, I., Lostaglio, S., Schneemann, M., Williams, L. et al. Junctional adhesion molecule: a novel member of the immunoglobulin superfamily that distributes at intercellular junctions and modulates monocyte transmigration. *J. Cell Biol.* 142: 117–127.

Pang, K.S. (2003). Modeling of intestinal drug absorption: roles of transporters and metabolic enzymes (for the Gillette review series). *Drug Metabol. Dispos.* 31: 1507–1519.

Pond, S.M. and Tozer, T.N. (1985). First-pass elimination: basic concepts and clinical consequences. *Clin. Pharmacokinetics* 9: 1–25.

Renwick, A.G. and George, C.F. (1989). Metabolism of xenobiotics in the gastrointestinal tract, in *Xenobiotic Metabolism in Animals: Methodology, Mechanisms and Significance*, Huston, D.H. et al., Eds., Taylor & Francis, London, pp. 13–40.

Ritter, J., Moore, P., Rang, H.P., and Dale, M.M. (2003). Absorption and distribution of drugs, in *Pharmacology*, 5th ed., Ritter, J. et al., Eds., Churchill Livingston, London, chap. 7.

Rozman, K.K. and Klaassen, C.D. (2001). Adsorption, distribution, and excretion of toxicants, in *Casarett & Doull's Toxicology: The Basic Science of Poisons*, 6th cd., Klaassen, C.D., Ed., McGraw-Hill, New York. p. 107–132.

Shargel, L. and Yu, A.B. (1999). *Applied Biopharmaceutics and Pharmacokinetics*, 4th Ed., McGraw-Hill, New York.

Watts, T., Berti, I., Sapone, A., Gerarduzzi, T., Not., T., Zielke, R., and Fasano, A. (2005). Role of the intestinal tight junction modulator zonulin in the pathogenesis of type I diabetes in BB diabetic-prone rats. *Proc. Natl. Acad. Sci. USA* 102: 2916–2921.

Whitehead, K. and Mitragotri, S. (2005). Oral Delivery of Macromolecules. Drug Delivery Companies Report, Spring/Summer 2005, PharmaVentures, http://www.drug deliveryreport.com/articles/ddcr_s2005_article2.pdf.

Wilson, B. (2004). Fick's First Law, Connexions Web site: http://cnx.rice.edu/content/m11365/1.2/.

Wright, Stephen (2005). Human Physiology 801, University of Arizona, Tucson. http://human.physiol.arizona.edu/.

6 Gastrointestinal Function and Toxicology in Canines

Charles Spainhour

CONTENTS

INTRODUCTION AND OVERVIEW

According to *Dorland's Medical Dictionary*, gastrointestinal means "pertaining to or communicating with the stomach and intestine." The broadest and most encompassing definition of the gastrointestinal (GI) tract can include the mouth, throat, esophagus, stomach, duodenum, pancreas, jejunum, liver, ileum, cecum, colon, rectum, and anus. However, for the purposes of this chapter the working definition of the GI tract will refer to the esophagus, stomach, small intestine, and large intestine.

The major function of the GI tract is to process and absorb water and nutrients while food is physically moved from the mouth to the colon where nonabsorbable wastes are stored for periodic elimination. The mucosal surface of the GI tract is composed of a highly dynamic population of epithelial cells that are specialized for transmembrane absorption and secretion. This epithelial lining comprises a huge surface area approximating the size of a tennis court and interacts with food, water, and xenobiotics from the external environment as well as with the intestinal microflora.

135

The secretory and absorptive abilities of the mucosa facilitate digestion and nutrient uptake, all of which must be accomplished while keeping potentially harmful pathogens and mutagens at bay in the gut lumen. The epithelium allows the absorption of fluid, electrolytes, and nutrients in health and the secretion of huge volumes of fluids and electrolytes in pathologic states. The lifetimes of epithelial cells in the GI tract vary with region and cell type, but can be almost as long as a week. Such a lifespan allows a period of environmental interaction with genes that may lead to the development of neoplasia. However, cellular turnover can occur as quickly as over a couple of days, thereby facilitating rapid recovery of function following acute insult.

It is important to note that the small intestine rarely develops epithelial neoplasia. However, the slower turnover of colonic epithelium, the slower movement of colonic luminal contents, and the bacterial modifications of chemical structures of xenobiotics in the luminal contents of the colon appear to support the existence of higher rates of neoplasia in the colon.

A very important and fundamental feature of the GI mucosa is the spatial segregation of the proliferative cellular compartment from terminally differentiated cells, especially in the small intestine where a gradient of differentiation exists from the depths of the crypts of Lieberkühn to the tips of the villi. This organization has a strong effect on the histology and pathophysiology of the GI tract.

The gastrointestinal epithelial mucosa, while very dynamic in nature, also serves a barrier function. This activity is accomplished through both the physical integrity of the mucosal surface and the extensive population of resident immune cells. Clinical consequences of physical disruption of the mucosal epithelial layer can include blood loss, fluid loss, pathogenic invasion, impaired digestion, and altered nutrient absorption. The intestinal lymphoid system must maintain a balance between dampening immune reactivity at the mucosal surface in order to prevent the constant and unrestrained activation of the immune system and the amplification of an appropriate immune response when surface defenses have been breached. Derangements in this balance of suppression and stimulation can predispose the GI tract to inflammation.

Proper GI function also depends on the coordinated propulsion of food through the gastrointestinal space via smooth muscle contractions. Dysfunction of smooth muscle contraction can of itself result in major pathology of the GI tract. The local and distant neural and endocrine factors that contribute to the regulation of intestinal motility are complex and the disruption of motility can alter the frequency of stool elimination and cause nausea, anorexia, abdominal pain, flatulence, constipation, and abdominal distension.

There is a tendency to view the GI tract as only a muscular tube with an epithelial lining, but such a view is myopic and incorrect. The GI tract can be affected directly or indirectly via secreted hormones, paracrine mediators, and its own enteric nervous system that contains 10 to 100 million neurons, an aggregation equal to the total number of neurons in the spinal cord. Immune cells collectively constitute the GI tract's associated lymphoid system (GALT) — the largest immune organ of the body.

Collectively, all of these systems must work together in a well coordinated and harmonious fashion to permit the smooth integration of the functions of this complex organ system. However, this same complexity presents multiple foci of potential interruption of function and subsequent dysfunction. To fully appreciate and understand the potential for toxicity to and the dysfunction of the GI tract, it is important to completely understand its structures, activities, and functions.

GROSS AND MICROSCOPIC ANATOMY

The esophagus is the first part of the GI tract [13, 16, 60, 73, 80, 94, 96, 124, 127, 174, 192, 199, 266, 277]. It is a connecting tube between the pharynx and stomach. In the collapsed state in a dog about medium size, it is approximately 30 cm in length and 2 cm in diameter. Due to its length it is divided into cervical, thoracic, and abdominal portions. The esophagus is not uniform in either the thickness of its wall or the diameter of its lumen. The wall of the cervical portion averages about 4 mm in thickness, the thoracic portion about 2.5 mm in thickness, and the abdominal portion about 6 mm in thickness. As suggested by the longitudinal folds (approximately ten) the esophagus is capable of a great degree of distension. The least expandable portions are at the very beginning and end of the organ.

The esophagus starts at the level of the axial vertebra and ends at the cardia of the stomach. A plicated ridge of mucosa, the *limen pharyngoesophageum*, which is most prominent ventrally, is the demarcation between the end of the pharynx and the start of the esophagus. The termination of the esophagus lies immediately ventral to the last thoracic vertebra. The cervical portion of the esophagus is ventral and to the left of the trachea.

At its origin the esophagus starts to incline to the left, so that at the thoracic inlet it usually is found to lie to the left lateral side of the trachea. However, individual variation is not uncommon and the cervical esophagus can be found to be left ventral or dorsal and left of the trachea. In proximity to the esophagus on either side are the common carotids, vagosympathetic nerve trunks, and internal jugular veins.

The thoracic portion of the esophagus extends from the thoracic inlet to the esophageal hiatus of the diaphragm. At the point of the thoracic inlet it usually is to the left of the trachea, but eventually obliquely crosses the left surface of the trachea to gain a dorsal position at about the same point as where the trachea bifurcates into bronchi ventral to the fifth and sixth thoracic vertebrae. The dorsal branches of the left and right vagal nerves run dorso-caudally across the sides of the esophagus and unite with each other on the dorsum of the esophagus at a point approximately 2 to 4 cm cranial to the dorsal part of the esophageal hiatus. The dorsal vagal trunk that is formed continues and passes through the dorsal part of the esophageal hiatus. The ventral vagal trunk follows a similar course.

The abdominal portion or terminal part of the esophagus is wedge-shaped. Dorsally, this portion of the esophagus immediately joins the stomach, but ventrally it notches the thin dorsal edge of the caudate lobe of the liver.

The esophagus has four coats. Moving from the superficial to the deep, these are the fibrous, muscular, submucous, and mucous coats. In the cervical region, the fibrous coat or adventitia blends with the deep cervical fascia. The adventitia of the thoracic and abdominal portions of the esophagus blends with the endothoracic and transversalis fascia, respectively. The esophagus is largely covered by pleura in the thorax and peritoneum in the abdomen. At those points where the esophagus is not covered by serosa, its adventitia blends with that of the organs with which it comes in contact.

The muscular coat is composed of two oblique layers of striated muscle fibers — an inner coat and an outer coat. While muscular fiber patterns are somewhat complex and possibly random in direction at the beginning and end of the esophagus, the main musculature of the esophagus is in the form of well-defined spiral fibers that start about 5 cm from the origination of the esophagus and end at a point about 5 to 10 cm from the cardia of the stomach. Fibers that are superficial on one side become deep on the other, kind of like a weaving pattern. These apparently continuous obliquely oriented bundles spiral around the axis of the esophagus in such a fashion as to cross each other at right angles, eventually comprising the two muscular coats of the organ. Lines of decussation are located both dorsal and ventral to the esophagus. In addition to the two oblique coats, several poorly developed groups of longitudinal fibers exist. The best developed of these bands are about 1 to 2 mm in width, located to the left and to the right of the esophagus, and typically fade away to nothing on the caudal portion of the cervical portion of the esophagus.

The submucous coat loosely connects the mucous and muscular coats and this allows the relatively inelastic mucous coat to be cast into prominent longitudinal folds when the esophagus is in the contracted or nondistended state. Blood vessels, nerves, and mucous glands reside in this layer.

The mucous coat is composed of a superficially cornified, stratified squamous epithelium that contains the openings at about 1-mm intervals of the esophageal glands. In the collapsed esophagus, this coat is notable for forming the large and numerous longitudinal rugae and folds observed upon gross examination. Cardiac glands are noted to occur in the distal part of the esophagus.

Most nerve branches to the esophagus are too small to be seen with gross examination and a degree of overlap or redundancy is known to exist. However, for each nerve source, a focal or primary area of innervation does appear to exist. The craniocaudal innervation of the esophagus involves as many as 23 paired spinal ganglia located between C1 and L2. Two peak areas of innervation — C2 to C6 and T2 through T4 — serve the cervical sector of the esophagus. Similarly, two peak areas of innervation — T2 through T4 and T8 through T12 — serve the thoracic region. Generally speaking, the cervical portion of the esophagus is thought to be supplied by the paired pharyngoesophageal and paired pararecurrent laryngeal nerves, the cranial thoracic region by the left pararecurrent laryngeal nerve, and the caudal thoracic and abdominal portions by the vagal trunks.

The blood supply to the cervical portion of the esophagus is from small branches originating from the cranial and caudal thyroid arteries. The cranial two-thirds of the thoracic portion of the esophagus is supplied by the broncho-esophageal artery. The blood supply of the remaining portion of the thoracic esophagus comes from branches emanating from the dorsal intercostal arteries. The terminal portion of the esophagus receives its blood from a branch of the left gastric artery. The veins that drain the esophagus basically form a satellite vasculature of the arteries that supply it. However, veins that drain the thoracic portion of the esophagus for the most part empty into the azygous vein.

The stomach is a highly variable in size, musculoglandular organ located between and connecting the esophagus and small intestine. In its dilated state, it is the largest organ of the entire GI tract. When empty, the stomach does not make contact with the abdominal wall, but when moderately filled, it presses against the xiphoid and left hypochondriac areas of the abdominal wall caudal to the liver. In its completely filled state, the stomach lies in contact ventrally with the xiphoid and umbilical portions of the abdominal wall as well as the right and left lateral portions of the abdominal wall, and reaches to a point just caudal to the umbilicus. An imaginary axis placed through the stomach traces the letter C rotated 90 degrees in a counterclockwise direction. It is therefore simple to visualize that the stomach is positioned essentially in a transverse fashion, but more to the left than the right of a median plane. The stomach forms a deep impression into the caudal surface of the liver, however, when the stomach is completely empty it can be located cranially to the thoracic outlet.

The stomach does not increase in size in a uniform fashion as it accumulates ingesta. In fact, when the stomach increases its size as a result of filling, the first part that expands is the fundus. As the fundus grows in size, it pushes caudally and dorsally, displacing the liver ventrally. The second part of the stomach to fill and expand is the body — the largest part of the stomach, capable of the greatest degree of expansion.

As the body fills, the stomach moves caudally and ventrally, makes extensive contact with the abdominal wall, and can crowd or displace the intestinal mass and spleen. The pylorus varies least in its position and shape as the stomach fills with ingesta and is the last to expand. Within the pyloric part, the pyloric antrum expands more than the pyloric canal. The most likely reason for this limited expansion is that the pyloric portion is designed to work essentially as a magazine or ejection mechanism by which the partly digested stomach contents (chyme) are squirted into the duodenum.

The capacity of the stomach is somewhat variable; its volume ranges from 0.5 to 8 liters. Typically, the capacity of the stomach is considered to be normalized to 100 to 250 ml of volume per kilogram of body weight. It is noteworthy that a normal stomach is capable of adjusting its size and capacity with only minimal changes in intragastric pressure.

The average empty stomach of a 15-kg dog weighs only about 100 g. Most commonly, food remains in a dog's stomach for 10 to 16 hours. The functions of the stomach are accepting and storing food and partly mixing the ingesta with enzymes, mucus, and hydrochloric acid coming from gastric glands. The inlet to the stomach is referred to as the cardia and the outlet is the pylorus. The stomach is divided into four areas, the cardiac portion, fundus, body, and pyloric portion. The stomach also has two curvatures, the greater and lesser, and two surfaces, a visceral and parietal.

The visceral surface of the stomach is the convex outer surface that faces chiefly dorsally, but also caudally and to the right. It lies in contact with the left lobe of the pancreas and is separated from the intestinal mass and left kidney by a fat-filled peritoneal sheet known as the greater omentum. The parietal surface of the stomach faces cranially, to the left, and ventrally. The greater curvature of the stomach is convex in shape and extends from the cardia to the pylorus. In a moderately filled state, the greater curvature is approximately 30 cm in length. The lesser curvature also runs from the cardia to the pylorus, but by the shortest path connecting the two parts. The lesser curvature forms an uneven concavity containing an angular notch into which the papillary process of the liver juts. The pyloric antrum and the pylorus lie to the right of the papillary process of the liver and the body of the stomach lies to the left of it.

The cardiac portion of the stomach actually unites with the esophagus. While the four coats of the stomach and esophagus blend together well, there are differences in the muscular and mucous layers of each organ. The fundus is the large blind outpocket of the stomach located to the left and dorsal to the cardia. The large middle portion of the stomach is referred to as the body. It extends from the fundus on the left to the pyloric region on the right. The shortest path that ingesta can take in moving from the cardia to the pyloric region of the stomach is known as the gastric groove. This path essentially follows the lesser curvature of the stomach. The pyloric portion represents about the distal one-third of the stomach, as measured along the lesser curvature. It is lightly sacculated as it joins the body of the stomach to the duodenum and eventually assumes an irregular funnel shape moving toward the cranially oriented pylorus.

The initial part of the pyloric portion has expandable thin walls and is referred to as the pyloric antrum. The distal third of the pyloric portion referred to as the pyloric canal is contracted and bent due to the presence of a heavy encircling double sphincter. The presence of this musculature also leads to the formation of the narrowest confine of the cavity of the stomach. The exit from the stomach to the duodenum is through the muscular sphincter, the pylorus.

The stomach has four coats: serous, muscular, submucous, and mucous. The serosa of the stomach is very thin and elastic and closely adheres to the stomach musculature by a small amount of subserous tissue. This serous coat covers virtually the entire surface of the stomach. The muscular coat is composed of an outer longitudinal layer and an inner circular layer of smooth muscle fibers to which is added a layer of oblique fibers in the region over the body of the stomach. The outer longitudinal layer is essentially continuous with the longitudinal layers of both the esophagus and duodenum. The inner circular layer of the stomach is better defined and more specialized than the longitudinal layer and is thickened to form the relatively weak cardiac sphincter at the area of the cardia. The inner circular layer is very well developed in the pyloric canal.

The pylorus is also surrounded by a distinct circular muscle referred to as the pyloric sphincter. The oblique fibers are adjacent to the submucosa and spread a pattern much like that of a fan. The submucous coat consists of a strong but thin elastic layer of tissue that attaches more firmly to the mucosa than to the muscularis and contains the finer branches of the gastric vessels and nerves. The mucous coat consists of a columnar-type of surface epithelium, a glandular lamina propria, and a lamina muscularis mucosae, with the latter consisting of irregularly woven or stratified muscular fibers.

In the empty or slightly distended organ, the mucosa and much of the underlying submucosa are observed to be thrown into folds known as the *plicae gastricae*. These folds are for the most part longitudinal in orientation and very twisted and contorted in form, except in the area adjacent to the lesser curvature where the folds are less crowded and relatively straight in form. In an empty stomach, the folds may approach 1 cm in height and lie closely adjacent to one another. The normal color of the mucosa in the body and the fundus of a fresh, perfused, normal stomach is pink to red-gray. The color is the same but lighter in hue in the pyloric portion. It should be mentioned that color can vary with the degree of freshness of the specimen and the adequacy of blood supply.

With some magnification, the mucosa can be observed to contain approximately 40 very small, mountain-like raised areas in every square centimeter of tissue. These areas are referred to as *areae gastricae*. Their surfaces and sides are stippled, with numerous minute, pinprick-like openings, termed *foveolae gastricae*. These structures are deepest in the pyloric region, where they average about 0.68 mm in length. They gradually decrease in size moving toward the cardia and eventually disappear, so that none are observed in the cardiac gland region. The stomach of a dog contains approximately one million foveolae, and each foveolae contains about sixteen gastric glands opening into it. Folds called *plicae villosae* may be observed between the gland openings.

The stomach has numerous gastric glands. These glands have necks and bodies, are branched and tubular in form, and extend all the way to the lamina muscularis mucosae. The three types of glands found in dogs are cardiac glands, pyloric glands, and gastric glands. It should be noted that the gross divisions of the stomach do not match exactly the populations of glands of the same or similar nomenclature. While cardiac glands are typically found in a narrow area encircling the cardia, they can also be found to occur along the lesser curvature. Pyloric glands inhabit the pyloric part of the stomach. Approximately two-thirds of the gastric mucosa of the fundus and body of the stomach is occupied by gastric glands or fundic glands. However, a zone of intermediate glands lies between the gastric glands and the pyloric glands.

This intermediate zone is approximately 2 to 3 cm in width as observed on an incised, opened, and laid-flat stomach. These glands differ by the types of cells that they contain and hence the secretions they produce. There are no strict lines of anatomic or histological demarcation separating the different types of glands found primarily in one area from those found in an adjacent area. Actually the intermediate gland zone mentioned earlier is probably typical of the merging of two different glandular populations.

The primary function of the glands of the cardiac, intermediate, and pyloric regions is to produce mucus, but the gastric glands produce hydrochloric acid and the pepsin enzyme. It should be noted that lymphoid tissue is scattered throughout the mucosa of the stomach, with some extension of it penetrating deeply through the lamina muscularis mucosae into the submucosa.

The four main types of glandular cells found in the stomach mucosa are parietal, chief, mucous, and enterochromaffin cells. Parietal cells are the sources of the hydrochloric acid in the gastric juice. Chief or zymogenic cells contain granules containing pepsinogen, the precursor to the main gastric enzyme, pepsin. Mucous cells are found in the necks of the gastric glands, occupying spaces between the parietal cells; they produce mucus. Enterochromaffin cells are mostly found in the gastric glands, to an extent in the pyloric glands, and also in the small and large intestines and pancreas. These cells are known by many different names, some based upon their histological staining characteristics, but all secrete polypeptides and biogenic amines. Alternate names for these cells include gastrointestinal endocrine cells, argentaffin cells, argyrophilic cells, and gastroenterohepatic (GEP) cells.

The nerve supply of the stomach comes from parasympathetic fibers running from the vagi and from sympathetic fibers coming from the celiac plexus. Sympathetic fibers arise from the celiacomesenteric plexus and reach the stomach by traveling on the numerous gastric branches of the celiac artery. Sensory innervation of the stomach comes from about 25 paired spinal ganglia (C2 through L5), with peak innervation of the stomach coming from the T2 through T10 area. The dorsal vagal trunk sends branches to the lesser curvature and ventral wall of the stomach. The ventral vagal trunk sends out small branches to the pylorus and the lesser curvature of the stomach.

The two main sets of arteries providing blood supplies to the stomach are the left and right gastric arteries. These vessels run along the lesser curvature and the right and left gastroepiploic arteries that travel along the greater curvature. The veins draining the stomach are satellites of the arteries supplying the organ. Blood leaving the stomach enters the liver via the portal vein and the lymphatic vessels of the stomach drain into the hepatic lymph nodes.

The small intestine consists of three parts: the duodenum, jejunum, and ileum. The initial portion of the small intestine is a short, relatively fixed-in-place loop called the duodenum. The next segment is freely movable and is known as the jejunum. The very short terminal portion is the ileum. The intestine extends from the pylorus of the stomach to the ileocecal orifice that marks the start of the large intestine. The small intestine is the longest part of the GI tract, having an average length in a normal living dog of approximately 3.5 times the length of the body. It should be noted that the length of the small intestine in a dead dog is significantly longer due to cessation of peristaltic contractions and a loss of muscular tone.

The duodenum is approximately 25 cm in length and originates in the upper right hypochondriac region opposite the ninth intercostal space. Running in a caudal fashion to the tuber coxae, the duodenum then turns back upon itself and travels cranially and obliquely to the left, eventually connecting with the jejunum at a position to the left of the root of the mesentery just beneath the spine. The duodenum can be subdivided into the cranial, descending, caudal, and ascending portions. Both the pancreatic and bile ducts open into the duodenum and accordingly in this area the acid contents of the stomach are then mixed with the alkaline secretions coming from the pancreas and the liver along with the small intestine.

The duodenum originates from the pylorus in such a fashion that its right wall is longer than the left wall, which results in the formation of the cranial duodenal flexure. This portion of the duodenum lies in contact medially with the pancreas, ventrally with the stomach, and dorsally and laterally with the liver. The descending portion of the duodenum moves caudad and is approximately 15 cm in length. The right lobe of the pancreas is dorsal to it and at its caudal extent the cecum is medial to it. The caudal portion of the duodenum connects the descending portion and the ascending portions, is approximately 5 cm in length, and typically is located ventral to the sixth lumbar vertebra.

Ventral to this segment is the terminal portion of the ileum and the jejunum. As the colon and urinary bladder fill, this portion of the duodenum can be pushed cranially. The curvature of the caudal portion is not sharp, but rather gradual in nature. The ascending portion of the duodenum is observed to course cranially, obliquely, and to the left from this caudal flexure. Dorsal to this segment of the duodenum are the ureters, caudal vena cava, aorta, and various nerve trunks, while ventral to it are coils of the jejunum. On the left, it lies in close proximity to the descending colon and eventually terminates in a ventral curve to form the duodenojejunal flexure.

The jejunum and ileum comprise the largest amount of the small intestinal mass by far. The jejunum starts with the duodenojejunal flexure located just caudal and to the left of the root of the mesentery. The jejunum is ventral and caudal to the empty stomach. Dorsal to it are the pancreas, kidneys, large intestine, aorta, and vena cava. The ileum ends as the ileal papilla, opening into the initial portion of the ascending colon. This papilla has an orifice and a sphincter muscle. The orifice is typically located between the descending and ascending portions of the duodenum. The jejunum and ileum are very mobile — probably the most mobile portions of the GI tract. This is a result of their suspension from the cranial portion of the sublumbar region via a large drape-like sheet of tissue called the mesentery.

No distinguishable gross or microscopic features in the walls of the small intestine definitely demarcate the division between the jejunum and ileum, but significant differences distinguish the mucosa of the jejunum and the mucosa of the ileum. Typically in a dog, the ileum comprises approximately the last 15 cm of the small intestine. By convention, only the terminal and highly thickened and contracted part of the small intestine is considered to be ileum. One easy way to identify the ileum is to look for the ileocecal fold and its antimesenteric (opposite the side of the attached mesentery) ileal vessels. The ileocecal fold is a narrow (1 cm in width) and long (2 to 30 cm) piece of peritoneum that connects the ileum to the cecum.

As with other parts of the GI tract, the small intestine has four different layers or coats: serous, muscular, submucous, and mucous. The serous coat covers virtually the entire small intestine and is peritoneum. The muscular coat consists of a thin outer longitudinal coat and a thicker inner circular layer of smooth muscle. The submucous coat resembles the coats of the stomach and large intestine. It loosely interconnects the muscular and mucous layers and smaller nerves, lymphatics, and blood vessels are located within it. The mucous coat has a velvet-like appearance throughout the entire small intestine that results from the presence of a large number of intestinal villi. These villi significantly increase the absorptive surface area of the small intestine; the ratio of mucosal area to serosal area for the entire small intestine of the canine is approximately 8.5 to 1. Two different types of cells comprise this surface. One produces mucus and is called a goblet cell and the other is a columnar-type cell that functions in absorption.

The deeper part of the mucosa contains intestinal glands and lymphoid tissue. Duodenal glands in the dog are different from general intestinal glands in that they closely resemble the pyloric glands of the stomach and are located only around a narrow zone of the duodenum contiguous to the pylorus. While the glands reside mostly in the submucosa, portions of them may extend into the lamina propria of the mucosa. Lymphoid tissue is aggregated together in about 22 different areas throughout the small intestine to form structures referred to as follicles. These follicles are readily visible during inspection of the intestine from the serosal surface in a distended bowel and are more frequently found in intestinal side walls as opposed to those portions of the wall attached to or opposite the mesentery. Many of these follicles are found in the duodenum and they are persistently found throughout the entire length of the small intestinal tract. They are reasonably well defined, circumscribed elevations approximately 2 by 1.5 cm in size.

Nerve fibers to the small intestine arise from the vagus and splanchnic nerves, via the celiac and cranial mesenteric plexuses. The small intestine receives its sensory innervation from as many as 15 paired ganglia (T2 through L3), with peak innervation coming from T6 through L1.

The duodenum receives its blood supply from both the cranial and caudal pancreaticoduodenal arteries. The jejunum receives its blood supply from 12 to 15 jejunal arteries that originate from the cranial mesenteric artery. The ileum receives its blood supply on its antimesenteric side via branches extending from the ileocecal artery and on the mesenteric side by the accessory cecal artery. It should be mentioned that the duodenum receives a richer blood supply than the ileum. Perhaps this is because the duodenum produces more fluid than the ileum, an amount approaching ten times as much. The veins draining the small intestine are satellites of the arteries supplying the organ. Lymph vessels from the duodenum drain into the hepatic lymph nodes and the variably present duodenal lymph node, while lymphatics from the jejunum drain into the right and left mesenteric lymph nodes. The ileum's lymphatics empty into the right and left mesenteric lymph nodes and the colic lymph nodes.

The large intestine of the dog more closely resembles those of humans than those of other domestic animals. It is of a slightly larger diameter than the small intestine, relatively short, has no striking structural features, and is relatively unspecialized in nature. Its most important functions are the absorption of water and electrolytes from the fecal stream, conversion of the fecal stream into solid mass, fermentation, and storage of the fecal stream until it can be expelled. Fermentation in the large intestine does not occur to the degree found in ruminants.

The large intestine harbors numerous bacteria, especially bacilli, and these microbes can digest substances like cellulose and perform various biochemical transformations. End products of the activities of various microbes residing in the large intestine include vitamin K, vitamin B_{12}, thiamin, and riboflavin. The production of vitamin K is critical to the organism because the amount present in normal food is insufficient to maintain a normal blood coagulation profile.

The large intestine can be subdivided into the cecum and colon. The cecum is typically considered the first part of the large intestine, but it should be emphasized that in dogs the ileum communicates with the colon and not the cecum. The cecum is simply a blind sac, extending off the proximal portion of the colon. The cecum can be of either sigmoid or corkscrew shape, with a large U-shaped bend extending to the left from its ileal attachment. The cecum is situated to the right side of a median plane and is partially encircled by the duodenal loop. It is generally intimately applied to the coils of the jejunum and ventral to the second to the fourth lumbar vertebrae. The openings of the cecum and ileum are in close apposition to each other — only about 1 cm apart. In a normal dog, the cecum is approximately 2 cm in diameter at its colic end, 5 cm in length, and ends as a blunted cone of approximately 1 cm diameter.

The middle portion of the cecum is the body. The cecum is mobile and can assume a variety of different orientations within the abdomen, but typically is aimed transversely or caudally and ventrally. It is connected to the ileum via peritoneum and is capable of expanding to twice its normal size. It is only able to communicate with the colon through the cecocolic orifice that limits access via the cecocolic sphincter, a specialized portion of the inner circular muscular coat.

The colon is generally divided into three different portions and their interconnecting flexures. The subdivisions are ascending, transverse, and descending. This organ is approximately 2 cm in diameter and 25 cm in length. The colon occupies the dorsal part of the abdominal cavity and because of a shorter sheet of mesenteric attachment does not shift around as much as the small intestine. It is shaped much like an inverted letter J. The small arm of the J represents the ascending colon; the curved portion, the transverse colon; and the long arm, the descending colon. The ascending colon is on the right side of the body; the descending colon is on the left side; and the transverse colon is cranial to the root of the mesentery. The ascending and transverse colons are connected via the right colic flexure and the descending and transverse colons are connected via the left colic flexure. The ascending colon originates at the ileocolic sphincter and is typically about 5 cm in length. From its origin, the ascending colon travels in a cranial fashion to its terminus at the right colic flexure. The ascending colon lies ventral to the right kidney and is bound on the right by the descending duodenum. The jejunal mass is generally ventral and to the left of the ascending colon. Cranially, the ascending colon touches the stomach. It should be noted that it is not uncommon for the ascending colon of a dog to be absent or found lying in a different spatial relationship to other organs. In cases of altered geography, the positional change has resulted from a failure of the entire gut to adequately rotate about the cranial mesenteric artery as should normally happen during development.

The transverse colon is approximately 7 cm in length and travels from right to left in a slightly curved fashion, cranial to the cranial mesenteric artery and the root of the mesentery. It lies cranially and dorsally to the left limb of the pancreas and cranially and ventrally to the stomach and is also not uncommonly found to be absent or lying in a different-from-normal spatial relationship to other organs. The descending colon is approximately 12 cm in length and traverses from the left colic flexure to and through the pelvic inlet, at which point it merges without gross distinction to the rectum. The descending colon travels in a relatively straight line along the left lateral abdominal wall, from approximately the left costal arch to the sacrum and also lies in close apposition to the left kidney. The ascending portion of the duodenum lies medial to the descending colon and the urinary bladder lies ventral to its most terminal portion.

The large intestine has the same four coats as the small intestine: mucous, submucous, muscular, and serous. The serous coat resembles that of the small intestine and while the muscular coat is similar to that found in the small intestine, is uniform in thickness, and consists of a thin outer longitudinal coat and a thicker inner circular layer of smooth muscle if observed to be present. The submucous coat does not differ significantly from that observed in the small intestine. Small nerves, lymphatics, and blood vessels are located within it. The mucous coat however is significantly different from that observed in the small intestine as it has no intestinal villi or aggregations of lymphoid tissue. However, solitary lymph nodules do exist and can be observed by viewing the dilated gut from the serosal aspect.

Folds occur in the large intestine, but are only noticeable when it is highly contracted; a minimal amount of distension is sufficient to remove them. The folds can be either circular or longitudinal in orientation, depending upon the type of contraction that the large intestine has undergone. The intestinal glands of the large intestine are longer and straighter than those found in the small intestine. The large intestine contains a significantly greater population of mucus-producing cells than is found in the small intestine. A columnar epithelium lines the intestinal glands and is continuous with the epithelium that lines the mucosal surface of the lumen of the gut.

The nervous supply of the large intestine arises from vagal general visceral afferents and vagal parasympathetics, with sympathetic fibers also supplying the large intestine via the cranial mesenteric plexus. The large intestine receives its blood supply from the caudal mesenteric and colic arteries. The veins draining the large intestine are satellites of the arteries supplying the organ with lymphatics from the jejunum draining into the mesenteric and right, middle, and left colic lymph nodes.

HISTOPHYSIOLOGY AND SECRETORY ACTIVITY

Numerous glands are located throughout the entire length of the GI tract and the secretions from these glands include enzymes to accomplish digestion and mucus for protection and lubrication [2, 4, 6, 47, 61, 65, 66, 72, 78, 79, 82, 86, 97, 98, 111, 112, 116, 133, 145, 147, 158, 166, 167, 170, 178, 205, 233–235, 242, 246, 248, 250, 287, 295, 299, 300, 306, 311]. The nature of the secretions can also vary with the type of luminal contents present. Production is in response to the anticipation or presence of food in the alimentary canal and interestingly only in amounts sufficient to perform and complete their intended function.

The production of mucus is especially important. In its purest form, mucus is a thick secretion composed of various glycoproteins, water, and electrolytes. While the character of mucus can change, depending upon the region of the GI tract that produces it, certain characteristics make it an ideal lubricant and protectant. Mucus has surface tension characteristics that promulgate a strong, even coating ability of and adhesion to both intestinal luminal contents and gastrointestinal epithelium. It has a low resistance to slippage and permits the facile sliding of material along or past the gastrointestinal epithelium. It is resistant to digestion by gastrointestinal enzymes and due to the chemical properties of inherent glycoproteins is capable of providing buffering action against both acid (hydrochloric acid) and alkali (bicarbonate ion). Mucus contains bicarbonate ion that contributes to the neutralization of hydrochloric and other acids. Finally, its presence causes the fecal stream to adhere to itself, causing the consolidation of fecal particles into a fecal mass.

The glands that produce these different secretions are various. In the stomach and upper portion of the duodenum, the glands that produce acid and pepsinogen are observed to be deep and tubular in shape. The intestinal epithelium has deep invaginations that reach down to the submucosa. These deepened pits are referred to as crypts of Lieberkühn and contain specialized secretory cells. Mucus or goblet cells are also prevalent and they respond to stimulation or irritation of the gastrointestinal epithelium with the production of mucus. The mucus produced by these glands extends all over the surface of the stomach and remaining GI tract and protects the mucosal epithelium from injury due to frictional abrasion, the caustic effects of acid, and the degradative effects of various enzymes.

As mentioned, the mechanical presence of food in the GI tract is in and of itself a sufficient stimulus to initiate secretory activities of the various glands in the area that the food occupies and in adjacent areas of the tract. This stimulation is the result of direct contact of food with the gastrointestinal epithelium and the glands. Distension of the gut wall, chemical interactions, and the presence of material can also activate the enteric nervous system. The resulting reflexes stimulate both mucous cells on the epithelial surface of the GI tract and glands located deep in the tract wall to increase their levels of secretory activity.

Stimulation of parasympathetic nerves innervating the GI tract also produces an increase of secretory activity. This response is especially vigorous in the upper portion of the tract where vagal parasympathetic nerves affect esophageal glands, gastric glands, the pancreas, and Brunner's (mucus-producing) glands of the duodenum. Similarly, pelvic parasympathetic nerves stimulate glands in the distal part of the large intestine. Secretion in the remainder of the small and large intestines occurs essentially in response to local neural and hormonal stimuli. Stimulation of sympathetic nerves in some parts of the GI tract can result in a small degree of increase in secretion, but sympathetic stimulation also causes vasoconstriction of the blood vessels supplying the epithelium and glands. Because of this restriction of blood supply, sympathetic stimulation in the presence of parasympathetic or hormonal-induced stimulation will generally result in a decrease of secretory activity.

Mention has been made to the importance of various hormones in the regulation of the amount and character of gastrointestinal secretions. These hormones are polypeptides or polypeptide-like and are released from the mucosa of the GI tract in response to the presence of food. Upon release, the hormones are absorbed into the blood where they are carried to different glands and secretion is stimulated. The complete picture of hormonal stimulation of gastrointestinal secretion is very complex and still not totally elucidated.

All of the steps of the processes of glandular secretion are not completely known, but certain basic steps undoubtedly apply in all cases. Secretory substances are produced in the endoplasmic reticulum and Golgi complex of a glandular cell using adenosine triphosphate generated by mitochondria and specific nutrients absorbed or actively transported into the cell. Ribosomes attached to the endoplasmic reticulum are essential for the formation of protein material. Secretory materials move through the endoplasmic reticulum to the Golgi apparatus, where they are packaged in special secretory vesicles. The vesicles are then moved to and stored in an area of the cell contiguous to a portion of the cell membrane from which secretion will take place. Appropriate nervous or hormonal stimulation increases the permeability of the cell membrane to calcium, which enters the cell. The presence of this increased local concentration of calcium causes the membranes of the secretory vesicles to fuse together with the cell membrane, break open, and release their contents into the extracellular area. However, for this secretion to be effectively delivered, permitting complete function, sufficient water and electrolytes are necessary to wash or carry away the organic substances secreted and released through the secretory border of the cell. It is generally believed that this washing or sweeping activity is accomplished in response to appropriate neural stimulation.

Signals from nerve endings terminating on the bases of glandular cells cause the active transport of chloride ions to the interiors of cells through the basal portions of the cell membranes. The build-up of negatively charged ions inside a cell in turn causes positively charged sodium ions to also move into the cell to preserve electric neutrality. The accumulation of sodium and chloride ions within the cell drives the accumulation of water inside the cell via osmosis. The cell swells and the interior hydrostatic pressure increases. This eventually causes small breaks in the cell membrane along the secretory aspect that permit the movement of water and electrolytes out of the cell. This rush of water and electrolytes moves the secreted organic material away from the border of the cell.

Although the secretion of saliva will not be specifically discussed because it is beyond the scope of this chapter, its production is nonetheless a very important component of the normal function of the GI tract. If saliva is not secreted, food becomes very difficult to swallow, even after the administration of copious amounts of water. Saliva contains large amounts of potassium and bicarbonate ions and lesser amounts of sodium and chloride ions; its typical pH range is between 6 and 7. Saliva contains two different types of protein secretions: serous and mucous. The serous portion contains ptyalin, an alpha-amylase carbohydrate digestive enzyme; the mucous part contains mucin, a surface protectant.

The main esophageal secretion is mucus, the character of which changes with region of the esophagus. Mucus secreted by the upper portion of the esophagus acts essentially as only a lubricant. Mucus arising from the distal portion of the esophagus must also provide protection from refluxing acidic gastric juices in addition to providing lubrication. To accomplish this, the main body of the esophagus is populated with simple mucous glands, but at the gastric end of the esophagus the glands are of a different type and complex in nature.

With regard to the process of secretion in the stomach, it is important to realize that gastric secretion has cephalic, gastric, and intestinal phases. In the cephalic phase, the sight, odor, taste, or memory of food can cause stimulation of the hypothalamus, amygdala, and/or cerebral cortex and in turn sends signals via the vagus nerves to the stomach so that gastric secretion initiates before food even enters the stomach. The relative contribution of this phase to gastric secretion is approximately one-fifth of the total amount of secretions produced by the ingestion of a bolus of food. The gastric phase is initiated as food enters the stomach; gastric juice is secreted in response to local enteric reflexes, vagal–vagal reflexes, and the gastrin hormonal cycle. This phase of gastric secretion can generate over a liter of gastric secretion within the course of a day and contribute the majority of total secretions.

The last or intestinal phase starts commences with the entry of food into the duodenum. As the duodenum undergoes distension, small amounts of gastrin are released by G cells located in the duodenal mucosa. Gastrin causes the stomach to continue to secrete a small amount of gastric juice to further digestion.

The entire surface of the stomach is populated with mucous cells and collectively these cells produce a continuous, very viscous, relatively insoluble coating of alkaline mucus about 1 mm in thickness that acts as a lubricant and protectant, preserving the gastric mucosa from abrasive or acid-induced injury. While it should be obvious, it is important to repeat that as a result of the presence of mucus, the gastric mucosa is never actually exposed to ingesta and the secretions of acid and enzymes produced by other glands in the gastric mucosa. Indeed, even the slightest direct contact of the mixture of food, acid, and enzymes with the gastric mucosa will trigger the secretion of additional amounts of viscous alkaline mucus.

The stomach has two other common and different types of glands in addition to the mucous glands and these are the gastric and pyloric glands. Pyloric glands located in the antral portion of the stomach are tubular in shape and secrete mainly mucus for protection of the pyloric gastric epithelium along with the enzyme pepsinogen and the hormone gastrin. Gastric or oxyntic glands are tubular in shape, located in the mucosa of the body and fundus of the stomach, and produce pepsinogen, mucus, intrinsic factor, and hydrochloric acid. In terms of relative populations, gastric glands outnumber pyloric glands by a ratio of almost 4:1.

The typical gastric gland is composed of parietal, peptic, and mucous neck cells. The mucous neck cells produce mostly mucus and small amounts of pepsinogen. Peptic or chief cells produce large quantities of pepsinogen. Parietal or oxyntic cells secrete hydrochloric acid and intrinsic factor. The parietal cells on their secretory borders have large numbers of deep, highly branched invaginations (canaliculi) that are freely open to and communicate with the lumen of the gastric gland.

Hydrochloric acid formed in the recesses of these canalicular lumina moves through these spaces to mix with other secretions of a gastric gland and then eventually mix with gastric contents. The acid solution secreted by parietal cells contains approximately 150 mmol of hydrochloric acid per liter. This concentration is essentially isotonic with body fluids, but at solution pH of about 0.8 and this level of hydrogen ion, concentration is higher than that found in arterial blood by a multiple of approximately three million. Although several proposed mechanisms exist with regard to the production of hydrochloric acid, one commonly accepted mechanism is presented here. Chloride ions are moved via an active transport process from the cytoplasm of a parietal cell into the lumen of the canaliculus.

While this process proceeds, sodium ions are actively transported from the lumen of the canaliculus. This combined action creates an electronegative sink that consequently attracts the diffusion of potassium ions and some sodium ions from the cytoplasm of the parietal cell into the lumen of the canaliculus. Thus the contents of the canaliculus early in a secretory cycle are essentially composed of potassium chloride with a small amount of sodium chloride. Water normally exists in equilibrium with its component hydrogen and hydroxyl ions and a membrane-bound $H^+/K^+/ATPase$ pump actively transports and exchanges hydrogen ions from the cytoplasm into and potassium ions out of the canalicular lumen while at the same time a separate sodium ion pump removes sodium ions from the canalicular space. The end result is that eventually all the sodium and potassium ions initially in the canaliculus are replaced by hydrogen ions.

Water persistently moves via osmosis into the canalicular space as a result of the secretion of ions into the canaliculus. The resulting concentrated hydrochloric acid solution is then secreted outward through the open end of the canaliculus into the lumen of the gastric gland. The final hydrochloric acid solution secreted into the gastric space contains approximately 150 meq/l of hydrogen chloride, 15 meq/l of potassium chloride, and a small amount of sodium chloride. In the final step of this cycle, carbon dioxide, an end product of normal metabolism, with the assistance of carbonic anhydrase, combines with hydroxyl ion in the cytoplasm to form bicarbonate ions. Bicarbonate ions diffuse out of the cytoplasm of the parietal cell into the extracellular fluid of the body in exchange for the chloride ions that enter the parietal cell and are eventually secreted into the canaliculus. In this fashion, electrical balance is maintained between the parietal cell and its extracellular microenvironment.

Various types of pepsinogens are secreted by the peptic or chief cells and mucous cells of the gastric glands, but despite differences, all pepsinogens perform the same biochemical activity. Nascent pepsinogen (molecular weight approximately 42,000) has no enzymatic activity, but when it comes in contact with hydrochloric acid, it becomes activated to pepsin (molecular weight 35,000). This process is accelerated in the presence of previously formed pepsin. Pepsin is a proteolytic enzyme exhibiting maximal hydrolytic activity within a pH range of 1.8 to 3.5 and is essentially inactive at pH values above 5.0. Other enzymes are found in gastric juices and these include but are not limited to gelatinase, gastric lipase, and gastric amylase; however these enzymes play relatively minor roles in the process of digestion.

The intrinsic factor substance mentioned earlier is essential for the absorption of vitamin B_{12} in the ileum and is secreted by parietal cells along with hydrochloric acid. Pyloric glands are basically identical to gastric glands, but instead contain mostly mucous cells and few or no parietal and peptic cells. The pyloric glands secrete the gastrin hormone and a small amount of pepsinogen along with a large amount of thin nonviscous mucus that aids the movement of ingesta along the GI tract.

Essential neurotransmitters and hormones that can bring about secretion by the gastric glands are gastrin, histamine, and acetylcholine. These substances bind to specific receptors, the process of which triggers a cascade of events culminating in secretion. Gastrin and histamine stimulate the production of acid, but exert few other stimulatory effects on secretory cells of the stomach. Acetylcholine, on the other hand, stimulates secretion by all cell types in the gastric glands and secretory products can include hydrochloric acid, pepsinogen, and mucus.

The secretion of acid from parietal cells is under the control of both neural signals and hormones. Parietal cells operate in close association with histamine-producing enterochromaffin cells located deep within the stomach mucosa, contiguous to the gastric glands. The production of histamine by these cells is elicited for the most part by the gastrin hormone and the acetylcholine neurotransmitter. Gastrin is produced almost completely by cells in the antral portion of the stomach mucosa in response to the presence of protein. Histamine is produced by parietal cells in intimate contact with hydrochloric acid and the amount of histamine produced by parietal cells is proportional to the amount of histamine produced by enterochromaffin cells. Acetylcholine is the end product of vagal nerve stimulation.

Gastrin is produced in two different equally important forms. One is a 34-amino acid polypeptide called G-34 and the other a 17-amino acid polypeptide referred to as G-17. The G-17 form is the more abundantly produced substance. Gastrin is produced by G or gastrin cells that reside in the pyloric glands of the distal stomach. As protein enters the antral portion of the stomach, its presence directly evokes a stimulatory response from the gastrin cells of the pyloric glands, resulting in the release of gastrin into the stomach lumen. The mixing of the gastric luminal contents promotes the interaction of gastrin with the enterochromaffin cells in the body of the stomach and histamine is released from the enterochromaffin cells. This histamine in turn stimulates the production of hydrochloric acid from parietal cells.

Pepsinogen production occurs in response to the presence of hydrochloric acid and acetylcholine. The hydrochloric acid most likely does not elicit its effect on pepsinogen production directly, but rather indirectly via interaction with the enteric nervous system and the initiation of enteric reflexes. Acetylcholine is produced as a result of the stimulation of the vagus nerves or the gastric enteric nervous plexus. While pepsinogen production appears to be essentially under nervous control, the rate of secretion of pepsinogen is significantly affected by the presence of hydrochloric acid in the stomach.

The gastric secretion of both hydrochloric acid and pepsinogen can be negatively modulated by excess acid. When the pH level of gastric contents falls below 3, the gastrin mechanism for the stimulation of gastric secretion becomes nonfunctional because the presence of hydrochloric acid seems to generate an inhibitory neural signal, ceasing gastric secretion and directly blocking the secretion of gastrin by G cells. This acid-mediated feedback inhibition protects the stomach from excess acidity or pepsin that could consequently damage the gastric mucosa. This control mechanism also ensures that the pH of stomach contents lies within a range supportive of optimal enzymatic function. The optimal pH of stomach contents is about 3.

While material in the stomach generally stimulates the production of gastric secretions, it can also inhibit the production during gastric secretion. Indeed, inhibitory hormones and the enterogastric reflex work together to reduce gastric motility at the same time gastric secretions are reduced. The benefit of intestinal-mediated inhibition of gastric secretion is probably to slow the release of chyme from the stomach when the small intestine is already filled or overly taxed. The presence of irritating substances, hyper-osmotic fluid contents, fats, certain protein break-down products, hypo-osmotic fluid contents, or acid can stimulate the release of a number of different intestinal hormones, including but not limited to gastric inhibitory peptide, somatostatin, vasoactive intestinal polypeptide, and secretin.

The roles played by these hormones, except for secretin, are relatively minor. Secretin is very important in the control of generation and release of pancreatic secretions, while at the same time reducing gastric secretions. The presence of food in the small intestine is capable of initiating a reverse enterogastric reflex that inhibits gastric secretion. This reflex is mediated through the vagus nerves, sympathetic nervous system, and myenteric nervous system and is elicited by a number of potential factors including distension of the bowel wall, mucosal irritation, or the presence of certain protein digestive products or acid.

Gastric secretions in the stomach persist between the introduction of food loads, but at very low levels. The gastric secretions at these times consist essentially of mucus, with little pepsinogen and no acid present. However, stress working via a mechanism similar to that described for the cephalic phase can significantly increase gastric secretions and alter their character from that observed with baseline levels.

Within the proximal few centimeters of the duodenum is a large population of compound mucous glands called Brunner's glands located essentially between the pylorus and the entry points of the ducts from the gallbladder and pancreas. Brunner's glands produce large amounts of alkaline mucus in response to secretin and various other gastrointestinal hormones, vagal stimulation, and direct stimulation. This alkaline mucus protects the sensitive intestinal mucosa from potential injury from very acidic gastric secretions. The copious amounts of bicarbonate ions in the mucus also help neutralize the acid in the chyme entering the proximal small intestine. Sympathetic stimulation inhibits the secretion of mucus by the Brunner's glands.

The entire surface of the small intestine is covered with what appears to be stippling or small pits that are openings to structures referred to as crypts of Lieberkühn. These crypts are interposed between intestinal villi. The mucosa covering both crypts and villi is populated with two visibly different types of cells: enterocytes and goblet cells. Enterocytes are present in large numbers and serve two different functions. Crypt enterocytes secrete copious quantities of water and electrolytes, but no enzymes.

The stimulus for this secretion is not completely understood, but is thought to be largely based in local enteric nervous reflexes stimulated by direct contact of substances with the mucosa, gastrointestinal movement, and the movement of gastrointestinal contents. There is some degree of hormonal regulation similar to that described for more proximal regions of the GI tract and this control is for the most part due to cholecystokinin and secretin hormones. Enterocytes located in the crypts can produce over 1.5 liters of alkaline (pH 7.5 to 8.0) fluid per day. This fluid acts as a solvent for the end products of digestion, decreases the viscosity of the chyme, increases the fluidity of the chyme, and improves the contact of substances with the absorptive surface of the intestinal mucosa, thereby enhancing absorption.

Villous enterocytes, on the other hand, contain substantial quantities of digestive enzymes that act to hydrolyze various food substances during the digestive process. These enzymes are located in the brush borders of the cells and include lactase, maltase, sucrase, isomaltase, intestinal lipase, and various peptidases. In addition to the absorption of the end products of digestion, villous enterocytes also absorb water and electrolytes. Goblet cells occur in moderate numbers and produce mucus for purposes of protection of the mucosa and lubrication. A very important aspect of the crypts of Lieberkühn is that cells in the deepest recesses of the crypts are continually undergoing mitosis. Newly produced cells migrate along the basement membrane away from the valley of the crypt to the tip of the villus. In this fashion, the cells covering each villus are constantly replaced. As cells move along in an escalator-type fashion, they mature in size and function. The complete life cycle of an intestinal epithelial cell is approximately 5 days. The failure or inadequacy of this regenerative system to compensate in a timely fashion for damage to intestinal epithelium can result in substantial pathologic consequences to the organism.

Enteroendocrine and Paneth's cells are also found deep in the intestinal glands. Paneth's cells have not been previously mentioned. They have the appearance of protein-secreting zymogenic cells and secrete antimicrobial substances into the bottom area of the crypt.

Repeated reference has been made to the presence of various digestive enzymes in the GI tract. Many of these enzymes come from the pancreas. When the pancreas is mentioned, the first thing that comes to mind is insulin hormone. However, insulin is produced by a different population of pancreatic cells — not by digestive enzyme-producing cells. Furthermore, insulin is introduced into the blood and not the intestinal lumen. While the structure and function of the pancreas will not be addressed, the nature of the secretory process and the secretions delivered to the intestine will be briefly discussed.

With proper stimulation, digestive enzymes are secreted and delivered in copious amounts and in an alkaline aqueous solution through two long ducts from the pancreas. Known as the pancreatic duct and the accessory pancreatic duct, they open into the duodenum through the major and minor duodenal papillae, respectively. The main stimulus for pancreatic secretion is essentially the presence of chyme in the duodenum. However, similar to the stomach, the pancreas has three phases of secretion: cephalic, gastric, and intestinal. In the cephalic phase, the release of acetylcholine from nerve endings embedded in the pancreas is initiated by the same stimuli that promote gastric secretion.

About 20% of a total postprandial bolus of enzymes is produced as a result of this initial stimulation, but little water and electrolytes are concurrently produced. This is because pancreatic enzymes are produced by compound acinous glands that deliver their contents into acini and a system of ducts increasing in diameter that eventually terminate in the confluence and formation of the pancreatic duct. The aqueous bicarbonate solution produced by the pancreas as the solvent for the protein component is secreted by the duct epithelium. In the absence of appropriate stimulation and an adequate supply of fluid, the enzymes remain stored in the acini and ducts until flushed into the duodenum with an adequate flow of water with its electrolytes and bicarbonate.

In the gastric phase of pancreatic secretion, neural stimulation of the secretion of enzymes continues, adding about an additional 10% contribution to the total postprandial bolus production of enzymes. However, again as with the cephalic phase, there is little production of fluid to wash the protein material into the duodenum. As the stomach empties its contents into the duodenum, the chyme initiates the release of the secretin and cholecystokinin hormones from the intestinal mucosa along with acetylcholine from parasympathetic vagal nerve endings and other cholinergic nerves. The acetylcholine and cholecystokinin act together to stimulate further enzyme production from appropriate acinar cells of the pancreas, with little stimulation of the bicarbonate-producing epithelial cells of the pancreas and its ducts.

Secretin, while not stimulating the production of any enzymes, does stimulate pancreatic ductal epithelium to generate copious amounts of a watery and non-viscous bicarbonate solution. This alkaline solution contains bicarbonate at a concentration of approximately 145 meq/l, very little chloride ion, and almost no enzymes. Secretin is a 27-amino acid polypeptide produced by S cells of the mucosa of the duodenum and jejunum in an inactive form called prosecretin. Upon mixture with the intestinal luminal contents where the pH is below 5.0, the prosecretin is converted into active secretin and absorbed into the blood. The critical reagent for this conversion of prosecretin to secretin is hydrochloric acid. It is important to note that secretin is released only from the mucosal epithelium of the small intestine when the pH of the intestinal contents falls below 5. Indeed, the production of secretin increases as the pH falls below 3.

As the pancreatic juice mixes with the chyme, the hydrochloric acid that is present and the added sodium bicarbonate react to form sodium chloride and carbonic acid. The carbonic acid quickly breaks down to form carbon dioxide and water. The carbon dioxide is rapidly removed via absorption and transport in the blood to the lungs for discharge, leaving a neutral aqueous salt solution behind in the gut lumen. With this simple mechanism, acidity from the stomach is effectively controlled and additional peptic activity in the duodenum ceased. This is very significant because the mucosa of the small intestine cannot withstand a prolonged insult of gastric acid. Furthermore, the presence of bicarbonate in the pancreatic secretion causes an average pH of 8.0 of the secretion, which works to create an environment with a pH range of 7.0 to 8.0, which is optimal for the highest degree of activity of pancreatic enzymes.

Cholecystokinin, a 33-amino acid polypeptide, is produced by I cells in the mucosal epithelium of the small intestine. The long chain fatty acids, peptones, proteoses, and to some degree hydrochloric acid initiate the secretion of this hormone, which moves via the blood to the pancreas where it causes the secretion of large quantities of digestive enzymes. Approximately 75% of the total post-prandial bolus production of enzymes results from cholecystokinin stimulation.

The total pancreatic secretion is capable of hydrolyzing fats, proteins, and carbohydrates. The character of pancreatic secretion can be modified by the character of the chyme. Disaccharides and trisaccharides are products of the action of pancreatic amylase on such substrates as glycogen, starches, and most other carbohydrates. Neutral fats are reduced to fatty acids and monoglycerides via the action of pancreatic lipase. Pancreatic phospholipase and cholesterol esterase produce fatty acids and phospholipids and fatty acids and cholesterol, respectively. The most important and abundant pancreatic proteolytic enzyme is trypsin.

Carboxypeptidase and chymotrypsin are also proteolytic enzymes of importance, but are found in lesser amounts than trypsin. Nucleases and elastases are also present in pancreatic secretions in small amounts, but are of lesser importance. Proteolytic enzymes produced by the pancreas are in enzymatically inactive forms that are activated only upon entry into the GI tract. This activation is achieved by kinases produced by the gastrointestinal mucosa and to a lesser degree by autocatalysis. The actions of nucleases and elastases are obvious. Trypsin and chymotrypsin cleave proteins and large polypeptides in such a fashion as to produce smaller peptides, but not individual amino acids. Carboxypeptidase, however, does hydrolyze peptides into individual amino acids.

Bile is another substance added to the intestinal stream to aid in the process of digestion. It is highly concentrated and primarily composed of a variety of different compounds classified as bile salts. These substances comprise almost half the total solutes found in bile, along with bilirubin (the principal break-down product of hemoglobin), lecithin, excess unused cholesterol, sodium ions, potassium ions, calcium ions, chloride ions, and bicarbonate ions. The secretion of bile by the liver is a two-part process. Hepatocytes contribute the bile salts, bilirubin, lecithin, and cholesterol to bile secretion.

Secretory epithelial cells lining the ductules and ducts of the biliary tree secrete water along with sodium and bicarbonate ions into the bile, which is injected into the duodenum after passage through a long duct, the bile duct, that opens into the duodenum through the major duodenal papilla. It should be noted that both the bile duct and pancreatic duct open into the duodenum through the major duodenal papilla.

The aqueous component of bile can equal in volume the very concentrated organic component. Stimulated by the presence of fatty foods entering the duodenum, I cells in the mucosa of the upper small intestine release cholecystokinin, which acts as the main source of stimulation of contraction of the gallbladder, injecting bile into the intestinal lumen. A smaller contribution to this contraction comes from stimulation of the gallbladder by vagal nerves and the intestinal enteric nervous system. It is noteworthy that when no fat is present in a meal, the gallbladder ejects very little of its content into the duodenal lumen. The secretion of the alkaline aqueous and electrolyte components is stimulated by the presence of secretin hormone.

About half a liter of bile is secreted every 12 hours and the gallbladder can maximally store only about 50 ml at any one time. A half to a full liter of bile can be released into the small intestine each day. In response to a fatty meal, the gallbladder can essentially empty itself completely in about 60 minutes. The quantity of bile secreted each day by the liver is closely tied to the amount of bile salts available. As much as 2.5 g of bile salts can be trapped in enterohepatic circulation and if this amount increases, the production of bile increases. Indeed, if bile salts are exogenously administered, the daily production of bile will increase; it can increase by as much as a factor of ten. As bile is stored in the gallbladder prior to its release into the small intestine, it is persistently concentrated by the epithelium of the gallbladder. This concentration effect can range up to a factor of almost 20-fold.

While bile contains no enzymes, it nevertheless plays a prominent role in the digestion and absorption of fat through the presence of bile acids. These substances promote the emulsification of large fat droplets into tiny little particles that can be readily attacked by pancreatic lipases and aid in the absorption of the end products of fat digestion. As the digestive process initiates in the upper GI tract, the gallbladder begins to empty its contents. This emptying is especially effective in response to a fatty meal and occurs 20 to 30 minutes after a meal.

The epithelial cells of the mucosa of the large intestine do not secrete any enzymes, acids, or factors into the lumen and are essentially of four different types including undifferentiated, immature absorptive, and mucus-producing goblet cells. The predominant population is composed of cells that produce mucus, the main secretion of the large intestine. Nonmucus-secreting cells located near the mucus-secreting cells produce bicarbonate ions that give the mucus of the large intestine an alkaline character.

There are no villi in the large intestine as are present in the small intestine, but it contains many crypts of Lieberkühn that are heavily populated with mucous cells. Epithelial cells of the large intestine are replaced approximately every 6 days by the proliferation and differentiation of cells residing in the lower third of the crypt. Secretion in the large intestine is initiated or controlled by local nervous reflexes acting upon the mucus-secreting cells and direct stimulation of the mucus-secreting cells. Parasympathetic innervations arising from the pelvic nerves supply the distal half of the large intestine and can significantly increase the amount of secretion of mucus and also motility. The mucus in the large intestine provides lubrication for the movement of the fecal stream, promotes the formation of the fecal mass, provides protection of the mucosa from the high level of microbial activity in the lumen, and as a result of its alkaline character (pH 8.0) provides protection of the mucosa from attack by acids and formed in the feces.

We have talked about a number of different endocrine cell secretions along the digestive tract. It seems appropriate to summarize the geography and distribution of these types of secretions in the GI tract at the close of this section. Gastrin is present in the intestinal stream, abruptly appearing at its highest levels in the pyloric antrum and persistent at those concentrations in the proximal part of the duodenum, at which point its concentration slowly falls to an almost immeasurable level by the end of the jejunum. Secretin is present in the intestinal stream, abruptly appearing at its highest levels in the proximal duodenum and persistent at those concentrations through the jejunum, at which point its concentration slowly falls to an almost immeasurable level by the end of the ileum. Cholecystokinin is present in the intestinal stream in a pattern that essentially mirrors that of secretin. Glucagon-like substances, although not specifically discussed here, are found in increasing amounts along the length of the entire GI tract through the end of the jejunum, at which point the concentration of these substances reaches a zenith and then persists at that level through the end of the large intestine.

TABLE 6.1
Enteroendocrine Cells of the Canine GI Tract

Cell Type	Location	Hormone Produced	Hormone Action
A-cell	Stomach	Glucagon	Hepatic glycogenolysis
D-cell	Pyloric stomach Duodenum	Somatostatin	Inhibition of other entero- endocrine cells
D1-cell	Entire GI tract	Vasoactive intestinal polypeptide	Ion flow Water secretion Enhanced gut motility
EC-cell	Entire GI tract	Serotonin Substance P	Enhanced gut motility
G-cell	Pyloric stomach	Gastrin	Gastric acid secretion stimulation
I-cell	Small intestine	Cholecystokinin	Gall bladder contraction Secretion pancreatic enzymes
K-cell	Small intestine	Gastric inhibitory Polypeptide	Inhibition of gastric acid secretion
L-cell	Small intestine	Glucagon-like substance	Hepatic glycogenolysis
Mo-cell	Small intestine	Motilin	Enhanced gut motility
S-cell	Small intestine	Secretin	Pancreatic bicarbonate secretion Pancreatic water secretion Gall bladder water secretion

Finally, somatostatin-like substances although not discussed here, are also found throughout the entire length of the GI tract. They appear abruptly at high levels in the fundic portion of the stomach and persist at these levels to the proximal portion of the duodenum, at which point they rapidly fall to about half their initial levels. These reduced levels of somatostatin-like substances then persist through the remainder of the GI tract.

Table 6.1 lists the principal enteroendocrine cells of the GI tract by type, location, hormone produced, and major action.

Only the cells that make major, well defined contributions to the function of the GI tract have been discussed in this chapter. Other cell types and their secretions have been mentioned as a matter of completeness.

DIGESTION AND ABSORPTION

Substances that enter the GI tract include minerals, water, electrolytes, carbohydrates, vitamins, proteins, fats, and xenobiotics. Certainly the majority of these substances fit into the general category of foods and nutrition. Compounds such as fats, proteins, and carbohydrates are macromolecules and of little nutritional value without digestion. To fully appreciate the function of the GI tract, it is important to first understand the processes of normal digestion and absorption [15, 18, 21–23, 28, 31, 33, 41, 42,

57, 59, 67, 68, 76, 81, 88, 91, 97, 101, 102, 119, 120, 134, 143, 157, 162, 198, 203, 204, 209, 214, 215, 224, 254, 256, 270, 276, 281, 282, 288].

Certainly xenobiotics are at least subject to the same biochemical processes of digestion and absorption as food and so an appreciation of the details of these activities as they pertain to food is important. Furthermore, xenobiotics have the potential to interfere with the normal processes of digestion and absorption, again making an understanding of the core processes important for better understanding and predicting the toxic responses of the GI tract. To put the process of absorption in perspective, each day the small intestine can absorb 50 to 100 g or more of carbohydrates, fats, amino acids, and ions in addition to about 7.5 liters of water. However, this level of absorption constitutes only 10 to 20% of the total absorptive capacity of the small intestine. The large intestine can absorb even more water, but only limited nutrients. This large capacity of the small intestine for absorption indicates the importance of absorption for sustenance of the organism. Vitamins and minerals have numerous and very specific mechanisms for uptake and these will not be discussed here.

One very important process represents a common thread of digestion and that process is hydrolysis. While the enzymes that perform hydrolysis change with the type of substrate, the basic reaction is the same and this reaction is the introduction of water into linkages that are specific for different types of substrates. The water is introduced not as molecular water, but rather as hydroxyl and hydrogen ions into a chemical bond that was previously formed in a condensation type of reaction during which water was extruded in the form of hydroxyl and hydrogen ions.

The most common form of fat is the triglyceride or neutral fat, composed of a molecule of glycerol and three fatty acids. Triglycerides are partly digested in the stomach via lingual lipase secreted from glands in the mouth and then swallowed with saliva. The degree of digestion from this lipase is small and the overwhelming degree of fat digestion occurs in the small intestine. The first step in digestion by the small intestine is emulsification or the break-down of the fat globules into small droplets. This allows the relevant enzymes to operate on a greater amount of fat per unit of volume and per unit of time since the surface area is increased. Indeed, as the droplets become smaller, the surface area of a unit of fat can increase by a factor as large as a thousand.

Gastric mixing contributes to the emulsification process, but the bulk of it occurs in the duodenum with the admixing of bile salts and lecithin that interact with the fat globules. Lecithin is a phospholipid and its presence is critical to the process. The polar portions of lecithin and bile salts interact with water and enhance solubility. The nonpolar portions of bile salts and lecithin are highly lipid-soluble and readily dissolve in fat. The fat-soluble portions of these hepatically produced molecules dissolve in the surface layers of the fat globules, with the polar parts oriented so as to orthogonally extend outward from the fat globules into the surrounding aqueous medium. This conglomeration or arrangement reduces the surface tension that normally exists at the interface between fat and water, facilitating emulsification and fragmentation of the fat globules. Lipases, which are water-soluble enzymes, can now more readily and effectively attack the fat. However, this attack can take place only on the surfaces of the tiny fat particles, emphasizing the importance of the process of emulsification.

The most important intestinal enzyme for fat digestion is pancreatic lipase, which breaks triglycerides down into free fatty acids, diglycerides, and 2-monoglycerides. The accumulation of fatty acids and monoglycerides in the microenvironment of the digesting fat inhibits further digestion. Accordingly, it is essential that these materials be moved quickly away from the globule-associated digestive processes. Compounds known as bile salts serve this important function. Bile salts are produced by hepatocytes in an amount equal to about 600 mg per day.

Dietary or endogenously produced cholesterol is the starting material for the synthesis or production of bile salts. In the first step, cholesterol is converted to chenodeoxycholic or cholic acids that in turn combine with glycine or taurine amino acids to form bile acids, which are nothing more than amino acid conjugates of the original acids, chenodeoxycholate or cholate. The sodium salts of these bile acids are the substances that are actually secreted into the bile. Bile acids and their salts can remove the fatty acids and monoglycerides away from the digesting globules of fat almost as quickly as the hydrolytic products are formed. A bile acid or salt is composed of a highly lipid-soluble sterol nucleus and a water-soluble polar group at the end of a hydrocarbon side chain.

For reasons of thermodynamics, bile acids and their salts at high concentrations aggregate to form structures known as micelles. A micelle is a collection of 20 to 40 molecules of bile acids and salts in a spherical arrangement. The central portion of the sphere is composed of sterol nuclei; the surface of the sphere consists of polar groups on connecting hydrocarbon side chains. The micelles incorporate into their lipid cores the very tiny products resulting from fat emulsification and digestion and quickly and efficiently move these tiny fat droplets away from the sites of hydrolysis. Micelles are approximately 3 to 6 nm in diameter. Because of the negative charges on the exterior polar groups, the micelle globule is readily dissolved in aqueous digestive fluid in stable fashion until absorption. These bile salt micelles also work to carry the free fatty acids and monoglycerides to the brush borders of the intestinal epithelial cells, where they press deeply into the valleys of the undulating microvilli and are eventually absorbed into the blood.

Cholesterol in the diet is generally found in the form of an ester composed of one molecule of cholesterol and one molecule of fatty acid. Cholesterol ester hydrolase, which comes from the pancreas, hydrolyzes cholesterol esters into their components: free fatty acids and cholesterol. Phospholipids also found in the diet are small molecules constructed of fatty acids and glycerol. However, only two of the alcohols of phospholipids are connected to fatty acid chains; the third is connected to a hydrophilic phosphate group that is in turn connected to a small hydrophilic compound like choline. A phospholipid can be hydrolyzed into a diglyceride (hydrolysis of carboxyl ester at position 2 of the glycerol) by the pancreatic enzyme phospholipase A_2. For both cholesterol esters and phospholipids, bile acid and salt micelles perform the same vital functions as for cholesterol in the processes of digestion and absorption.

Before leaving the topic of digestion and absorption of fats and bile acids and salts, we should mention enterohepatic circulation of bile salts. Indeed approximately 95% of all bile acids and salts are reabsorbed into the circulation from the small intestine. The same bile compounds can recycle themselves approximately 18 times before they are eventually eliminated from the body in the feces. This reabsorption is accomplished via an active transport type of process in the mucosa of the distal ileum and diffusion through the mucosa of the proximal part of the small intestine. Upon absorption into the blood, bile salts move via the portal blood back to the liver and into the hepatic venous sinusoids, where they are absorbed by hepatocytes and secreted again into the bile. Any bile compounds that are lost in the feces are replaced by the synthesis of new bile compounds.

The majority of ingested carbohydrates are mainly of three types: starches, sucrose, and lactose. Starches are large complex polysaccharides; lactose and sucrose are disaccharides. Other types of carbohydrates that are ingested in much smaller amounts include cellulose, glycogen, amylose, dextrins, pectins, and insignificant amounts of various carbohydrate derivatives. Mastication initiates the process of digestion of carbohydrates with the introduction of ptyalin to a bolus of food. This enzyme is secreted by the parotid salivary glands and hydrolyzes starch into the disaccharide maltose and various other 3- to 9-unit polymers of glucose. However, only a small amount of the total starch load will have been hydrolyzed by the time the food bolus has entered the stomach.

After the food bolus enters the stomach, this digestion will continue for approximately 1 hour, after which the ingesta is thoroughly mixed with gastric secretions that are added to the mixture. The acidity of the gastric secretions inactivates the salivary amylase, but approximately half of the available starch will have been hydrolyzed into maltose by the time this happens. Hydrolysis of carbohydrates continues in the small intestine with the introduction of pancreatic secretions. Pancreatic amylase performs the same activity as oral amylase, but has a much higher throughput or turnover number. Indeed, almost all remaining starches are converted to maltose and other very small polymers of glucose while the ingesta transits the duodenum. The small polymers of glucose and disaccharides produced as a result of prior hydrolytic cleavage must be further reduced to monosaccharides for intestinal absorption to occur.

Four enzymes critical to achieving these chemical breakdowns are sucrase, maltase, alpha-dextrinase, and lactase. These enzymes are found in the enterocytes lining the microvilli brush border of the small intestine. As materials come in contact with these enzymes, further hydrolysis takes place. Lactose is split into a molecule of glucose and one of galactose; sucrose is split into a molecule of glucose and a molecule of fructose. Maltose and other glucose polymers are reduced to single units of glucose. The final hydrolytic product of carbohydrate digestion is a monosaccharide and most commonly glucose. These terminal products are all very water-soluble and readily absorbed.

Proteins are macromolecules that are polymers of amino acids joined together via peptide linkages. These linkages are broken down via hydrolysis by means of the pepsin enzyme to produce compounds like peptones, polypeptides, and proteoses. Pepsin can also hydrolyze collagen, a significant component of meat that is very resistant to degradation by a number of other enzymes. If collagen is not hydrolyzed, the effectiveness of hydrolysis or digestion of protein in materials like meat is highly impaired and hence so is absorption. The products resulting from the break-down of proteins by pepsin enter the small intestine, the chief site for the digestion of protein.

As soon as stomach contents are moved into the duodenum, the chyme is attacked by several pancreatic enzymes including proelastase, chymotrypsin, and carboxypolypeptidase. Proelastase is converted into elastase, which degrades elastin. Trypsin and chymotrypsin degrade protein into polypeptide fragments of varying size. Carboxypolypeptidase trims amino acids off of the carboxy termini of the various polypeptide products produced by previous enzymatic cleavage. Unlike carbohydrates, only a small component of protein is completely hydrolyzed to component amino acids by pancreatic enzymes. Indeed, protein for the most part is reduced only to dipeptides, tripeptides, tetrapeptides, etc.

The total amount of fluid that must be absorbed by the intestines on a daily basis is approximately 9 liters, and this volume is comprised of up to 1.5 liters of ingested fluid and 7.5 liters of secreted fluid. Approximately 80 to 90% of this fluid is absorbed in the small intestine, leaving the remainder to be absorbed in the large intestine. The stomach lining lacks a villus absorptive surface and has very tightly woven junctions between apposed epithelial cells, making the gastric mucosa a poor area for absorption. Exceptions to this are highly lipid-soluble materials, salicylates, and ethanol, which can all be directly absorbed through the stomach wall in small quantities.

The entire surface of the mucosa of the small intestine, basically from the point at which the common bile duct empties into the duodenum to the terminus of the ileum, contains millions of very small villi that project approximately 1 mm from the surface of the mucosa. While the villi are somewhat less populous near the end of the small intestine, their density is such that they exist in very close apposition to one another. Their presence increases the surface available for absorption by a factor of almost 10. In addition to this gross anatomic adaptation of the gut that acts to increase and facilitate absorption, a microscopic adaptation increases the surface available for absorption by a factor of almost 20. This feature is the brush border found on the free surface of each intestinal epithelial mucosal cell on each villus.

The brush border is a series of multiple invaginations or evaginations of the enterocytic membrane that result in the formation of microvilli. As many as 1000 microvilli may be present on the free surface of each intestinal enterocyte. These microvilli are approximately 0.1 μm in diameter and 1 μm in length. Collectively these adaptations work together to enhance the intestinal surface area available for absorption by a factor of almost 500.

The basic mechanisms of absorption include diffusion, active transport, and solvent drag. The two different kinds of diffusion are simple and facilitated. In simple diffusion, kinetic molecular motion moves molecules or ions through a membrane, pore, gate, opening, or any intermolecular space without the necessity of binding with a carrier protein in the membrane. The rate of diffusion is dependent on the concentration of the substance, its kinetic energy, and the numbers and sizes of openings through which the substance can pass. Facilitated diffusion requires the participation or help of an ancillary or carrier protein that chemically binds with the substance being moved and shuttles it through a membrane.

Active transport is the process of moving or transporting materials against a concentration gradient. It is important to appreciate that energy is imparted to the substance transported via active transport. The two types of active transport are primary and secondary, both of which utilize carrier proteins that span or access both sides of a membrane. For primary active transport, the process energy is derived directly from the break-down of adenosine triphosphate or an alternate high energy phosphate bond compound. However, for secondary active transport, the energy for the process comes from energy stored in the form of ionic concentration differentials between two sides of a membrane; the difference is created by the process of active transport. In the case of solvent drag, dissolved substances can be pulled along as a solvent is absorbed because of various physicochemical forces that exist between the solvent and solute.

Transport systems exist not only in the surface membranes of cells, but also in intracellular membranes and intercellular membranes or junctions. Transport through the intestinal epithelium must occur through a sheet of cells and not simply through one cell membrane. The basic mechanism for the transport of a substance through a cellular sheet is active transport of the substance through the cell membrane on one side of a cell followed by simple or facilitated diffusion through the cell membrane on the opposite side of the cell. A variety of different combinations and locations of transport systems for the absorption process exist throughout the gut, but the basic principles remain the same, regardless of the nature of the substance involved.

In addition to the above processes, a very small contribution is made to absorption by pinocytosis, a physical process that occurs continually in most cells, but at widely differing rates according to cell type. This process is the means by which most macromolecules and proteins enter cells; however, the process can involve large carbohydrates, lipids, and other substances. Indeed the degree of pinocytosis significantly increases as macromolecules attach themselves to a cell membrane.

Particles of several thousand nanometers in diameter were reported to have been taken up by the duodenum. Latex particles of 22 microns in diameter have been carried through the cytoplasm of intestinal epithelium and deposited into the lamina propria, with subsequent absorption into the lymphatics. For this process to occur, proteins bind to specialized receptors embedded in a cell membrane; the receptors are specific to that type of protein or sequence within a protein. They are located in miniscule depressions called coated pits on the cell surface. Deep in the coated pits and on the interior surfaces of cell membranes are net-like arrays of clathrin and other proteins, possibly including actin and myosin.

When the binding between protein and receptor is adequate and complete, the pit invaginates, enveloping the entire protein and a small amount of extracellular fluid. At the completion of this process, the invaginated portion of the cell membrane pinches off in such a fashion as to maintain cell membrane integrity and form a totally sealed vesicle (pinocytotic vesicle) inside the cell. The pinocytotic vesicle then combines with a lysosome and is digested or broken down by the machinery of the cell. Small degradation products such as sugars, amino acids, etc. can diffuse through the membrane of the digestive vesicle into the cytoplasm where they can be immediately utilized or follow the paths of similar substances being absorbed via other mechanisms. Undigested residual material is excreted directly through the cell membrane in a process known as exocytosis.

Each intestinal villus is almost finger-like in shape. A cross-section cut transversely mid-level through a villus appears somewhat like a small onion. The outermost layer is the brush border, discussed previously. Immediately below this layer are the enterocytes that are firmly anchored to the deeply underlying basement membrane. The inner area of each villus is a network of vasculature embedded in loose connective tissue. Capillaries connect a supplying artery with a draining vein. At the innermost central core is the very important central lacteal located approximately along the central axis of each villus that collects the lymphatic fluid draining the villus.

The lymphatic system is an accessory route by which fluid can flow from interstitial areas, eventually back into the blood. However, the lymphatic fluid can also carry whole proteins, large molecules, fat, and particulate matter away from a local tissue space, eventually back into the blood. This alternative route compensates for the fact that none of these materials can be directly absorbed into the bloodstream.

Water is absorbed from the small intestine by diffusion and obeys the laws of osmosis. However, water can move in different directions. It can flow from the fluid intestinal contents into the villous blood or from the plasma of the blood into the lumen of the small intestine. The latter can occur when the chyme is hyper-osmolar in character.

A variety of ions are absorbed from the small intestine and they include but are not limited to sodium, calcium, potassium, magnesium, iron, chloride, bicarbonate, and phosphate. A significant deficit exists between sodium secreted into the intestinal lumen (influx) and sodium absorbed from the intestinal contents (efflux). This differential strongly favors the loss of sodium. Accordingly, under normal conditions with no intervening pathology or toxicology, an amount of sodium equal to about 10 to 20% of the total body sodium must be absorbed each day. Fortunately, sodium is rapidly absorbed through the mucosal epithelium of the intestine. Sodium ion concentration in intestinal contents averages approximately 142 meq/l and approximates that of plasma, but intracellular sodium ion concentration is only approximately 50 meq/l. Consequently, sodium follows the concentration gradient and moves by facilitated diffusion from the liquid intestinal contents through the brush border of the epithelium of the small intestine into the cytoplasm of the enterocytes. This sodium is then moved from the cell interior through the basolateral aspect of the cell (base of cell rests on basement membrane; brush border side of cell is exactly opposite and lies in contact with the chyme) by means of active transport and the energy of adenosine triphosphate into a paracellular space.

Paracellular spaces are small areas located between adjacent enterocytes. They are bound deeply by the basement membrane and superficially by the tight junctions welding adjacent intestinal epithelial cells together at points on the lateral walls just beneath the brush border. Some chloride ion can be absorbed simultaneously with sodium ion, as the opposing electrical charges work in an attractive fashion causing a drag effect. Additional sodium is also absorbed as a consequence of the necessary and required activity of the sodium–potassium pump. As the sodium ions accumulate in the paracellular spaces, water moves by osmosis into these same areas. The water for the most part enters these paracellular spaces through the tight junctions mentioned earlier, but a small portion arises from or through the cell membranes of the enterocytes. As the water flows into and through the paracellular spaces, the ions and water eventually enter the blood circulating in the villus. Before leaving the topic of sodium ion absorption, it should be mentioned that under certain physiologic conditions the adrenal cortical hormone aldosterone can be released and this hormone can significantly enhance the absorption of sodium by the intestinal epithelium.

Chloride absorption occurs rapidly in the duodenum and jejunum and also occurs via diffusion. As sodium ions follow the path described previously, an electric potential is established and the intestinal contents become more negative. Chloride ions follow the electrical gradient, trailing the sodium ions and moving from the more negative area to the more positive area. Chloride ions are absorbed by enterocytes located on the villi of the ileum and large intestine in a process that secretes a bicarbonate ion for each chloride ion absorbed. The purpose of this activity is most likely to provide some degree of basification of the acidic products present in the intestinal stream contents as well as to maintain the electrochemical gradient.

Bicarbonate ions are present in large numbers in the small intestine, not only as a result of intestinal secretory activity, but also through secretions from the liver and pancreas. It is important to recapture these ions to maintain a normal acid–base homeostasis in the body. The reabsorption occurs somewhat indirectly in the duodenum and jejunum. Bicarbonate ions combine with existing hydrogen ions to form carbonic acid, which is relatively unstable and decomposes rapidly to form carbon dioxide and water. The water remains as part of the intestinal contents and can follow the absorptive path described previously. The carbon dioxide is very soluble, readily absorbed, and quickly moved to the blood in the villi. It is eventually cleared from the body through the lungs with expiration.

In general, monovalent ions are absorbed from the lumen of the gut with great ease, but bivalent ions are absorbed in only small amounts. Indeed the maximal absorption of bivalent ions can be as little as only 2% of the maximal absorption of monovalent ions. Potassium (monovalent), magnesium, and phosphate are most likely actively absorbed through the intestinal mucosa. Calcium absorption is very highly regulated and calcium is absorbed heavily from the duodenum. Other factors controlling calcium absorption are vitamin D, parathyroid hormone, and the degree of physical activity of the organism (Wolf's law).

Absorbed nutrients fall into three general classes: proteins, fats, and carbohydrates, the same general classes cited for digestion. For the most part, carbohydrates are ultimately absorbed as monosaccharides and the most common monosaccharide is glucose. The sugar monomers of fructose and galactose are also absorbed, but they exist in smaller amounts. Absorption of glucose is via an active transport process. Disaccharides are absorbed in only small amounts and sugar polymers of greater numbers are virtually not absorbed at all. A fact that is not commonly appreciated is that no glucose absorption can occur in the absence of sodium ion because glucose is co-transported with sodium ion.

We mentioned earlier that sodium follows a concentration gradient and moves by facilitated diffusion from the liquid intestinal contents through the brush border of the mucosal epithelium of the small intestine into the cytoplasm of the enterocytes. This sodium is then in turn moved from the cell interior through the basolateral aspect of the cell by means of active transport into the paracellular space. The facilitated diffusion is accomplished with the aid of a transport protein, but sodium ion will not be transported into the interior of the cell unless the transport protein combines with another appropriate moiety, glucose. In this process, both glucose and sodium are co-transported into the interior of the enterocyte. The low concentration of intracellular sodium ion is the energy driving this process. Once inside the enterocyte, the glucose is moved outside the cell through the basolateral membrane of the intestinal epithelial cell into the paracellular space by means of facilitated diffusion. From this space, the glucose is readily taken up by the blood circulation of the villus. Galactose is absorbed by the same exact mechanism as glucose, but fructose is not. Fructose moves through the enterocyte by means of facilitated diffusion, but the movement is not coupled with sodium ion transport. As fructose enters the cell, most of it is phosphorylated, converted to glucose, and then transported as glucose into the paracellular space. This lack of co-transportation with sodium ion leads to a significantly reduced rate of transport when compared to that of glucose.

Most proteins are absorbed as dipeptides, tripeptides, and amino acids directly through the enterocytic membranes that line the lumen of the gut, chiefly in the areas of the duodenum and jejunum. Again, a sodium ion co-transport mechanism works in the same fashion as that for sodium and glucose. The enterocytes have brush borders composed of hundreds of microvilli projecting from the surface of each cell. Anchored in the membranes of these microvilli are peptidases that extend into the milieu of the intestinal luminal space. Two classes of peptidases are worthy of note: dipeptidases and aminopolypeptidases. These enzymes degrade large polypeptides into dipeptides, tripeptides, and amino acids. The small peptides or amino acids then bind to a specific transport protein in the enterocyte's microvillus membrane that requires sodium ion binding as a prerequisite to transport.

The amino acids, dipeptides, and tripeptides are readily transported through the membrane of the microvilli into the interiors of the enterocytes. As a sodium ion moves down the electrochemical gradient into the enterocyte, it pulls along an amino acid or small peptide. Some amino acids do not require a sodium ion co-transportation mechanism, but rather move via facilitated diffusion and specialized membrane transport proteins.

While much still remains to be elucidated with regard to the absorption of amino acids and small peptides, we know of at least five different types of amino acid and peptide transport proteins in the luminal or free surface membranes of enterocytes that are reflective of the different chemical characteristics of different amino acids. When in the enterocytic cytosol, additional peptidases specific for different types of amino acids act to degrade the small polymers of amino acids into individual amino acid components. This process occurs within seconds to minutes and the single amino acids are moved from the enterocyte most likely via facilitated diffusion or active transport processes to enter the villus blood. It can be seen from this that almost all the digestion products of proteins that are absorbed are taken up in the form of amino acids. Only rarely are peptides and whole proteins absorbed into the blood. Indeed, the absorption of proteinaceous material can result in the development of serious allergic or immunologic disorders.

Because of their lipid solubility, the monoglyceride and fatty acid end products of fat digestion diffuse readily from their transporting micelles through the membrane of the enterocyte into the interior of the cell when contact is made between the micelle and the microvillus membrane. The unloaded micelles remain in the chyme where they accumulate more monoglycerides and fatty acids to repeat this ferrying or transport cycle until fat absorption is complete.

The importance of micelles to this whole process is illustrated by the fact that almost 100% of the fat in any food load is absorbed in their presence. In the absence of micelles, only about half the fat in a particular food load is absorbed. When the monoglycerides and fatty acids are inside enterocytes, they are taken up by the endoplasmic reticulum where they are recycled to form new triglycerides that are extruded into the lymph. These triglycerides then become parts of lymph chylomicrons — small structures that transport triglycerides through the lymphatic system to a point at which they are eventually mixed with the blood of the circulatory system. It should be noted that some proportion of very short-, short-, and medium-chain length fatty acids can be absorbed directly into the portal venous blood supply of the villi rather than following the processing path and journey through the lacteals and lymphatic system as just described. The reason for this difference is probably the greater degrees of water solubility of these types of compounds.

The large intestine is the major site for the absorption of water and electrolytes in the GI tract and can absorb up to a maximum of approximately 5 to 8 liters of fluid containing electrolytes daily. However, if this maximum capacity is exceeded, watery stool or diarrhea can result, with a loss of water and electrolytes. Similar to the small intestine, the mucosa of the large intestine has a large capacity for absorption of both sodium and chloride ions. Indeed, by the time large intestinal contents are ready for excretion, only a couple of milliequivalents each of sodium and chloride ions remain in the feces.

The principles of absorption for ions and water are the same for both the small and large intestines, with one important difference. The tight junctions between the epithelial cells are much tighter in the large intestine than in the small intestine. This closer apposition establishes a much stronger barrier because any diffusion back into the intestinal lumen is prohibited. This increases the extent of absorption of ions, especially sodium and chloride, and establishes a greater concentration gradient of ions.

When the aldosterone hormone is secreted, the absorption process becomes even more stringent or efficient. Similarly, as in the small intestine, the mucosa of the large intestine secretes bicarbonate ion into the intestinal lumen to counteract the acidity of microbial end products produced by bacterial fermentation. As bicarbonate ions are secreted by the mucosa of the large intestine, equal milliequivalent amounts of chloride ion are absorbed via the same mechanism described previously. As observed more proximally in the GI tract, both sodium and chloride ions exist in osmotic and electrochemical gradients across the barrier of the epithelial mucosa of the large intestine and the energy of these gradients indirectly drives the absorption of water from the intestinal fecal stream.

Unless there is a direct-acting pharmacologic or toxic effect, xenobiotics present in the GI tract do not produce effects until they are absorbed into the system [2, 141, 243, 244, 271, 272, 274, 293]. Agents can be absorbed anywhere along the GI tract via any mechanism described. These mechanisms include but are not limited to passive diffusion, facilitated diffusion, active transport, and cotransport. The specific details with regard to each of these mechanisms have already been addressed.

A number of factors must be appreciated with regard to the absorption of xenobiotics from the GI tract regardless of the method of administration or introduction. The fat content of a diet can produce a significant effect on the absorption of individual xenobiotics and an understanding of these potential effects must be achieved for any test. Similarly, fasting can also affect the profile of absorption. Specialized transport systems commonly exist in the gastrointestinal system, and it is not rare for a xenobiotic to be absorbed solely or partly via one of these types of systems. While much still remains to be learned with regard to these systems, a greater understanding has developed in recent years. It is now thought that there are a number of different families of xenobiotic transporters.

One transporter family consists of the multidrug-resistant (mdr) proteins or p-glycoproteins. This transporter moves chemotherapeutic drugs out of neoplastic cells and thereby contributes to the development of neoplastic resistance. Additionally, the mdr transporter system is responsible for the movement of chemicals out of hepatocytes, renal epithelial cells, intestinal epithelial cells, and brain endothelial cells along with protection of the fetus. The multi-resistant drug proteins (mdp) are also responsible for the movement of xenobiotics out of cells, but favor phase II conjugates like glucuronides and glutathione adducts as substrates.

Acids, bases and neutral compounds can be transported by organic anion-transporting peptides (oatps), which also play a prominent role in the hepatic absorption of xenobiotics. The organic anion transporter (oat) group is very important in the uptake of anions, especially in the kidney. The organic cation transporter plays a significant role in the absorption of xenobiotics and is of special importance in renal and liver cells. Metals, nucleotides, and di- and tri-peptides are absorbed with the assistance of the divalent metal ion transporter (dmt), nucleotide transporter (nt), and peptide transporter (pept), respectively. Thallium, cobalt, and manganese are absorbed by the same system that absorbs iron and lead is absorbed by the calcium uptake system.

Congeners of various pyrimidines can be transported by pyrimidine transport systems. Co-transport systems exist also, but are most common for metals and metal-containing compounds. In such systems, the presence of one moiety can affect the absorption of another in a positive or negative fashion. Despite the broad spectrum of systems available for absorption, it is important to emphasize that the number of xenobiotics that are actively absorbed or absorbed via co-transportation by the GI tract is low. Most xenobiotics enter the body via the process of simple diffusion across the gastrointestinal mucosal epithelial barrier.

If one looks at the locations of these specialized transport systems in the small intestine and colon, the following general observations can be made. The specialized transport of calcium, iron, fatty acids, and chloride is at a high level in the proximal small intestine, moderate level in the mid small intestine, low in the terminal small intestine, and nonexistent in the colon. Bile salts and vitamin B_{12} are transported only to a small degree in the mid portion of the small intestine and a large degree in the terminal small intestine. Sodium is actively transported at a high level throughout the entire length of the GI tract. Pyrimidines are transported only in small amounts and only in the proximal and mid portions of the small intestine. Sugars and neutral amino acids are transported in moderate to high amounts through the entire length of small intestine, but not in the large intestine. Basic amino acids and triglycerides are transported in moderate amounts throughout the entire length of the small intestine, but not in the large intestine. Gamma globulins are transported in increasing amounts through the length of the small intestine only, reaching their zenith of absorption in the terminal ileum. Hydrogen ion transport occurs at low levels in the middle portion of the small intestine and at moderate levels in the distal portion of the small intestine and the entire large intestine.

Generally speaking, if a test compound has a molecular weight below 10,000, at least some degree of absorption will occur [1, 17, 46, 54, 75, 83, 87, 95, 107, 138, 202, 211, 222, 228, 230, 251, 252, 273, 280, 296, 298, 308, 309, 314]. How much absorption takes place will depend in part upon the physical and chemical properties of a molecule (solubility, water partition coefficient, dissolution rate, etc.) as well as the characteristics of the formulation in which the xenobiotic is delivered. If xenobiotics are delivered as large particles, absorption can be very low. Similarly, insoluble solids have little opportunity to make contact with the intestinal mucosa.

Animal physiology can also have a profound effect on absorption. It is not uncommonly assumed that the gastrointestinal absorption of xenobiotics is similar or even identical across species. This is not the case and numerous studies demonstrating significant differences in bioavailabilities of species are supported with adequate distribution, metabolism, elimination, and excretion data. For example, it has been suggested that the rate limiting step in the absorption of any xenobiotic is the removal of the xenobiotic from the very thin static or non-agitated water layer that lies in intimate contact with the lipophilic membranes of the epithelium of the gastrointestinal mucosa. Species differences in the absorption of xenobiotics may well be due to differences in the thickness of this water layer.

Differences of GI tract size, anatomy, histology, and histophysiology may also contribute in a profound fashion to differences in the absorption of xenobiotics across species. Considerations of size alone may be of paramount importance, considering the fact that most xenobiotics are absorbed via the process of passive diffusion. To that point, gastrointestinal absorption is highly dependent on local pH values within the GI tract, and again important differences between species have been found.

Neonates have poorly developed intestinal mucosal barriers that permit facile absorption of a wide variety of substances. Inflammation and parasitic infestation can also lead to enhanced or altered absorption. Scarring and thickening of the intestinal wall can lead to decreased absorption. It is important to remember that digestive fluids, microbial flora, and other moieties in the gastrointestinal stream may modify the structure of a chemical or bind to it in some fashion, thereby radically changing the absorptive profile of the test article as well as its anticipated pharmacology and toxicology.

Secondary amines can be converted under certain circumstances into carcinogenic nitrosamines.

One interesting observation is that the dilution of a xenobiotic typically results in an increased rate and degree of absorption. We do not know whether this increase in absorption is a direct result of dilution or merely a consequence of increased dose volume, more rapid emptying of the stomach, and the increased transit of material into the small intestine where the absorptive surface area is greater. It bears repeating that one of the most important aspects of the absorption of xenobiotics from the GI tract is the fact that lipid-soluble compounds are absorbed more readily than water-soluble compounds. This is because the former are in a nonionized state and the latter are in an ionized state.

Two general rules burgeon from this concept. The first is that weak organic acids exist in the nonionized and lipid soluble form in the stomach. Accordingly, one might expect significant absorption of weak organic acids to take place in the stomach, but as a result of differences in the characteristics of gastric mucosa and the intestinal mucosa, increased residence time in the intestine, and exposure of the weak organic acid to significantly greater surface area in the intestine, the greatest degree of absorption of weak organic acids takes place in the intestine. This is because blood flow rate and absorptive surface area are more important than pH for the absorption of weak acids. The second rule is that weak organic bases exist in a nonionized and lipid-soluble form in the intestine and as a direct result of this are indeed absorbed in the intestine. It was mentioned previously that the lipid-soluble form of any substance is the preferred form for absorption. Ethylenediaminetetraacetic acid (EDTA) is thought to increase the absorption of some compounds by improving lipophilicity and thereby enhancing intestinal permeability. However, the degree of lipid solubility apparently has an upper limit since some exceedingly lipid-soluble compounds do not dissolve in the gastrointestinal contents and their absorption can be extremely low.

Not surprisingly, organic acids and bases of small molecular weight are typically absorbed by simple diffusion. Remember that gastric juices are acidic and intestinal contents are essentially neutral to very slightly basic, and the degree of lipid solubility of weak organic acids or bases varies with the proportions of populations of ionized and nonionized forms of the xenobiotic. The proportions of these populations can differ markedly within different regions of the GI tract, because of changes in the pH of the milieu. Davis and Morris reported the approximate average values of pH in different regions of the canine GI tract: anterior stomach, 5.5; posterior stomach, 3.4; proximal small intestine, 6.2; terminal small intestine, 7.5; cecum, 6.4; large intestine, 6.5; and feces, 6.2. For compounds that are organic in nature and either acidic or basic, the relative proportion of ionized and nonionized species is of paramount importance. This is best appreciated through the Henderson–Hasselbalch equation:

For a weak acid: $pKa - pH = \log \{[\text{nonionized}]/[\text{ionized}]\}$

For a weak base: $pKa - pH = \log \{[\text{ionized}]/[\text{nonionized}]\}$

A derivation of this equation is not appropriate for this text, but can be found in any biochemistry textbook. However, some examples of the application of this equation may be useful. For the case of a weak base having a $pKa = 5$ and residing in the stomach at a gastric environmental pH = 2,

$$pKa - pH = \log \{[\text{ionized}]/[\text{nonionized}]\}$$

$$5 - 2 = \log \{[\text{ionized}]/[\text{nonionized}]\}$$

$$3 = \log \{[\text{ionized}]/[\text{nonionized}]\}$$

$$10^3 = [\text{ionized}]/[\text{nonionized}]$$

$$1000 = [\text{ionized}]/[\text{nonionized}]$$

In this case, the equilibrium does not favor absorption.

For the case of a weak acid having a pKa = 4 and residing in the intestine at an intestinal environmental pH = 6,

$$\text{pKa} - \text{pH} = \log\{[\text{nonionized}]/[\text{ionized}]\}$$

$$4 - 6 = \log\{[\text{nonionized}]/[\text{ionized}]\}$$

$$-2 = \log\{[\text{nonionized}]/[\text{ionized}]\}$$

$$10^{-2} = [\text{nonionized}]/[\text{ionized}]$$

$$1/100 = [\text{nonionized}]/[\text{ionized}]$$

In this case the equilibrium does not favor absorption.

To this point we have focused on the absorptive capabilities of the GI tract and tacitly assumed the presence of no other confounding processes. However, it is important to point out that the GI tract is not simply a flexible tube capable of absorption, but is a metabolically active organ. The flow of blood from and to the GI tract serves as a vehicle for the transport of substances to the body as a whole and also as a means for the delivery of vital nutrients to the GI tract for the performance of all of its functions. Using a human as an example, the GI tract devoid of contents comprises approximately 2% of the total body weight of an average human and is very well perfused by the circulation system. In fact, the human GI tract as defined in this chapter (esophagus, stomach, small intestine, large intestine) receives approximately 20% of the total cardiac output and has a blood flow in a resting normal subject of about 1050 ml/min. To put this into perspective, this amount of blood flow is greater than that of the brain or skeletal muscle and about equal to the flows of the liver and kidney. The metabolic activities of the liver and kidney are well appreciated and so the potential for metabolism in the GI tract should not be ignored. It should be emphasized that the above figures are provided for purposes of relative comparison only and should not be taken as exact values for the canine GI tract.

This potential for metabolism leads us to mention the first pass effect. Under most circumstances, substances are absorbed into the body system via mechanisms and routes previously described. However, for some xenobiotics a first pass effect can be quite significant. In this process, xenobiotics are removed in normal fashion from the intestinal stream and then either metabolized by intestinal epithelial cells directly or hepatocytes after delivery to the liver by the portal blood supply that drains the intestinal bed. The important aspect of this process is that parent compound can be significantly reduced in amount by metabolism before it even enters the systemic circulation. Indeed, this effect can be quite substantial for some compounds and in some cases can essentially obliterate the total amount of parent compound administered.

With regard to the metabolic transformation of xenobiotics, the intestines are considered to have a moderate level of metabolic activity, equal to that of the kidney and second only in amount to that of the liver. While a variety of phase I enzymes can be found in the GI tract, the most common phase I enzymes found in the canine small intestine are from the CYP2C subfamily. The most phase II reactions that take place in the canine intestine are glucuronidation, ethereal sulfation, methylation, acetylation, and sulfation. While the first pass effect may be a formidable protection mechanism, it can at the same time present a substantial barrier to pharmacotherapy. The biotransformation of xenobiotics is addressed in more detail elsewhere in this reference.

In summary, it is fair to state that much has been learned about the principles of gastrointestinal absorption of xenobiotics from the mechanisms of absorption of nutrients, carbohydrates, proteins, and fats. Xenobiotics penetrate the gastrointestinal epithelium to a degree and facility related to the chemical structure of the substance and its physicochemical properties. Gastrointestinal absorption of xenobiotics occurs mostly by diffusion and is highly dependent upon the values of local pH within the GI tract.

A very important physicochemical property of a xenobiotic is its pKa, which governs how much of a compound will exist in a lipophilic, nonionized, and absorptive form versus a hydrophilic, ionized, nonabsorptive form at a specific pH. Keep in mind that a difference of only a single unit of pH can translate into a change of concentration of ionized versus nonionized species of one order of magnitude.

The discussion of absorption to this point has focused on the movement and transport of nutrients and xenobiotics into the system. However, what about the movement of xenobiotics out of the system? It is commonly assumed that the presence of xenobiotics, whether in parent form or not, in the feces is the result of either lack of absorption or excretion into the bile. While this is true for many compounds, it is not true for all. Indeed, for some substances, there appears to be a direct transfer from the blood through the gastrointestinal mucosal epithelium into the lumen of the GI tract. Again, passive diffusion is probably the most common mechanism for this transfer, but cellular exfoliation may well be another mechanism for the elimination of some xenobiotics into the intestinal stream. The exfoliation of gastrointestinal epithelial cells into the gastrointestinal lumen or intestinal excretion is a slow process. Accordingly, this mode is only a pathway of significance for xenobiotics that exhibit low rates of biotransformation or low rates of hepatic (biliary) or renal clearance. Not surprisingly, it has been found that as the lipophilicity of gastrointestinal contents increases, the rate of intestinal excretion increases.

Another way in which xenobiotics can enter the GI tract and be excreted in the feces is the ingestion of secretions that contain the xenobiotic. Such secretions include those that move up the tracheobronchial tree and are swallowed, secretions from salivary glands, and secretions from the stomach, intestines, liver, or pancreas. With the exception of liver secretions, these contributions are generally small amounts and of little concern; still the potential for the recirculation of xenobiotics nonetheless exists via these routes. The liver, however, can be involved in a not-so-insignificant recirculation process termed enterohepatic cycling. In this process, xenobiotics secreted into the bile and excreted into the intestinal contents are reabsorbed efficiently and quickly from the chyme and redirected via the portal blood back to the liver for secretion again into the bile. Substances can persist in this cycle for a large number of iterations. The end result of this cyclic process is that the elimination half-life of a given xenobiotic can be significantly prolonged and toxicity to the GI tract and other organs can be amplified.

GASTROINTESTINAL MOTILITY

As substances are permitted entry into the GI tract, a variety of secretions are added and for their presence to be effective, mixing must occur [12, 24, 35, 37, 43, 49, 50, 51, 58, 70, 71, 89, 92, 93, 97, 103, 109, 115, 117, 121, 130–132, 136,139, 140, 149–151, 153, 160, 161, 171, 175, 180, 183, 186–188, 190, 191, 226, 238, 239, 259, 260, 266–268, 278, 283, 284, 289, 292, 302, 307]. The proper and adequate degree of mixing of gastrointestinal contents facilitates both diges-tion and absorption. Materials must also be moved along the length of the GI tract to optimize absorption, use the different regional absorptive capabilities of the tract, and eventually eliminate the waste stream. For these activities to take place, the GI tract must be a very physically active organ.

The GI tract is in a continuous state of contractile activity, mixing ingesta via segmental contractions and then moving the material along in an aboral fashion by a series of peristaltic contractions. The overall control of these activ-ities is very complicated and not totally understood. However, it is known that contributions are made by the enteric nervous system, central nervous system, humoral agents, and muscles. The central nervous system achieves its effects by means of autonomic nerves, somatic nerves, and humoral pathways.

As described previously, the GI tract is invested with smooth muscle that extends both longitudinally down the tract and circularly enwraps it. The fibers within each bundle of muscle are interconnected via large numbers of gap junc-tions that permit the facile transfer of electrical currents and communication due to the low-resistance movement of ions from one cell to the next. Accordingly, electrical signals that initiate muscular contraction can spread readily from one muscular fiber to another. While the smooth muscle fibers are separated from one another by loose connective tissue, they are still joined together at many points, forming a woven-like mass that functions as would be seen in a syncytium. When an action potential is initiated anywhere within a muscle, it radiates outward in all directions, but more quickly along the long axis of a muscle fiber as opposed to the transverse axis of the fiber. However, the distance that the action potential travels is dependent on the excitability of the muscle. If a muscle is not in an electronically excitable state, it will not respond to stimulation. Connections also exist between the circular and longitudinal muscle layers, so that different layers can excite each other as well.

The smooth muscle of the GI tract has a slow continuous level of electrical activity taking place along its membranes. The two types of activity are slow waves and spikes. The resting membrane potential of gastrointestinal smooth muscle is not fixed and is capable of change, which can translate into changes of the motor activity of the GI tract. Gastrointestinal contractions are rhythmic in nature and the character of this rhythm is determined essentially by the frequency and character of the slow waves. The cause of slow waves is not really known, but may result from cyclical variations in the action of a sodium–potassium pump. Slow waves are not true action potentials causing muscle contraction except possibly in the stomach, but rather are slow persistent sinusoidal-like cycling changes of the resting membrane potential that can shift to become more hyperpolarized or depolarized in nature. The more depolarized the voltage about which the cycling takes place will dictate the frequency of appearance of spike potential waves that in turn stimulate muscle contraction. The intensities of contractions vary with region of the GI tract.

Spike waves are action potentials and generally occur when the resting membrane potential of gastrointestinal smooth muscle becomes more positive than approximately –40mV. Again, the more the slow wave potential rises above this level, the greater the frequency at which spike potentials occur. Spike potentials can occur at frequencies of about 1 to 10 per second and in gastrointestinal muscle are of greater duration than action potentials observed in nerve fibers by a factor of 10 to 40. It is worth noting that the mode of generation of action potentials in nerve fibers is different from that in gastrointestinal smooth muscle. In nerves, action potentials are caused by the rapid flow of extracellular sodium into the fiber, whereas in gastrointestinal smooth muscle, large amounts of calcium along with smaller amounts of sodium enter the cells.

The gates through which this flux occurs are termed calcium–sodium channels and they open and close more slowly than the channels of nerve fibers. This slowness of action explains the long duration of action potentials in gastrointestinal smooth muscle. As expected, the flux of calcium plays a significant role in muscle contraction. As noted earlier, the resting membrane voltage can also change. Under general conditions, the normal resting membrane potential is about –56 mV. Factors that can make a membrane less negative than this baseline value or more excitable are stimulation by gastrointestinal hormones, parasympathetic nerve stimulation, physical stretching of the muscle, and acetylcholine. The presence of epinephrine and norepinephrine and the stimulation of the sympathetic nerves can make a membrane more refractory or negative. It is of sufficient importance to bear repeating that the peaks of slow waves generate spike or action potentials and that the large quantities of calcium that concomitantly enter the muscle fibers cause most of the contractile activity.

The GI tract has a self-contained nervous system, known as the enteric nervous system, located in the wall of the alimentary canal, starting in the esophagus and extending through the colon, that controls gastrointestinal movements and secretion.

This system is composed of an outer or myenteric plexus and an inner or submucosal plexus. The myenteric plexus lies between the circular and longitudinal muscle layers and the submucosal plexus resides in the submucosa. Gastrointestinal movements such as the intensity of contraction, increased tonicity of contraction, rate of contractile rhythm, and velocity of conduction of excitatory waves along the GI tract wall are controlled mostly by the myenteric plexus. The myenteric plexus also releases through fiber endings vasoactive intestinal polypeptide. This inhibits intestinal sphincter muscle activity and accordingly slows the movement of gastrointestinal contents along the tract, the emptying of contents from the stomach into the intestine, and the emptying of contents from the small intestine into the large intestine.

Blood flow, secretion, local absorption, and local contraction that modulate the degree of in-folding of the gastrointestinal mucosa are controlled by the submucosal plexus. Some degree of intercommunication exists between the two systems and sympathetic and parasympathetic fibers connect with both plexuses. While the enteric nervous system can and does function independently, signals from the parasympathetic or sympathetic systems can activate or inhibit gastrointestinal functions. Stimulation of the parasympathetic nerves causes a general increase in activity of the complete enteric nervous system, enhancing the activity of most gastrointestinal functions. Stimulation of the sympathetic nerves inhibits activity of the GI tract, generally causing a decrease in the activity of most gastrointestinal functions. Sensory nerve fibers originating in the mucosal epithelium send fibers to both enteric plexuses, the vagus nerves, the paravertebral ganglia, and the spinal cord.

The stomach has three motor functions. The first of these is storage of food until it can be processed in the lower GI tract. The next is mixing food with gastric secretions to turn it into chyme. The final function is slowly emptying the chyme into the small intestine at a rate that permits adequate digestion and absorption by the small bowel. If the stomach is empty, intense contractions can occur and the contractions generally start 12 to 24 hours after the last ingestion of food. These aborally moving rhythmic peristaltic contractions in the body of the stomach can sustain themselves in tetany for up to 3 minutes. They can be influenced by low levels of blood sugar.

When the stomach contains food, constrictor or mixing waves originate in the middle portion of the stomach wall and travel toward the antrum at an approximate frequency of one every 15 to 20 seconds. As these waves move from the body to the antrum, they become ring-like constrictions of the gastric wall and their increasingly greater intensity force the gastric contents under high pressure toward the pylorus. These contractions can create forces of 50 to 70 cm of water pressure; each time a peristaltic wave moves toward the antrum, it presses firmly against the antral contents. However, the opening of the pylorus is small enough to allow only a few milliliters of chyme into the duodenum with each compressing peristaltic wave.

In its normal resting state, the pyloric sphincter usually remains sufficiently open for liquids to empty from the stomach without resistance. However, this formidable barrier prevents the passage of food into the small bowel until it has been adequately mixed. Keep in mind that as each peristaltic wave approaches the pylorus, the pyloric muscle contracts. This activity inhibits the expulsion of gastric contents into the duodenum and accordingly antral contents are ejected upstream through a peristaltic ring back toward the body of the stomach. This process is repeated over and over, permitting a great degree of mixing in the stomach and reduction of a food mass to a fluid-like consistency. As the stomach slowly begins to empty, contractions initiate further up the body of the stomach wall, gradually isolating the food into the lower portions. This mixing and pro-pelling activity is sometimes referred to as the pyloric pump.

The rate of emptying of the stomach is controlled via signals from the stomach and duodenum, with the latter providing the more significant level of control, which assures adequate digestion and absorption in the small intestine. The gastric factors that stimulate emptying of the stomach are the volume of gastric contents and the presence of the gastrin hormone. Duodenal-based factors that inhibit gastric emptying are osmolarity of the chyme, degree of distension of the duode-num, acidity of the chyme, irritation of duodenal mucosa, degradation products of proteins, and the degradation products of fats and hormones released from the small intestine (cholecystokinin, gastric inhibitory peptide, and secretin).

Similar to the stomach, the small intestine possesses muscular contracting activities that facilitate the mixing and propulsion of its contents. Segmental contractions ensure proper mixing, whereas peristaltic contractions move the chyme along the tract in an aboral direction. The mixing and propulsion are not separate activities; they overlap to a great extent. Reduced segmental activity can speed transit time while reduced peristaltic activity can prolong it. As the wall of the small bowel becomes distended, the stretching stimulates the initiation of local ring-like contractions at various locations and intervals along the small intestine. Each of these contractions resembles a hand squeezing a sausage-shaped balloon. The contractions can be isolated, irregularly spaced, regularly spaced, or weak and irregularly spaced. They occur at a frequency of about 12 per minute in the duodenum and jejunum and about 9 per minute in the ileum. The slow waves in the smooth muscle of the intestinal wall play an important role in the maintenance of segmental contracting activity, but the assistance of and contri-bution from the enteric nervous system are essential for normal function.

Peristaltic waves can occur in any part of the small intestine, producing a net aboral movement of contents at an average velocity of about 1 (0.5 to 2.0) cm/sec. Movement is somewhat faster in the more proximal segment of the small intestine. This means that 2 to 5 hours are required for chyme to enter the duodenum and reach the ileocolic sphincter. These waves are also initiated by distension of the intestinal wall and typically travel 3 to 5 cm and only rarely travel further than 10 cm. They are characterized by the formation of ring-like contractions that move aborally, pushing the intestinal contents along the long axis of the GI tract. These contractions resemble the actions of a pair of pinched fingers working to extrude toothpaste from a tube.

With the proper type of stimulation (toxins, irritation, etc.), peristaltic and segmental contractions can significantly increase in magnitude and frequency. Peristalsis moves contents along the small intestine toward eventual elimination and also spreads out the chyme along the intestinal mucosa, facilitating digestion and absorption.

Peristalsis is significantly increased after a meal and subject to both neural and hormonal control. The stimuli initiating peristalsis are the entry of chyme into the duodenum and more significantly the gastroenteric reflex. This reflex is started with distension of the stomach and impulses sent from the stomach through the myenteric plexus to and along the walls of the small intestine. Gastrin, serotonin, insulin, and cholecystokinin enhance intestinal motility; secretin and glucagon inhibit it. Other neurotransmitters have been implicated in gastrointestinal function, but little is known about their roles. These substances include somatostatin, bombesin, dopamine, adenosine triphosphate, leu-enkephalin, and met-enkephalin.

The muscularis mucosa mentioned in the section on anatomy can cause folds of varying length to appear in the intestinal mucosa. The folds increase the absorptive surface area and hence the rate of absorption. These same muscularis mucosa fibers also extend into the intestinal villi, causing them to extend or contract, again increasing or decreasing the available absorptive surface of the small intestine. Local nervous reflexes mediate the mucosal and villous contractions. The repeated cycle of villus elongation and contraction aids in the drainage of lymph from the central lacteal of the villus to the lymphatic system.

As chyme moves along the small intestine, it may eventually become blocked at the ileocolic sphincter. The consumption of an additional meal can stimulate the gastroileal reflex and propulsion of the chyme through the ileocolic sphincter valve into the large intestine, which receives approximately 1500 ml of chyme each day. The ileocolic sphincter has two main functions. The first is to prevent the backwash of colonic contents into the small intestine and the second is to prolong the residence time of intestinal contents so as to enhance absorption. The ileocolic sphincter is of sufficient strength to withstand anterograde pressures of approximately 50 cm of water.

The proximal half of the colon is designed for absorption and the distal half primarily for storage. Accordingly, the movements of the colon are very slow. Despite this sluggish nature, the same movements exhibited in the small intestine occur in the large intestine. The mixing contractions can almost momentarily obliterate the colonic lumen and the combined actions of the circular and longitudinal muscles work to persistently turn over the fecal contents, much like the tilling of a garden, constantly exposing new material to the colonic absorptive surface. Propulsive contractions progressively move the increasingly more solid fecal stream toward the rectum over a period of 8 to 15 hours. Typically about 80 to 200 ml of feces are expelled each day.

Mass movement is a modified type of peristalsis by which distal colonic contents are forced into the rectum. As the colon becomes distended, constrictive rings form and travel as they do in the small intestine to move colonic contents further along. These constrictive rings propagate for about 20 cm, with the propulsive activity lasting about 30 seconds. After 2 to 3 minutes of relaxation, the cycle begins anew. Mass movements typically last about 30 minutes and do not recur until 12 to 24 hours later. Mass movements are stimulated by the gastrocolic and duodenocolic reflexes, which in turn are initiated by distension of the stomach and duodenum, respectively. Davies and Morris reported transit times for dogs to be about 96 minutes through the stomach, approximately 110 minutes through the small intestine, and about 770 minutes through the entire length of gut.

Reference was made earlier to the enterogastric, gastrocolic, duodenocolic, and gastroileal reflexes that can affect motility of the GI tract. There are basically three types of gastrointestinal reflexes. The first group of reflexes are contained within the enteric nervous system and involve such activities as contraction, peristalsis, local effects, mixing, and secretion. The second class of reflexes travels from the wall of the gastrointestinal system to the paravertebral sympathetic ganglia and then back to the wall of the gut. These reflexes send signals over long distances and are involved in functions such as signals from the stomach to elicit evacuation of the colon. The third and last group of reflexes are cycles that involve the travel of impulses from the wall of the GI tract to the spinal cord or brain stem and then back to the gut wall. These reflexes can initiate gastric motor or secretory activity via the vagus nerves, defecation, or the sensing of pain and the development of a response to it. Pain reflexes typically invoke a general inhibition of GI tract activity. A number of reflexes such as the peritoneointestinal, vesicointestinal, renointestinal, and somatointestinal not referenced in this chapter can all inhibit gastrointestinal motility.

BACTERIAL FLORA

Any discussion of the GI tract would not be complete without some attention to its bacterial flora [26, 163, 172, 182, 185, 227, 231, 232, 253, 285]. The digestion and absorption of carbohydrates, fats, proteins, peptides, amino acids, and vitamins are all highly influenced by the presence of a healthy microbial population. Indeed, some short-chain fatty acids produced by bacteria can even stimulate secretory activity.

The resident microbial population works to prevent the colonization of pathogens and provides a low level of stimulation for the enteric immune system. Indeed, the presence of a normal, functioning, and healthy population of intestinal bacteria can affect such characteristics as intestinal motility, rate of enterocyte turnover, rate of microvillous enzyme turnover, and even the size of villi. The total population of microbial flora increases as one travels aborally from the duodenum to the colon. The maintenance of this gradient of microbial numbers is the result of many factors including patency of the ileo–ceco–colic valves, degree of intestinal motility, amounts of bacteriostatic or bacteriocidal secretions (gastric acid, pancreatic secretions, bile), substrate type, substrate availability, and intestinal lumen size and patency. An imbalance of any of these factors or extreme divergence from the normal homeostatic state can cause the overgrowth of small intestinal bacteria — an undesirable situation with adverse consequences. The loss of tolerance of the normal population of flora can initiate inflammation and dysfunction of the intestine and even neoplasia.

The normal canine small intestinal microbial population includes but is not limited to aerobes, anaerobes, and facultative anaerobes. *Proteus* spp., *Escherichia coli, Bacillus* spp., *Staphylococcus* spp., *Corynebacterium* spp., *Enterococcus* spp., *Streptococcus* spp., and Enterobacteriaceae are common aerobes. *Clostridium* and *Bacteroides* spp. are common anaerobes. A healthy dog has approximately 10^9 colony-forming units of aerobic and anaerobic bacteria per milliliter of undiluted gastrointestinal juice in the proximal portion of the small intestine. Xenobiotics, especially antibiotics, can affect both the total count of bacteria in the small intestine and also the relative populations of microbes. However resident bacterial populations in the small intestine appear to be relatively resistant to changes in the diet.

While qualitative and quantitative differences exist, microflora in animals are strikingly similar, but exceptions to this general rule have been noted. First, the number of bacteria in the canine intestinal tract exceeds by several orders of magnitude the number found in humans, so caution should be used when comparing matters impacting bacterial flora in humans and dogs. As microbes can be expected to contribute to the break-down, metabolism, and modification of xenobiotics, species differences in bacterial populations can be important. An example might be the presence of bacterial beta-glucosidase activity in the proximal portion of the small intestine. If this activity is nonexistent or significantly decreased due to low numbers of relevant microflora, the aglycone portion of a xenobiotic may not be absorbed or may be absorbed at a significantly reduced level.

The large intestine, however, contains the greatest number of bacteria of any region in the canine GI tract. Typically 10^{11} organisms can be found per gram of feces. *Streptococci* spp. *and Enterobacteria* spp. are the predominant aerobes found in the large intestine. *Lactobacilli* spp., *Clostridia* spp., *Bacteroides,* spp., and Bifidobacteria are the predominant anaerobes. However, over 90% of the microbial population in the large intestine is anaerobic. As in the small intestine, a variety of factors are necessary to maintain proper balance to prevent bacterial overgrowth and the development of ensuing pathology. These factors include normal intestinal motility, normal coating of mucus on the mucosa, adequate dietary nutrients and levels of oxygen, and bacterial interactions suitable to fostering a normal stable microbial population. The presence of xenobiotics, especially antibiotics, can upset this balance, as can increased levels of bile salts.

The microflora present in the large intestine serve an important function in the digestion of remaining undigested proteins and carbohydrates. Luminal bacteria degrade protein and carbohydrate nutrients to short-chain fatty acids like butyrate, acetate, and propionate that are quickly absorbed by the intestinal mucosa. The acetate and propionate are utilized by hepatocytes for the synthesis of triglycerides and cholesterol as well as for the production of energy. Butyric acid is the preferred energy source for colonic epithelial cells and is essential for their normal growth and function. Collectively, the short-chain fatty acids contribute to the maintenance of the acidic luminal pH. Such acidification prevents the formation of potential large intestinal corrosive agents and irritants such as ammonia, ionized bile acids, and ionized long-chain fatty acids which, if present in significant amounts, can lead to dysfunction of the large intestine and the development of pathology.

We have mentioned the potential of xenobiotics for direct killing effects on microbes in the GI tract and the development of ensuing pathology. This killing can be selective, favoring a particular species of bacterium or group or, alternatively, can be broad spectrum, thereby eradicating the bacterial population as a whole. In the former case, bacterial overgrowth can occur and lead to a loss of the homeostasis in the gut. At the other extreme is the total obliteration of bacteria. Neither of these options is desirable and both can lead to overgrowth of pathogenic organisms.

Other toxicology-related consequences should be considered with regard to xenobiotics and their potential interactions with gastrointestinal microflora. Bacteria can function in such a fashion as to produce toxic metabolites of xenobiotics and even active carcinogens. These metabolites can be very different from those found in tissues and the system of an organism as a whole and their concentrations can be highly variable. Even insignificant levels can lead to the development of notable toxicities. Alternatively, xenobiotics can be detoxified by microbes in the GI tract or even converted into other pharmacologically active metabolites with similar or different types of activities. The microbial metabolism of xenobiotics can lead to the production of metabolites that are able to undergo enterohepatic circulation, thereby resulting in increased exposure to the break-down products of the parent.

Finally, as a result of differences in the genetics and metabolic activities of varying components of the total population of gastrointestinal bacteria, different toxicity profiles may emerge and may be noted as differences in the character or degree of toxicity between species or between individuals within a species. One example is the reduction of aromatic nitro groups to aromatic amines by bacterial flora. These compounds can be goitrogenic or carcinogenic in nature.

PATHOPHYSIOLOGY AND TOXICOLOGY OF GASTROINTESTINAL TRACT

As stated earlier, the GI tract communicates with the external environment and is exposed to a wide variety of substances. Indeed, the GI tract is not surpassed by any other organ of the body in terms of exposure to a broad spectrum of materials. Because the GI tract is a dynamic organ that plays a key role in the absorption of nutrients and facilitates the passage of ingesta, digesta, chyme, and feces through the body, it finds itself very susceptible to injury via the same processes that permit it to provide nutrition.

A variety of mechanisms can damage the GI tract. They include immune reactions, enterocyte necrosis, accelerated apoptosis of epithelial cells, destruction or impairment of function of mucosal stem cells, stimulation of division of mucosal stem cells, direct cytotoxicity, genetic toxicity, corrosion, irritation, reduction in the supply of oxygen (ischemia or hypoxia), reduction in blood supply, generation of reactive oxygen moieties, hypersensitivity, damage to the enteric nervous system, compromise of the brush borders of enterocytes, enzyme inhibition, enzyme activation, disruption of intracellular signaling processes, altered permeability of the mucosal layer, destruction of the mucus barrier, increased susceptibility to acid, inhibition of production of important humoral agents (e.g., prostaglandins), stimulation of production of important humoral agents (e.g., gastrin), and alteration of transport mechanisms. Toxic exposure can also produce delayed consequences such as the development of neoplasia [3, 5, 8, 11, 17, 53, 64, 90, 108, 110, 113, 129, 135, 163, 181, 189, 211, 212, 217, 217, 225, 229 237, 240, 247, 258, 261, 263, 297, 304, 310, 312, 313].

While some agents can cause toxicity of the GI tract by means of a single mechanism, most involve multiple mechanisms that can be concurrent or sequential and can move toward single or different endpoints. Due to regional differences in structure and function within the GI tract, manifestations of toxicity can vary with the location of exposure. It is fair to state that toxic responses of the GI tract can generally be classified as inflammatory, erosive, or stimulatory. Obviously, the gross characterization of any toxic exposure depends upon a number of factors such as the duration of exposure, size of the dose, extent of gastrointestinal damage, types of cells or tissues involved in the damage, mechanism of action of the offending agent, and accommodation of injury or ability of the GI tract to implement repair in a timely fashion. At a microscopic level, the toxicity profile is dictated at least in part by the abilities of individual cells to retain viability, maintain internal homeostasis, generate energy, reseal damaged membranes, and replace lost, damaged, or nonfunctional components.

Most materials consumed, regardless of toxicity, are absorbed into the body by passing directly through enterocytes or around them via passive paracellular diffusion. This passage is not without challenge. An agent must move from the aqueous milieu of the lumen through the nonstirred water layer, mucus layer, and epithelial cells to gain access to the circulation. The physicochemical characteristics of a substance are very important to the successful navigation of this movement, with large polar molecules poorly penetrating uncompromised normal epithelium with functional tight junctions.

Tight junctions are of varying permeability, depending upon their location within the intestine, and become progressively more impermeable the farther aborally a material travels. Weak acids and bases as noted can exist in an equilibrium that permits or does not favor absorption. Electrically neutral and small molecules can quickly move around epithelial cells to accomplish absorption. While specific transporters can play important roles in absorption, a substance can be passively absorbed between epithelial cells through the tight junctions joining the cells together if no such system exists.

Moieties that gain access inside an enterocyte can be extruded via various transporter systems back into the intestinal lumen, permitted full absorption, metabolized, or eliminated. Metabolism, regardless of the site, can result in the manufacture of substances that are equally, more, or less toxic than the parent compound.

This brief review of the penetration of the gastrointestinal mucosal epithelial barrier function and associated absorptive activities serves to emphasize the complexity of gastrointestinal epithelial mucosal function and interaction. It would also appear that the profiles of toxicity of the GI tract may also be complex. The clinical signs of gastrointestinal toxicity are vomiting, diarrhea (with or without blood), and/or malabsorption. Strangely, while vomiting and diarrhea are considered primary responses to toxic agents, they also serve as the first lines of defense in protection against toxic insult.

Emesis or vomition can be a toxic response, but can also be thought of as a reflex to protect the stomach and intestines from the intromission of toxic substances and prevent deeper penetration into the alimentary canal and a greater degree of absorption [6, 153, 154, 168, 207, 262, 264, 265]. Typically associated with emesis is nausea, which is hard to assess in the canine. Typical signs of nausea in canines include excess salivation, dullness, lack of responsiveness, depression, lack of interest in food, and vomiting. Dogs are considered very susceptible to vomition and a somewhat detailed discussion is in order.

The emetic process consists of three phases: pre-ejection, retching, and ejection. In the pre-ejection portion, gastric relaxation and retrograde peristalsis occur. Retching involves the rhythmic action of respiratory muscles preparatory to the act of vomiting and involves the contraction of intercostal, abdominal, and diaphragmatic muscles and relaxation of the upper esophageal sphincter. Shivering and salivation driven by the autonomic system can accompany retching. If the activity is prolonged, behavioral changes along with the dullness and depression can occur.

These events are thought to be coordinated by a central emetic center residing in the lateral reticular formation of the middle portion of the brainstem adjacent to the chemoreceptor trigger zone in the area postrema, beneath the floor of the fourth ventricle and the vagal-fed nucleus tractus solitarius. It is important to mention no blood–brain barrier surrounds the chemoreceptor trigger zone (CTZ) and this permits persistent analysis of substances in the blood or cerebrospinal fluid by the CTZ. Upon proper stimulation, the CTZ can send signals to the emetic center to initiate the protective process of emesis. Splanchnic afferents and the vagus nerve also provide input to the emetic center along with the cerebral cortex and the vestibular apparatus generally associated with motion-related stimulation. The contribution of the cerebral cortex of the canine is not well defined, but is nonetheless felt to be involved.

The emetic center communicates via appropriate efferents to generate relevant smooth muscle, skeletal muscle, vasomotor, respiratory, and salivary activities that participate in the process of emesis. Specific efferent information sent to the GI tract results in the stimulation of retrograde duodenal contractions, retrograde gastric contractions, relaxation of the caudal esophageal sphincter, gastroesophageal reflux, opening of the proximal esophageal sphincter, and the evacuation of gastrointestinal contents.

High concentrations of norepinephrine, serotonin (5-hydroxytryptamine), acetylcholine, opioid, histamine, substance P, neurokinins, enkephalins, and dopamine receptors exist in the CTZ. Specific receptor subpopulation types within these groups are α_2 adrenergic, 5-hydroxytryptamine$_3$ (5-HT$_3$) serotinergic, M$_1$ cholinergic, H$_1$ and H$_2$ histaminergic, neurokinin 1 (NK$_1$) neurokininergic, enkephalin mu (ENK$_\mu$) and enkephalin delta (ENK) enkephalinergic, and D$_2$ dopaminergic. Associated with these neurotransmitters are various synthetic or degradative enzymes including 5-hydroxytryptophan decarboxylase, choline acetyltransferase, histidine decarboxylase, aminopeptidase, and enkephalinase, dopa decarboxylase, and dopamine-hydroxylase. The presence of all of these receptors and agonists/antagonists indicates that the emetic process is apparently very complex. Undoubtedly some sort of hierarchy exists among the myriad neurotransmitter and receptor pathways, but the relative levels of priority of the mechanisms of action are not yet unequivocally defined.

The emetic center has been found to contain primarily α_2-adrenergic (α_2) and 5-hydroxytryptamine$_{1A}$ (5-HT$_{1A}$) as the major receptors involved in the control of emesis exerted by the emetic center. The vestibular apparatus more than likely has a mixed population of histamine (H$_1$) and muscarinic (M$_1$) cholinergic receptors. Opioid (ENK$_\mu$) and benzodiazepine (ω_2) receptors are purportedly present in the cerebral cortex, but their contributions are not well recognized and may play only minor roles in the emetic process. The nucleus tractus solitarius is populated with many histamine, neurokinin (NK$_1$), and cholinergic receptors along with some 5-HT$_3$ receptors.

Specific toxins, corrosive activity, general irritation, mechanical irritation, inflammation, luminal distension, cell necrosis, accelerated apoptosis, or any loss of cells can cause emesis in the GI tract. Accordingly, many different types of receptors such as motilin (MOT), muscarinic$_2$ cholinergic (M$_2$), 5-hydroxytryptamine$_4$ (5-HT$_4$), neurokinin$_1$, and 5-hydroxytryptamine$_3$ (5-HT$_3$) are found in the GI tract. The 5-hydroxytryptamine$_3$ (5-HT$_3$) receptors more than likely play the most important role in the initiation of emesis in the GI tract. Drugs that are cytotoxic by nature bring about the release of 5-hydroxytryptamine from enterochromaffin cells in the tract. The 5-hydroxytryptamine activates 5-HT$_3$ receptors in vagal afferents that in turn stimulate the nucleus tractus solitarius, which then stimulates the emetic center. Whether the release of 5-hydroxytryptamine is associated with inflammation, irritation, corrosion, the presence of specific toxins, cell necrosis, cell loss, and luminal distension has not been unequivocally established.

The variety of motor activities performed by various parts of the GI tract that cause vomition are mediated by signals from vagal efferents and myenteric neurons. These signals cause excitation or inhibition of smooth muscle. Emptying of the stomach and intestinal transit are at least partially controlled by receptors located on myenteric neurons and gastrointestinal smooth muscle. They include neuronal-based, D_2-dopaminergic, and 5-hydroxytryptamine$_4$ receptors as well as those that are smooth muscle-based, motilin, and M_2 muscarinic cholinergic.

It is important to realize emesis can be induced in only two ways: via a humoral pathway and via a neural pathway. In the humoral pathway, the CTZ is stimulated by emetogenic substances in the blood. In the neural pathway, the emetic center can be stimulated by (1) vestibular input (motion) to the cerebellum, (2) sensory (pain, smell, sight) input to the cerebral cortex, (3) memories (fear) in the cerebral cortex, (4) mechanical stimulation such as pharyngeal gagging that sends signals through glossopharyngeal and trigeminal afferents to the nucleus tractus solitarius, and (5) vagal and sympathetic afferents from the stomach and small intestine that carry signals as a result of direct stimulation or irritation to the nucleus tractus solitarius.

With the inputs identified above, the cerebral cortex, cerebellum, and nucleus tractus solitarius can initiate activity in the emetic center that can result in vomition. Vestibular and sensory inputs as well as memory undoubtedly provide only small contributions to the emetic process of the canine. Antagonism of the of the CTZ can abolish emetic activity stimulated by the presence in blood of emetogenic substances, but emetic center antagonism, vagotomy, and sympathectomy are not helpful in abolition of emetic activity brought about by the presence of blood-borne emesis-inducing agents. Alternatively, gastrointestinal pathology or toxicity-induced emetic activity can be abolished via emetic center antagonism, sympathectomy, or vagotomy, but not by antagonism of the CTZ. This redundancy of pathways underscores the importance of this process as a method of protection. However, a complete, well defined, and uniformly accepted process for emesis has still not been defined.

Emesis may occur as a result of or in association with toxicity and also with a number of medical conditions such as infection or infectious conditions, inflammation, neoplasia, uremia, hepatic failure, hypercalcemia, septicemia, endotoxemia, systemic organ failure, hyperthyroidism, and hypoadrenocorticism. Chemical substances that can be associated with emesis include opioids, aminoglycosides, cytotoxic drugs, cholinergic mimetics, L-DOPA, bromocriptine, macrolide antibiotics, and digitalis glycosides. Radiation can also induce emesis.

Although diarrhea is a toxic response, it can also be considered a protective mechanism when potentially toxic materials evade emesis and penetrate into the GI tract beyond the stomach [38, 77, 84, 100, 159]. The pathophysiology of diarrhea can have a variety of etiologies. The onset and progression may result from many events occurring at the same time or consecutive events occurring in a sequential and dependent fashion. For example, pancreatic toxicity can lead to exocrine pancreatic insufficiency and the resulting intestinal bacterial overgrowth can lead to inadequate digestion of intestinal contents, hyperosmolarity, and irritation.

Another example is the administration of an antibiotic that can cause bacterial overgrowth or a shift in the relative proportions of populations of flora. If the *Escherichia coli* enteropathogenic bacteria take advantage of this situation, they will produce toxic amounts of a heat-stable enterotoxin that will stimulate the production of cyclic guanosine monophosphate (cGMP) in enterocytes via the activity of guanylate cyclase. cGMP in turn activates guanosine monophosphate-dependent protein kinases, resulting in a profuse secretory diarrhea. Consequently and concurrently, platelet-activating factor, prostaglandins, and leukotrienes are locally released and can contribute to the development of disturbances of permeability, intestinal motility, and malabsorption.

In any case of bacterial overgrowth, the potential exists for higher numbers of different types of microbes to bring about the bacterial degradation of enzymes admixed into the intestinal stream. If fat digestion and absorption are primarily affected, a fatty type of diarrhea or steatorrhea develops. Diarrheas of small intestinal origin are characterized by hypersecretion, altered mucosal permeability, and dysfunctional absorption or malabsorption. Diarrheas of large intestinal origin are characterized by mucosal injury, altered absorption or malabsorption, and hypersecretion.

If a substance is not completely or sufficiently expelled from the body via emetic activity or diarrhea and it establishes a presence in the GI tract, a variety of responses in addition to vomiting and diarrhea may be manifest. In some cases, generalized responses typical of the entire length of the GI tract may ensue. In other cases, the responses may be regionally specific. These responses generally can occur in conjunction with or exclusive of vomiting or diarrhea. However, vomiting and diarrhea commonly develop as each pathogenic mechanism pursues its course. Brief discussions of these responses follow [10, 25, 30, 32, 34, 36, 39, 62, 63, 74, 85, 104–106, 114, 118, 128, 137, 144, 146, 156, 169, 173, 176, 179, 194–197, 208, 210, 231, 236, 257, 269, 286, 294, 301, 305].

As stated previously, the mucosa of the GI tract comprises a protective barrier to external insult, while at the same time performing functions vital to complete digestion and efficient absorption. As part of its mucosal population the GI tract has extensive areas containing rapidly dividing stem cells. This is strange because of the hostile environment in which these cells reside. Other rapidly dividing stem cells in the body such as the hematopoietic cells of the marrow and sperm precursors in the testes exist in highly protected environments. However, despite this lack of protection, the stem cells and the mucosa of the GI tract are not as frequently sites of toxic injury as one might expect. Some possible explanations for this finding are the fact that intestinal contents are dilute, a protective mucus layer covers the entire mucosa, epithelial cell membranes are enriched with membrane strengthening glycosphingolipids, mucosal cell lifetimes are relatively short, and the large total surface area permits frequent and intimate contact of xenobiotics with cells capable of bringing about detoxifying biotransformation.

The effectors of biotransformation can be membrane-bound or cytosolic in location and comprise a variety of different types. Despite these protective mechanisms, if irritation of the mucosa does occur, increased levels of prostaglandins can be produced; they protect the mucosal cells by preserving blood flow and stimulating the secretion of bicarbonate into the small intestine. If mucosal cells are not terminally damaged, they can retain viability through a process of resealing their damaged membranes. In general, mucosal cells are very effective in modulating the basal rate of mucosal cell proliferation so as to maintain a fully competent mucosal epithelial barrier. Indeed, in the presence of toxic substances, the lifetime of an enterocyte is reduced and with the passage of a toxic threat, the parameters of epithelial mucosal replacement return to normal within 72 hours.

Toxic substances can cause the losses or deaths of enterocytes. Regardless of the cause, losses of cells from the epithelial population can impede the overall ability of the GI tract to transport chloride ion, conduct sodium–glucose co-transportation, and other aspects of absorption or secretion that are dependent on cellular signal transduction pathways. These activities are mediated by opioid, norepinephrine, 5-hydroxytryptamine, acetylcholine, and prostaglandin E_2 receptors located on enterocyte membranes.

Disruption of the intestinal mucosal barrier can result in a loss of tolerance and resistance of the intestinal epithelium to acids, bacteria, and enzymes, resulting in the development of inflammation, corrosion, ulcer formation, ischemia, and cytotoxicity. In cases of dysfunction and malabsorption in the small intestine, substances that are susceptible to fermentation are moved along to the large intestine, where they are converted to products that exhibit a greater degree of osmotic activity. This activity leads to the damage of large intestinal mucosa with subsequent inflammation. Mucosal damage results in the development of altered mucosal permeability and the exudation of fluids into the intestinal lumen. Inflammation leads to the release of prostaglandins, which in turn stimulates the release of histamine and the secretion of electrolytes. The consequences of inflammation include altered absorption or malabsorption and the development of altered gastrointestinal motility.

Damage to the brush borders of enterocytes can occur as a result of direct toxicity, inflammation, bacterial overgrowth, or enzyme inhibition. Anaerobic bacteria are extremely proficient in causing destruction of the brush borders and associated enzymes and transport proteins. Brush border damage can result in maldigestion, dysfunctional absorption, and possible bacterial overgrowth with complications of fermentation and the development of osmotic diarrhea.

Intestinal hypersensitivity can evoke the onset of diarrhea via the initiation of inflammation and the production of a wide variety of different chemical mediators. This topic is more completely discussed elsewhere in the section addressing immunology of the GI tract [200].

Inflammation or inflammatory response can occur as the sole component or complication of a toxic response of the GI tract and has been implicated in the development of diarrhea and malabsorption. The development of inflammation should be no surprise, considering the hostile environment that exists throughout the total length of the lumen of the GI tract. It contains damaging enzymes, acids, and millions of bacteria that can speed the development of serious lesions, most commonly seen as ulcers. Intestinal inflammation can be initiated by any of a number of factors including bacterial overgrowth, epithelial irritation or abrasion, cell necrosis, cell loss, or the presence of specific directly toxic agents.

While inflammatory responses associated with lesions of a pure toxicologic origin tend to not be severe, the complication of insult due to the persistent presence of acids, enzymes, and bacteria can radically change that pattern. Inflammation of the stomach is generally referred to as gastritis and that of the large intestine as colitis. Small intestinal inflammation is generally referred to as enteritis, but if regional specificity is found, it may be termed duodenitis, jejunitis, or ileitis. Stated simply, the various formed elements of the blood combined with appropriate levels of a whole host of chemical mediators work in a synergistic fashion to create an inflammatory response in the epithelial mucosa and submucosa. The inflammatory response incurs the presence of cellular infiltrates, accumulation of fluid (localized edema), and the alteration of epithelial barrier efficiency, intestinal motility, and mucosal permeability.

Inflammation in the GI tract is characterized by alterations in vascular diameter that lead to altered blood flow to the affected area, structural changes in the microvasculature that permit plasma proteins to leave the circulation (exudates or transudates), emigration of leukocytes from the microcirculation, accumulation of leukocytes at the focus of injury or insult, activation of leukocytes, secretion of large amounts of mucus, and development of ulcers, bleeding, and lymphoid hyperplasia. It should be obvious that pain and loss of function are involved. Loss of function can include the impairment of many different mechanistic processes and the severity of loss of function can be directly proportional to the severity of inflammation and the total amount of tissue damage sustained. Inflammation can be acute or chronic in nature and can be characterized by the populations of cells accumulating in the area of interest.

Chronic inflammation usually involves large numbers of lymphocytes, macrophages, and plasma cells in the affected area. Levels of arachidonic acid metabolites from the cyclooxygenase and lipoxygenase pathways become elevated during inflammation. Thromboxane A_2 formed by platelets is one of these compounds and is a potent vasoconstrictor that can bring about extensive mucosal damage as a result of induced hypoxia, especially in the presence of the taurocholate bile acid. Vascular thrombosis and local infarcts can also result from increased levels of thromoxane A_2, that cause aggregations of platelets. Leukotrienes are additional products of the arachidonic cascade and also promote vasoconstriction and decreased supply of oxygen. At a sufficient level of hypoxia or even ischemia, cells can become sloughed off the basement membranes and the formation of ulcers initiated. However, prostaglandins, prostacyclins, and lipoxins increase mucosal blood flow and improve the supply of oxygen, counteracting the oxygen deprivation actions of other compounds. It is easy to see that this process has a delicate balance that can be readily tipped to the disadvantage of the integrity of the GI tract.

Regardless of the cause, inflammation can involve the production of reactive oxygen species. While these free radicals can provide defensive protective effects, they can also create toxicity in the GI tract. Neutrophils and macrophages produce hypochlorous acid and hydroxyl, superoxide, and peroxyl radicals. Neutrophils, thrombocytes, and vascular endothelial cells produce nitric oxide. The generation of reactive oxygen species is an ongoing process in all tissues, but moieties are generated at very low levels and in the presence of protective measures. If the levels of reactive oxygen species rise above that for which adequate control can be provided, tissue damage naturally occurs.

Xenobiotics and the processes of inflammation can overwhelm the intracellular enzymes (catalase, superoxide dismutase, and glutathione(SH) peroxidase) and extracellular fluid-based antioxidants (vitamin A, vitamin E, selenium, β-carotenes, ascorbic acid, and α-tocopherols) normally present to prevent or limit the degree of oxidative damage to tissues and cells. Sequelae to reactive oxygen species include altered blood flow, alterations of vascular permeability, direct cell toxicity, cell death, fluid secretion into the intestinal lumen, and cell loss.

When the accelerated loss of enterocytes from villi or the reduced supply of enterocytes from stem cells located in the bottoms of intestinal crypts occurs, atrophy of the villi and hence total available absorptive surface area occurs. Toxicity can target mature cells, maturing cells, or stem cells located deep in the intestinal crypts. While cells can make accommodations to preserve the intestinal barrier and absorptive functions, such actions occur at the price of loss of absorptive function and capacity. The viral infections of dogs attract the most attention to this aspect of the development of diarrhea, but any substance that directly or indirectly results in the denudation of cells from a villus will produce the same end result, diarrhea. Immunosuppressive drugs such as azathioprene, cyclophosphamide, vincristine, and glucocorticoids can all cause severe atrophy of villi. Interestingly, some of these same compounds can facilitate epithelial cell renewal; the type of end result is dose-related and the undesirable result occurs only at high doses.

Enterocytes located on villi can in the face of decreasing numbers alter their morphology to cover or occupy a greater area over the basement membrane. Indeed, cells residing at the edges of ulcers and erosions are also stimulated to restore the gastrointestinal barrier by spreading out or migrating over vacant basal lamina. This is accomplished by means of an array of suitably anchored actin microfilaments that permit cells to become taller, plumper, thinner, broader, or flatter. These individual cellular changes working in concert with changes in the shape and extension of individual villi brought about by threads of smooth muscle located in the villous lamina propria work to preserve epithelial barrier integrity. Failure to maintain this barrier can result in severe inflammation and deleterious changes.

Not unlike other organs of the body that are engaged in substantial activities, the mucosa of the GI tract requires a persistent supply of oxygenated blood. Restriction of this flow can have disastrous consequences, including cell death and the complete sloughing of the gastrointestinal mucosa. The blood supply to the GI tract was discussed earlier. The blood flow is controlled by the central nervous system by means of sympathetic and parasympathetic nerves and also by the enteric nervous system, autoregulation, and sensory neurons contiguous to local blood vessels. A variety of neurotransmitters can bring about either vasoconstriction (norepinephrine, adenosine triphosphate, neuropeptide Y) or vasodilation (calcitonin gene-related peptide and vasoactive intestinal peptide).

Autacoids can also function in the control of flows and they include vasodilators such as nitric oxide, prostaglandin E_2, prostacyclin, and histamine and vasoconstrictors such as leukotriene C_4 and thromboxane A_2. Autacoids arise from vascular endothelial cells, smooth muscle endothelial cells, mast cells, and platelets.

It is important to appreciate that sensory nerves play an important role in the regulation of gastrointestinal blood flow. Calcitonin gene-related peptide and vasoactive intestinal peptide, both of which cause vasodilation, can be released from sensory nerves with stimulation. Calcitonin gene-related peptide is considered to be a major contributor to the development of increased gastric mucosal blood flow associated with increased levels of nitric oxide. Increased blood flow is associated with increased oxygen supply and is therefore thought to be connected with the protection of the gastrointestinal mucosa from injury.

When speaking of the GI tract, we naturally think of nutrition, but seldom consider water a nutrient. Water is essential for life, and death occurs much more rapidly in its absence than it occurs in the absence of food. Two very important functions of the GI tract are the absorption of water and also the secretion of aqueous fluid. The fluxes of water balance strongly favor absorption and the consequences of the development of diarrhea for any organism are simple: dehydration and electrolyte imbalance. The dehydration results from increased secretion of fluid into the intestinal lumen or decreased absorption of fluid from the intestinal stream or a combination of both. In any event, losses of extracellular and intracellular fluids from the body follow.

With regard to electrolyte imbalance, bicarbonate ions are lost in the diarrhea, which leads to an increase in the anion gap (difference between positive and negative charges in the body) and an accumulation of intracellular hydrogen ion with the development of acidosis. The increasing amounts of positively charged hydrogen ion cause the shedding and decrease in levels of intracellular potassium ion. The reduction in the level of potassium impairs the homeostasis of existing electrochemical gradients and the accumulation of intracellular hydrogen ion changes pH and accordingly alters the levels of function of many physiologic enzymes. All of these changes work collectively and synergistically to compromise the functions of cells, tissues, organs, and the system as a whole. As extracellular potassium levels increase, elimination of potassium is enhanced. Hyperkalemia can provoke cardiac arrest.

Neoplasia is not a common problem with laboratory canines and will not be discussed in detail here. However, it can produce diarrhea as a result of obstruction-induced fluid secretion or the release from tumors of physiologically active substances like histamine, gastrin, or 5-hydroxytryptamine [7, 9, 19, 20, 27, 40, 48, 55, 56, 122, 148, 218–221]. These chemical mediators can also cause changes that result in intestinal bacterial overgrowth, reduction in normal absorptive surface area, or exudation of proteins and lipids. Neoplasia is usually the result of exposure to agents that bring about altered states of proliferation of gastrointestinal mucosa. Mechanisms can involve hyperproliferation, promotion, and alterations of apoptosis.

Impairment of the flow of lymph as a result of inflammation or some advanced states of hypertrophy in the intestinal tract can lead to the development of diarrhea. Inadequate lymphatic drainage from the intestine secondary to right-sided heart failure can also lead to the development of diarrhea.

Constipation is the opposite of diarrhea, cannot be considered a protective activity, and can present a significant toxicologic or pathophysiologic event [303]. Indeed, constipation is one of two major toxicologic or pathophysiologic conditions of the colon or large intestine; the other is diarrhea. Constipation is characterized by lack of defecation, reduced defecation, painful defecation, or the passage of dry or concrete-like feces. The presence of blood in the stool resulting from mucosal irritation due to abrasion from the hardened intestinal stream is an additional and not infrequent clinical sign. Constipation is usually a transient event. If it becomes persistent or is irreversible, it is referred to as obstipation.

Obstipation can be associated with the permanent loss of function and can lead to the development of a condition known as megacolon or toxic megacolon, in which the body can begin to absorb toxic substances from the static fecal stream. The pathophysiology of this condition is not entirely understood. It appears to be neurally based, but could also be the result of impairment of smooth muscle (longitudinal and circular) function. Nerves of the autonomic or enteric nervous systems can be affected. In cases where megacolon has developed, no gross or histological findings are observed, but smooth muscle develops a weaker level of tone when compared to normal smooth muscle upon stimulation by acetylcholine, substance P, and cholecystokinin. The current view is that megacolon possibly results from a disturbance in the intracellular cascade of events that occur subsequent to occupancy of a membrane-bound receptor, resulting in weaker contractile activity.

Conditions or agents associated with constipation are inflammation of colonic epithelium, nerve dysfunction, myenteric plexus dysfunction, dehydration, hypokalemia, hypocalcemia, hypercalcemia, hypothyroidism, nutritional secondary hyperparathyroidism, barium sulfate, phenothiazines, cholinergic antagonists, diuretics, and opioid agonists.

The production of mucus and fluid is a benchmark response of toxicity that can occur throughout the entire length of the GI tract and is typically the result of increased levels of production of normal processes previously described in detail. Both responses are protective as well as toxic in nature.

Enterocytes possess a variety of different types of receptors on their surfaces. Some of these receptors appear to be specific for select toxins, such as that expressed by *Vibrio cholera*. The reason for this is unknown, but the disruption of intracellular signal transduction systems typically results in the development of a secretory diarrhea. This diarrhea is a function of both fluid secretion by enterocytes and nerve-mediated alterations of intestinal motility.

The GI tract is heavily invested with a nervous supply as previously described and has its own myenteric nervous system. Neural function in the GI tract is very complex and involves more than simple sensation and the stimulation of motor activities. The loss, impairment, or stimulation of motor function affects the efficiency of the digestive process as well as absorption. However, nerves are also intimately involved in the regulation of regional blood flow and the release of substances essential for proper digestion and absorption. Accordingly, neural damage can serve as a prelude to the development of diarrhea and malabsorption.

A variety of enzymes are present in the luminal space of the GI tract, in the mucosal brush borders, and in the mucosal epithelial cells. In the presence of injury or inflammation, even more enzymes can be added to the mix from cells such as neutrophils. These latter enzymes can include gelatinases, elastases, and collagenases that can bring about major structural damage to the scaffolding of the GI tract upon which the mucosal epithelium rests. In conditions of toxicity, enzymes can be activated or inhibited and these alterations can lead to the development of gastrointestinal pathology. As discussed previously, many enzymes are secreted in an inactive form, awaiting a proper set of conditions for activation. For example, reactive oxygen species are able to avert normal processes and are capable of prematurely converting inactive enzymes to active forms. This alternate pathway and avoidance of normal control mechanisms can predispose the gastrointestinal mucosa to enzymatic damage.

SPECIFIC TOXIC AGENTS

The final portion of this chapter includes a number of examples that demonstrate toxicity to and the responses of the GI tract to the presence of a variety of toxic agents. While the list of causative substances is by no means complete and the mechanisms of pathophysiology not all inclusive, the wide range of substances and responses serve to underscore the complexity of an organ system that does not attract the attention given to higher profile organs such as the heart, liver, hematopoietic, and central nervous systems.

Arsenic-containing compounds, when ingested, are readily absorbed by the mucosal epithelium of the intestine [241, 245]. After this occurs, enterocytes can rapidly die and are shed into the intestinal lumen. If this accelerated loss of enterocytes is of sufficient magnitude that normal protective compensatory actions cannot permit the maintenance of a complete, intact integral epithelial cell barrier, areas of exposed basement membrane on the villi will develop. This exposure will lead to an altered state of permeability of the villi, with movement of exudates, transudates, and blood from the circulation into the intestinal lumen. This significant influx of fluid into the intestine creates distension of the lumen that stimulates increased motor activity with associated pain and diarrhea. The normal replacement of cells is hampered by the persistent presence of arsenic; barring complications, the gastrointestinal epithelium will eventually be replaced by normal reparative processes.

Arsenates work by competing with phosphate ions, uncoupling oxidative phosphorylation and disrupting the production of energy necessary for the performance of normal enterocyte functions and cellular homeostasis. Arsenites react with the sulfhydryl groups in proteins, thereby altering active sites and the necessary specific three-dimensional structures required for activity. For example, arsenites inhibit alpha-keto oxidases that are involved in the oxidation of pyruvate. The function of lipoic acid is also impaired. Lipoic acid is an essential coenzyme for both pyruvic acid oxidase and alpha-glutaric acid oxidase. Elemental arsenic induces vasodilation and vascular endothelial damage, and organic pentavalent arsenic compounds may interfere with the functions of vitamins B_1 and B_6.

We are all familiar with the toxicity caused by exposure to lead as manifested in the central nervous, hematopoietic, and skeletal systems [255]. The gastrointestinal toxicity of lead is based primarily upon its ability to inhibit various enzyme systems. It too has an affinity for thiol groups and is also capable of competing with zinc and calcium in zinc- and calcium-dependent enzyme systems. Lead interferes with DNA transcription factors by binding to cysteine residues.

Lead can also interfere with the calcium-mediated exocytosis of neurotransmitters. Protein kinase C, a calcium-dependent enzyme system that regulates a variety of cellular activities including cell growth, is also adversely impacted by lead. While acute exposures to lead can result in vomiting and abdominal pain, chronic exposures can result in the development of constipation, most likely secondary to reduced motility. The reduction in motility is most likely due to the competition of lead with calcium in the contractile process.

Heavy metals can exhibit general corrosive effects on the mucosal epithelium of the GI tract. Iron, for example, can cause severe ulceration and erosion of the stomach lining with resulting dramatic losses of fluid into the lumen. The general themes of toxicity for agents of this type appear to be corrosion and enzyme inhibition.

Cholera toxin, although not a xenobiotic, is still considered a classical gastrointestinal toxin [14, 52, 142, 152, 279]. A discussion of its mode of action is valuable from the perspective of illustrating the consequences of alteration of intracellular signaling pathways. Cholera toxin is composed of a catalytic peptide unit (A) and five smaller peptide units (B). The B peptides bind to carbohydrates on G_{M1} gangliosides on the surfaces of intestinal epithelial cells. After binding, peptide A is delivered into a cell via calveolar-mediated endosomal entry. Upon entry into the cytoplasm, peptide A is cleaved by breakage of a disulfide bond into two fragments, A_1 and A_2. The A_1 fragment is the important catalytic component and is involved with the development of pathology. A_1 interacts with 20-kDa cytosolic proteins called ADP ribosylation factors. The resulting ADP ribosylation factor–A_1 complex catalyzes the ADP ribosylation of a 49-kDa G protein (G_s) which, upon binding with nicotinamide adenine dinucleotide (NAD) and guanosine triphosphate (GTP), leads to the generation of an activated G_s that then binds to and stimulates adenylate cyclase.

The ADP-ribosylated G_s is permanently in an active GTP-bound state, resulting in the persistent activation of adenylate cyclase. The activated adenylate cyclase generates high levels of intracellular cyclic adenosine monophosphate (cAMP) from adenosine triphosphate (ATP). cAMP stimulates the secretion of chloride and bicarbonate ions into the lumen of the intestine along with associated sodium ions and water, but sodium and chloride reabsorption also appear to be inhibited as part of this pathogenesis.

Cholera toxin also exerts effects on the enteric nervous system, with subsequent alterations of gut motility and additional changes in the mucosal transport of fluid and electrolytes. It is important to note that because the intestinal epithelium remains intact and essentially competent, most absorptive processes remain functional and competent as does the barrier function.

Nonsteroidal anti-inflammatory drugs (NSAIDs) in general are organic acids and local gastrointestinal tissue damage is caused as a result of the direct contact of dissolved drug with the gastric mucosa [29, 44, 69, 155, 164, 177, 184, 193, 206, 216, 223, 275]. NSAIDs increase gastric cell wall permeability and can uncouple oxidative phosphorylation, which collectively or individually can result in impaired cellular homeostasis and the development of cellular edema and apoptosis. While all areas of the GI tract may theoretically be susceptible to the development of NSAID-induced lesions, the most frequent sites of damage are the stomach and duodenum.

Ulcers (peptic) are the classic lesions with associated blood, fluid, and protein loss into the gastrointestinal stream. In advanced cases, ulcers can even progress into perforations of the gastrointestinal wall. However, the most important mechanism associated with exposure to NSAIDs and the development of subsequent pathology is the reversible inhibition of the cyclooxygenase-1 (COX-1) enzyme. The inhibition of COX-1 by NSAIDs initiates the development of pathology by blocking the production of prostaglandins in gastric tissues, which results in the decreased production of mucus and bicarbonate, the increased production of acid, and decreased flow of blood into the gastric mucosa. An underlying *Helicobacter pylori* infection can potentially worsen the toxic profile.

The inhibition of COX-2 activity, however, is generally associated with a lessening of the adverse effects that can be brought about with a triggering of the cyclooxygenase cascade. NSAIDs that are specific for inhibition of COX-2 activity provide the most beneficial and least troublesome toxicologic profiles.

The cyclooxygenase system (COX) is responsible for the synthesis and production of prostaglandins. Cyclooxygenases exist in two forms, COX-1 and COX-2, and both possess cyclooxygenase and hydroxyperoxidase activities. COX-1 is a constitutive, noninducible enzyme normally present in the stomach, intestine, and platelets. It functions in the synthesis of platelet aggregation agents and the regulation of regional blood flow, thereby providing gastrointestinal mucosal protection. In contrast, COX-2 is an inducible enzyme; its activity increases in response to a variety of inflammatory stimuli. Indeed, the prostanoids produced by COX-2 are segments of a typical inflammatory response. In general, COX-mediated prostaglandin synthetic activity can be initiated by a variety of stimulators including physical trauma, chemical exposure, cell proliferation, and inflammation. Arachidonic acid is the substrate for the COX enzyme system and is generated when phospholipase A_2 splits arachidonic acid from the phospholipid membrane of the cell.

Cyclooxygenases produce the unstable intermediate prostaglandin (PGG_2) that is quickly hydrolyzed via the same enzyme to prostaglandin H_2 (PGH_2). PGH_2 is unstable and rapidly metabolized by tissue-specific isomerases to multiple prostanoids such as prostacyclin (PGI_2), thromboxane A_2 (TXA_2), prosta-glandin D_2 (PGD_2), prostaglandin E_2 (PGE_2), and prostaglandin F_{2a} (PGF_{2a}). These prostanoids stimulate specific G protein-coupled receptors to induce various effects that range from protection of the GI tract to the aggregation of platelets (thrombus formation). PGI_2 is associated with vasodilation and the inhibition of platelet aggregation, while PGD_2, PGE_2, and PGF_{2a} are associated with vasodilation and potentiation of edema. TXA_2 causes aggregation of platelets and vaso-constriction.

It is worth noting that thromboxane A_2 may also be a mediator in the development of gastrointestinal food-allergen hypersensitivity. The COX-1-mediated production of prostacyclin PGI_2 and prostaglandin PGE_2 is considered protective of the gastrointestinal mucosa, essentially because of the vasodilation induction properties of the two compounds and the resulting ability to preserve or enhance mucosal blood flow and oxygen supply; the initiation of COX-2 activity is considered deleterious.

Mycotoxins are secondary fungal metabolites that exert toxic effects on a variety of systems and a broad spectrum of species [123, 291]. They are typically found as contaminants in grains and grain-based products. Although a variety of different types of mycotoxins exist, we will discuss only one, the trichothecenes.

Trichothecenes are produced by *Fusarium* spp. and include such compounds as deoxynivalenol (vomitoxin), T-2 toxin, and diacetoxyscirpenol. Gastrointesinal toxicity is typically manifest as vomiting, bloody diarrhea, dehydration, and weight loss. Trichothecenes generally inhibit protein synthesis, which eventually causes cell death. Deoxynivalenol can delay gastric emptying and intestinal motor activity, possibly through a serotonin-mediated pathway. The actively dividing tissues of the GI tract are most susceptible to the actions of T-2. It is important to note that even for certified feeds, mycotoxin presence and levels are not routinely determined by analysis.

The 5-fluorouracil (5-FU) pyrimidine analog is a halogenated derivative of pyrimidine and an antineoplastic agent of the antimetabolite class [125, 201]. 5-FU requires enzymatic conversion to the nucleotide in order to exert its cytotoxic activity. Incorporation of 5-FU into both RNA and DNA occurs, but the relevance or importance of the incorporation is unclear because normal excision repair processes may well remove the halogenated moiety before any toxic consequence can be elicited. Alternatively, incorporation of 5-FU into RNA causes toxicity resulting from the exertion of major effects on both the processing and functions of RNA, thereby inhibiting cell division.

Accordingly, the rapidly dividing cells of the GI tract are ideal targets for these types of compounds.

Steroid toxicity closely resembles the toxicity manifest by NSAIDs because steroids inhibit the function of phospholipase A_2, which generates arachidonic acid, the substrate for the COX enzymatic system described above. In the absence of substrate, adequate supplies of prostacyclin and prostaglandins cannot be sustained, and the beneficial and protective effects of prostaglandins are missing; this leaves the gastrointestinal mucosa susceptible to injury and compromise.

The ingestion of a variety of plants, plant materials, and plant extracts is followed by the development of nausea, vomiting, diarrhea, and bloody diarrhea.

The most common mechanism of gastrointestinal toxicity is direct irritation of the gastric or intestinal mucosa. Another mechanism for plant-induced gastrointestinal toxicity is antimitosis. Colchicine is probably the best known cause of this mechanistic type of toxicity. The antimitotic action is brought about by the blockage of formation of microtubules and subsequent failure to form a competent mitotic spindle.

Finally, glycoproteins, a group of compounds in a variety of plants, can interact with select carbohydrate moieties present on the membranes of mucosal epithelial cells. Once binding is complete, the function of the brush borders on the luminal surfaces of enterocytes is altered and a nonspecific inhibition of all absorption gradually develops. Among these glycoproteins is a group of compounds called lectins. Upon entry into cells, lectins inhibit protein synthesis, causing cell death.

The classic gastrointestinal toxin group includes the acetylcholinesterase inhibitors. Acetylcholine is a neurotransmitter present at synaptic and neuroeffector endings of cholinergic motor and secretomotor neurons of the enteric nervous system. Inhibition of the acetylcholinesterase enzyme leads to an accumulation of acetylcholine at synapses or effector sites and resultant persistent stimulation. Increased motor activity is the result of the interaction of acetylcholine with M_3 muscarinic receptors and the increase in gastric and intestinal secretions results from stimulation of both M_1 and M_3 muscarinic receptors. Inhibition of acetylcholinesterase activity causes the secretion of large volumes of fluids and electrolytes into the GI tract, with the development of a profuse watery diarrhea accompanied by a severe cramping pain.

Sucralfate is an oral antiulcer agent that acts by forming a protective barrier over the site of an ulcer and consists of a complex of sucrose octasulfate and polyaluminum hydroxide. In the local environment of the stomach, polymerization and cross-linking occur and result in the formation of a sticky, yellow-white gel that combines with proteinaceous exudates in the stomach to form an adherent barrier preventing the contact of gastric acid with the lesion, compromising the integrity of the mucosal barrier. Continued exposure can result in the slow release of aluminum into the system and the development of constipation by a mechanism that is unclear.

Ethanol is commonly used as a vehicle or excipient in a variety of concentrations and along with other alcohols can directly induce toxicity on the mucosal epithelial cells of the GI tract. This toxicity is characterized by the formation of hemorrhagic erosions in the gastric mucosa and is chiefly the result of a disordering of the lipid bilayer of the cell membrane, which results in altered membrane fluidity and subsequently cell damage, loss of cellular homeostasis, and cell death. Vascular injury can also develop concurrently as a result of direct cytotoxicity, which then leads to the degranulation of mast cells, release of leukotrienes, and enhanced mucosal permeability. In the presence of a sound oxygen supply and good flow of blood, restitution of the mucosal epithelial cells can occur on a timely basis.

Continued exposure to ethanol can result in the increased production of various growth factors such as epidermal growth factor that possibly protect the gastric mucosa from injury by stimulating the rate of cell proliferation, and also generate susceptibility to the possible development of neoplasia. Exposure to ethanol can inhibit the secretion of bicarbonate ion, impair the synthesis of mucus, increase luminal sodium ion concentration, enhance the permeability of the mucosa, permit the back-diffusion of hydrogen ion, and in a dose-response fashion deplete intracellular stores of glutathione. At high concentrations, exposure to ethanol can be associated with increased levels of synthesis of prostacyclin and prostaglandins that possibly offer protective effects to the gastrointestinal mucosa after ethanol-induced injury.

REFERENCES

1. Abou-Donia, MB, El-Masry, EM, and Abu-Qare, AW. Metabolism and toxicokinetics of xenobiotics, in *Handbook of Toxicology*, 2nd ed., Derelanko, MJ and Hollinger, MA, Eds., CRC Press, Boca Raton, 2002.
2. Adibi, SA. The oligopeptide transporter (Pept-1) in human intestine: biology and function. *Gastroenterology* 113, 332, 1997.
3. Allan, SG et al. *Cancer Res* 46, 3569, 1986.
4. Allen, A, Flemstrom, G, Garner, A, and Kivilaakso, E. Gastroduodenal mucosal protection. *Physiol Rev* 73, 823, 1993.
5. Allen, A and Garner, A. Mucus and bicarbonate secretion in the stomach and their possible role in mucosal protection. *Gut* 21, 249, 1980.
6. Andrews, PLR, Rapeport, WG, and Sanger, GJ. Neuropharmacology of emesis induced by anti-cancer therapy. *Trends Pharmacol Sci* 9, 334, 1988.
7. Anti, M et al. Effect of omega-3 fatty acids on rectal mucosal cell proliferation in subjects at risk for colon cancer. *Gastroenterology* 103, 883, 1992.
8. Appleton, GV et al. Effect of dietary calcium on the colonic luminal environment. *Gut* 32, 1374, 1991.
9. Appleton, GVN et al. Inhibition of intestinal carcinogenesis by dietary supplementation with calcium. *Br J Surg* 74, 523, 1987.
10. Arends, MJ and Wyllie, AH. Apoptosis: mechanisms and roles in pathology. *Int Rev Exp Pathol* 32, 223, 1991.
11. Aungst, B and Shen, DD. Gastrointestinal absorption of toxic agents, in *Gastrointestinal Toxicology*, Rosman, K and Hanninen, O., Eds., Amsterdam, Elsevier, 1986.
12. Azpiroz, F and Malagelada, JR. Intestinal control of gastric tone. *Am J Physiol* 249, G501, 1985.
13. Banks, WJ. *Applied Veterinary Histology*, 3rd ed., Mosby Year Book, 1993.
14. Banno, Y, Kobayashi, T, Kono, H et al. Biochemical characterization and biologic actions of two toxins (D-1 and D-2) from *Clostridium difficile*. *Rev Infect Dis* 6 (Suppl. 1), S11, 1984.
15. Bard, P. in *Medical Physiology*, 10th ed., Henry Kimpton, London, 1956.

16. Barker, IA et al. The alimentary system, in *Pathology of Domestic Animals*, Jubb, KVF et al., Eds., Academic Press, New York, 1993.

17. Barnett, HL, McNamara, H, Schultz, S, and Tomposett, R. Renal clearances of sodium penicillin G, procaine penicillin G, and inulin in infants and children. *Pediatrics* 3, 418, 1949.

18. Barnett, RJ. Demonstration with the electron microscope of end products of histochemical reactions in relation to the fine structure of cells. *Exp Cell Res Suppl* 7, 65, 1959.

19. Baron, JA and Greenberg, ER. Could aspirin really prevent colon cancer? *New Engl J Med* 325, 1644, 1991.

20. Baron, JA et al. Calcium supplementation and rectal mucosal proliferation: a randomized controlled trial. *J Natl Cancer Inst* 87, 1303, 1995.

21. Basora, N et al. Relation between integrin $\alpha7\beta1$ expression in human intestinal cells and enterocytic differentiation. *Gastroenterology* 113, 1510, 1997.

22. Bates, TR and Gibaldi, M. Gastrointestinal absorption of drugs, in *Current Concepts in the Pharmaceuticals Sciences: Biopharmaceutics,* Swarbrick, J., Ed., Lea & Febiger, Philadelphia, 1970.

23. Batt, RM and Morgan, JO. Role of serum folate and vitamin B_{12} concentrations in the differentiation of small intestinal abnormalities in the dog. *Res Vet Sci* 32, 17, 1982.

24. Bayguinov, O et al. Parallel pathways mediate inhibitory effects of vasoactive intestinal polypeptide and nitric oxide in canine fundus. *Br J Pharmacol* 126, 1543, 1999.

25. Bertam, T. Gastrointestinal tract, in *Handbook of Toxicologic Pathology*, Haschek, WM and Rousseaux, CG, Eds., Academic Press, Boston, 1991.

26. Binder, HJ and Sandle, GI. Electrolyte absorption and secretion in the mammalian colon, in *Physiology of the Gastrointestinal Tract*, Johnson, LR, Ed., Raven Press, New York, 1987.

27. Bird, RP. Effect of dietary components on the pathobiology of colonic epithelium: possible relationship with colon tumorigenesis. *Lipids* 21, 289, 1986.

28. Bivin, WS, Crawford, MP, and Brewer, NR. Morphophysiology, in *The Laboratory Rat,* Vol. 1, Baker, HJ et al., Eds., Academic Press, New York, 1979.

29. Bjarnason, I et al. Side effects of nonsteroidal anti-inflammatory drugs on the small and large intestine in humans. *Gastroenterology* 104, 1832, 1993.

30. Boeckxstrens, GE et al. Evidence for nitric oxide as mediator on non-adrenergic non-cholinergic relaxations induced by ATOP and GABA in the canine gut. *Br J Pharmacol* 102, 434, 1991.

31. Borowitz, JL, Moore, PF, Him GKW, and Miya, TS. Mechanism of enhanced drug effects produced by dilution of the oral dose. *Toxicol Appl Pharmacol* 19, 164, 1971.

32. Boyd, AJ, Sherman, IA, and Saibil, FG. Intestinal microcirculation and leukocyte behavior in ischemia-reperfusion injury. *Microvasc Res* 47, 355, 1994.

33. Browning, J, Gannon, BJ, and O'Brien, P. Microvasculature and gastric luminal pH of the forestomach of the rat: comparison with the glandular stomach, *Int J Microcirc Clin Exp* 2, 109, 1983.

34. Bruggeman, TM, Wood, JG, and Davenport, HW. Local control of blood flow in the dog's stomach, *Gastroenterology* 77, 736, 1979.

35. Bueno, L, Rayner, V, and Ruckebusch, Y. Initiation of the migrating myoelectric complex in dogs. *J Physiol* (Lond) 316, 309, 1981.

36. Burks, T F. Pathophysiological mechanisms of gastrointestinal toxicity, in *Comprehensive Toxicology*, Vol. 9, *Hepatic and Gastrointesinal Toxicology*, McCuskey, RS et al., Eds., Pergamon, Oxford, 1997.

37. Burks, TF. Neurotransmission and neurotransmitters, in *Physiology of the Gastrointestinal Tract*, 3rd ed., Johnson, LR, Ed., Raven Press, New York, 1994.

38. Burks, TF and Villar, H, in *Gastrointestinal Motility*, Christensen, J., Ed., Raven Press, New York, 1980.

39. Buset, M et al. Injury induced by fatty acids or bile acid in isolated human colonocytes prevented by calcium. *Cancer Lett* 50, 221, 1990.

40. Buset, M et al. Inhibition of human colonic epithelial cell proliferation *in vivo* and *in vitro* by calcium. *Cancer Res*, 46, 5426, 1986.

41. Buss, NE et al. Teratogenic metabolites of vitamin A in women following supplements and liver. *Human Exp Toxicol* 13, 33, 1994.

42. Calabrese, EJ. Gastrointestinal and dermal absorption: interspecies differences. *Drug Metab Rev*, 15, 1013, 1984.

43. Camilleri, M, Saslow, SB, and Bharucha, AE. Gastrointestinal sensation: mechanisms and relation to functional gastrointestinal disorders. *Gastroenterol Clin North Am* 25, 247, 1996.

44. Carson, JL and Willet, LR. Toxicity of nonsteroidal anti-inflammatory drugs: an overview of the epidemiological evidence. *Drugs* 46, 243, 1993.

45. Caulfield, MP. Muscarinic receptors: characterization, coupling and function. *Pharmacol Ther* 58, 319, 1993.

46. Chabra, RS, Pohl, RJ, and Fouts, JR. A comparative study of xenobiotic-metabolizing enzymes in liver and intestine of various species. *Drug Metab Dispos*, 2, 443, 1974.

47. Chang, EB. Intestinal water and electrolyte absorption and secretion. *Transplant Proc* 28, 2679, 1996.

48. Chang, WW. Mode of formation and progression of chemically induced colonic carcinoma. *Prog Clin Biol Res* 186, 217, 1985.

49. Christensen, J. Motility of the colon, in *Physiology of the Gastrointestinal Tract*, Johnson, LR, Ed., Raven Press, New York, 1987.

50. Christensen, J. Motility of the colon, in *Physiology of the Gastrointestinal Tract*, 3rd ed., Johnson, LR, Ed., Raven Press, New York, 1994.

51. Code, CF and Marlett, JA. The interdigestive myoelectric complex of the stomach and small bowel of dogs. *J Physiol* (Lond) 246, 289, 1975.

52. Cohen, MB et al. Age-related differences in receptors for *Escherichia coli* heat-stable enterotoxin in the small and large intestine of children. *Gastroenterology* 94, 367, 1988.

53. Conklin, JL and Christensen, J, in *Physiology of the Gastrointestinal Tract*, 3rd ed., Johnson, LR, Ed., Raven Press, New York, 1994.

54. Conney, AH. Pharmacological implication of microsomal enzyme induction. *Pharmacol Rev* 19, 317, 1967.

55. Craven, PA and DeRubertis, FR. Effects of aspirin on 1,2-dimethylhydrazine-induced colonic carcinogenesis. *Carcinogenesis* 13, 541, 1992.

56. Cross, HS et al. Growth control of human colon cancer cells by vitamin D and calcium *in vitro*. *J Natl Cancer Inst* 84, 1355, 1992.

57. Dantzig, AH, Duckworth, DC, and Tabas, LB. Transport mechanisms responsible for the absorption of loracarbef, cefixime, and cefuroxime axetil into human intestinal Caco-2 cells. *Biochem Biophys Acta* 1191, 7, 1994.

58. Dantzler, WH. Comparative physiology, in *Handbook of Physiology*, Oxford University Press, New York, 1997, sec. 13.

59. Davies, B and Morris, T. Physiological parameters in laboratory animals and humans. *Pharm Res* 10, 1093, 1993.

60. Dellmann, HD and Eurell, JA. *Textbook of Veterinary Histology*, 5th ed., Lippincott Williams & Wilkins, Baltimore, 1988.

61. DelValle, J and Yamada, T. Amino acids and amines stimulate gastrin release from canine antral G-cells via different pathways. *J Clin Invest* 85, 139, 1990.

62. Deschner, EE and Lipkin, M. Cell proliferation in normal, preneoplastic and neoplastic gastrointestinal cells. *Clin Gastroentol* 5, 543, 1976.

63. Deschner, EE and Lipkin, M. Proliferative patterns in colonic mucosa in familial polyposis. *Cancer* 35, 413, 1975.

64. DiPalma, JA et al. Occupational and industrial toxin exposures and the gastrointestinal tract. *Am J Gastroenterol*, 86, 1107, 1991.

65. Dockray, GJ, Varro, A, and Dimaline, R. Gastric endocrine cells: gene expression, processing, and targeting of active products. *Physiol Rev* 76, 767, 1996.

66. Dockray, GJ. Physiology of enteric neuropeptides, in *Physiology of the Gastrointestinal Tract*, 3rd ed., Johnson, LR, Ed., Raven Press, New York, 1994.

67. Donowitz, M and Welsh, MJ. Ca^{2+} and cyclic AMP in regulation of intestinal Na, K, and Cl transport. *Ann Rev Physiol* 48, 135, 1986.

68. Dreyfuss, J, Shaw, JM, and Ross, JJ. Absorption of the adrenergic-blocking agent, nadol, by mice, rats, hamsters, rabbits, dogs, monkeys and man: unusual species differences. *Xenobiotica* 8, 503, 1978.

69. Eberhart, CE and Dubois, RN. Eicosanoids and the gastrointestinal tract. *Gastroenterology* 109, 285, 1995.

70. Edmonds, B, Gibb, AJ, and Colquhoun, D. Mechanisms of activation of glutamate receptors and the time course of excitatory synaptic currents. *Annu Rev Physiol* 57, 495, 1995.

71. El-Sharkawy, TY, Morgan, KG, and Szurszewski, JH. Intracellular electrical activity of canine and human gastic smooth muscle. *J Physiol* (Lond) 279, 291, 1978.

72. Engel, E, Guth, PH, Nishizaki, Y, and Kaunitz, JD. Barrier function of the gastric mucus gel. *Am J Physiol* 269, G994, 1995.

73. Evans, HE. The digestive apparatus and abdomen, in *Miller's Anatomy of the Dog*, 3rd ed., W.B. Saunders, Philadelphia, 1993.

74. Feil, W et al. Rapid epithelial restitution of human and rabbit colonic mucosa. *Gastroenterology* 97, 685, 1989.

75. Ferguson, HC. Dilution of dose and acute oral toxicity. *Toxicol App Pharmacol* 4, 759, 1962.

76. Ferraris, RP, Lee, PP and Diamond, JM. Origin of regional and species differences in intestinal glucose uptake. *Am J Physiol*, 257, G689, 1989.

77. Field, M, Rao, MC, and Chang, EB. Intestinal electrolyte transport and diarrheal disease. *New Engl J Med*, 321, 800, 1989.

78. Flemstrom, G. Gastric duodenal mucosal secretion of bicarbonate, in *Physiology of the Gastrointestinal Tract*, 3rd ed., Johnson, LR, Ed., Raven Press, New York, 1994.

79. Forstner, JF and Forstner, GG. Gastrointestinal mucus, in *Physiology of the Gastrointestinal Tract*, 3rd ed., Johnson, LR, Ed., Raven Press, New York, 1994.

80. Frappier, BL. Digestive system, in *Basic Histology*, 7th ed., Junqueira, LC et al., Eds., Appleton & Lange, Norwalk, CT, 1992.

81. Frederick, CB, Hazelton, GA, and Frantz, LD. The histopathological and biochemical response of the stomach of male F344/N rats following two weeks of oral dosing with ethyl acrylate. *Toxicol Pathol* 18 247, 1990.

82. Fyfe, JC. Feline intrinsic factor (IF) is pancreatic in origin and mediates ileal cobalamin absorption. *J Vet Intern Med* 7, 133, 1993.

83. Gad, SC. *Drug Safety Evaluation*, Wiley-Interscience, New York, 2002.

84. Gaginella, TS et al. Reactive oxygen and nitrogen metabolites as mediators of secretory diarrhea. *Gastroenterology* 109, 2019, 1995.

85. Garland, C et al. Dietary vitamin D and calcium and risk of colorectal cancer: a 19-year prospective study in men. *Lancet* 1, 307, 1985.

86. Garret, JA, Ekstrom, J, and Anderson, LC. *Glandular Mechanisms of Salivary Secretion*, Karger, New York, 1998.

87. Gooringe, JAL and Sproston. The influence of particle size upon the absorption of drugs from the gastrointestinal tract, in *Absorption and Distribution of Drugs,* Binn, TB, Ed., Williams & Wilkins, Baltimore, 1964.

88. Gordon, J. Intestinal epithelial differentiation: new insights from chimeric and transgenic mice. *J. Cell Biol* 108, 1187, 1989.

89. Goyal RK and Hirano I. The enteric nervous system. *New Engl J Med* 334, 1106, 1996.

90. Granger, DN, Grisham, MB, and Kvietys, PR, in *Physiology of the Gastrointestinal Tract*, 3rd ed., Johnson, LR, Ed., Raven Press, New York, 1994.

91. Granger, DN, Kvietys, PR, Perry MA, and Barrowman, JA. The microcirculation and intestinal transport, in *Physiology of the Gastrointestinal Tract*, Johnson, LR, Ed., Raven Press, New York, 1987.

92. Greeley, GH. *Gastrointestinal Endocrinology*, Humana Press, Totowa, NJ, 1999.

93. Gregersen, H and Kassab, G. Biomechanics of the gastrointestinal tract, in *Neurogastroenterol Motil* 8, 277, 1996.

94. Griffiths, DFR et al. Demonstration of somatic mutation and colonic crypt clonality by X-linked enzyme histochemistry. *Nature* 333, 461, 1988.

95. Grisham, MR, VonRitter, C, Smith, BF, Lamont, JT, and Granger, DN. Interaction between oxygen radicals and gastric mucin. *Am J Physiol* 253, G93, 1987.

96. Guilford, WG and Strombeck, DR. Gastric structure and function, in *Strombeck's Small Animal Gastroenterology*, 3rd ed., Guilford, WG et al., Eds., W.B. Saunders, Philadelphia, 1996.

97. Guyton, AC and Hall, JE. *Textbook of Medical Physiology*, 10th ed., W.B. Saunders, Philadelphia, 2000.

98. Hakanson, R, Chen, D, and Sundler, F. The ECL cells, in *Physiology of the Gastrointestinal Tract*, 3rd ed., Johnson, LR, Ed., Raven Press, New York, 1994.

99. Hall, EJ and Batt, RM. Development of a wheat-sensitive enteropathy in Irish setters: biochemical changes. *Am J Vet Res* 51, 983, 1990.

100. Hall, EJ and Simpson, KW. Diseases of the small intestine, in *Textbook of Veterinary Internal Medicine Diseases of the Dog and Cat*, 5th ed., Ettinger, SJ et al., Eds., W.B. Saunders, Philadelphia, 2000, chap. 137.

101. Hall, JA. Diseases of the stomach, in *Textbook of Veterinary Internal Medicine Diseases of the Dog and Cat*, 5th ed., Ettinger, SJ et al., Eds., W.B. Saunders, Philadelphia, 2000, chap. 136.

102. Hall, JA, Burrows, CF, and Twedt, DC. Gastric motility in dogs: normal gastric function. *Compend Contin Educ Pract Vet* 10, 1282, 1988.

103. Hallikainen, A and Salminen, S, in *Gastrointestinal Toxicology*, Rosman K. et al., Eds., Elsevier, Amsterdam, 1986, p. 338.

104. Hauser, J and Szabo, S. Extremely long protection by pyrazole derivatives against chemically induced gastric mucosal injury. *J Pharmacol Exp Ther* 256, 592, 1991.

105. Hawkins, EC et al. Digestion of bentiromide and absorption of xylose in healthy cats and absorption of xylose in cats with infiltrative bowel disease. *Am J Vet Res* 47, 567, 1986.

106. Hayton, WL. Rate-limiting barriers to intestinal drug absorption: a review. *J Pharmacokin Biopharm,* 8, 321, 1980.

107. Heath, DF and Vandekar, M. Toxicity and metabolism of dieldrin in rats. *Br J Ind Med*, 21, 269, 1964.

108. Heddle, R, Miedema, BW, and Kelly, KA. Integration of canine proximal gastric, antral, pyloric, and proximal duodenal motility during fasting and after a liquid meal. *Dig Dis Sci* 38, 856, 1993.

109. Hermiston, ML et al., Simon, TC, Crossman, MW, et al., in *Physiology of the Gastrointestinal Tract*, 3rd ed., Johnson, LR, Ed., Raven Press, New York, 1994.

110. Hersey SJ and Sachs G. Gastric acid secretion. *Physiol Rev* 75, 155, 1995.

111. Hersey, SJ. Gastric secretion of pepsins, in *Physiology of the Gastrointestinal Tract*, 3rd ed., Johnson, LR, Ed., Raven Press, Raven, New York, 1994.

112. Hill, MJ et al. Faecal bile-acids and clostridia in patients with cancer of the large bowel. *Lancet* 1, 535, 1975.

113. Hills, BA, Butler, BD, and Lichtenberger, LM. Gastric mucosal barrier hydrophobic lining to the lumen of the stomach. *Am J Physiol*, 244, G561, 1983.

114. Hinder, RA and Kelly, KA. Canine gastric emptying of solids and liquids. *Am J Physiol* 233, E335, 1977.

115. Holst, JJ. Enteroglucagon. *Annu Rev Physiol* 59, 257, 1997.

116. Holzer, P and Holzer-Petsche, U. Tachykinins in the gut. Part II. Roles in neural excitation, secretion and inflammation. *Pharmacol Ther* 73, 219, 1997.

117. Holzer, P, Livingston, EH, and Guth, PH, in *Physiology of the Gastrointestinal Tract*, 3rd ed., Johnson, LR, Ed., Raven Press, New York, 1994.

118. Hopfer, U and Liedtke, CM. Proton and bicarbonate transport mechanisms in the intestine. *Annu Rev Physiol* 49, 51, 1987.

119. Houston, JB, Upshall, DG, and Bridges, JW. A re-evaluation of the importance of partition coefficients in the gastrointestinal absorption of nutrients. *J Pharmacol Exp Ther* 189, 244, 1974.

120. Hunt, JN and Stubbs, DF. The volume and energy content of meals as determinants of gastric emptying. *J Physiol* (Lond) 245, 209, 1975.

121. International Agency for Research on Cancer. *Monographs on the Evaluation of Carcinogenic Risk in Humans,* World Health Organization, Lyon, 1994, vol. 60.

122. International Agency for Research on Cancer. *Some Naturally Occurring Substrates: Food Items and Constituents, Heterocyclic Aromatic Amines and Mycotoxins*, World Health Organization, Lyon, vol. 56, 1993.

123. Iatropoulos, MJ. Morphology of the gastrointestinal tract, in *Gastrointestinal Toxicology*, Rozman, K. et al., Eds., Elsevier, New York, 1986.

124. Ijiri, K and Potten, CS. Further studies on the response of intestinal crypt cells of different hierarchical status to eighteen different cytotoxic agents. *Br J Cancer* 55, 113, 1987.

125. Isikawa, H et al, Studies on bacterial flora of the alimentary tract of dogs. III. Fecal flora in clinical and experimental cases of diarrhea. *Jpn J Vet Sci* 44, 343, 1982.

126. Ito, S. Functional gastric morphology, in *Physiology of the Gastrointestinal Tract*, Johnson, LR, Ed., Raven Press, New York, 1987.

127. Izzo, AA, Mascolo, N, and Capasso, F. Nitric oxide as a modulator of intestinal water and electrolyte transport. *Dig Dis Sci*, 43, 1605, 1988.

128. Jacobson, ED. Circulatory mechanisms of gastric mucosal damage and protection. *Gastoenterology*, 102, 1788, 1992.

129. Jankowski, JA et al. Maintenance of normal intestinal mucosa: function, structure, and adaptation. *Gut* 41 (Suppl. 1), S1, 1992.

130. Jergens, AE and Willard, MD. Diseases of the large intestine, in *Textbook of Veterinary Internal Medicine Diseases of the Dog and Cat*, 5th ed., Ettinger, SF et al., Eds., W.B. Sauncers, Philadelphia, 2000, chap. 138.

131. Jodal, M. Neuronal influence on intestinal transport. *J Intern Med Suppl* 732, 125, 1990.

132. Johnson LR. *Gastrointestinal Physiology*, Mosby, St. Louis, 1997.

133. Johnson, LR, Ed. *Physiology of the Gastrointestinal Tract*, 3rd ed., Raven Press, New York, 1994.

134. Jones, TC, Mohr, U, and Hunt, RD, in *Digestive System: Monographs on Pathology of Laboratory Animals*. Springer-Verlag, Berlin, 1985.

135. Kararli, TT. Comparison of the gastrointestinal anatomy, physiology and biochemistry of humans and commonly used laboratory animals. *Biopharm Drug Dispos* 16, 351, 1995.

136. Kaur, P and Potten, CS. Cell migration velocities in the crypts of the small intestine after cytotoxic insult are not dependent on mitotic activity. *Cell Tissue Kinet*, 19, 601, 1986.

137. Kelly, D and Kostial, K. The effect of milk diet on lead metabolism in rats. *Environ Res* 6, 355, 1973.

138. Kelly, KA and Code, CF. Gastric pacemaker. *Am J Physiol* 220, 112, 1971.

139. Kelly, KA. Gastric emptying of liquids and solids: roles of proximal and distal stomach. *Am J Physiol* 239, G71, 1980.

140. KernÈis, S et al. Conversion by Peyer's patch lymphocytes of human enterocytes into M cells that transport bacteria. *Science* 277, 949, 1997.

141. Keusch, GT et al. Pathogenesis of shigella diarrhea: serum anticytotoxin antibody response produced by toxigenic and nontoxigenic *Shigella dysenteriae*. *J Clin Invest* 57, 194, 1976.

142. Kienzle, E. Carbohydrate metabolism of the cat. 4. Activity of maltase, isomaltase, sucrase and lactase in the gastrointestinal tract in relation to age and diet. *J Anim Physiol Anim Nutr* 70, 89, 1993.

143. Kitahora, T and Guth, PH. Effect of aspirin plus hydrochloric acid on the gastric mucosal microcirculation. *Gastoenterology* 93, 810, 1987.

144. Kitamura, N et al. Endocrine cells in the gastrointestinal tract of the cat. *Biomed Res* 3, 612, 1982.

145. Konturek PC et al. Epidermal growth factor in protection, repair, and healing of gastroduodenal mucosa. *J Clin Gastroenterol* 13 (Suppl.), S88, 1991.

146. Kovacs, TA et al. Gastrin is a major mediator of the gastric phase of acid secretion in dogs: proof by monoclonal antibody neutralization. *Gastroenterology* 97, 1406, 1989.

147. Kroes, R and Wester, PW. Forestomach carcinogens: possible mechanisms of action. *Food Chem Toxicol* 24, 1083, 1986.

148. Kumar, D and Wingate, DL. *An Illustrated Guide to Gastrointestinal Motility*, 2nd ed., Churchill Livingstone, New York, 1994.

149. Kunze, WA and Furness, JB. The enteric nervous system and regulation of intestinal motility. *Annu. Rev. Physiol* 61, 117, 1999.

150. Lagniére, S et al. Digestive and absorptive functions along dog small intestine: comparative distributions in relation to morphological parameters. *Comp Biochem Physiol A Physiol* 79, 463, 1984.

151. Lai, CY. The chemistry and biology of cholera toxin. *CRC Crit Rev Biochem*, 9, 171, 1980.

152. Lang, IM et al. Videoradiographic, manometric, and electromyographic analysis of canine upper esophageal sphincter. *Am J Physiol* 260, G911, 1991.

153. Lang, IM, Sarna, SK, and Condon, RE. Gastrointestinal motor correlates of vomiting in the dog: quantification and characterization as an independent phenomenon. *Gastroenterology* 90, 40, 1986.

154. Lanza, FL. Gastrointestinal toxicity of newer NSAIDs. *Am J Gastroenterol* 88, 1318, 1993.

155. Lapre, JA et al. The antiproliferative effect of dietary calcium on colonic epithelium is mediated by luminal surfactants and dependent on the type of dietary fat. *Cancer Res* 53, 784, 1993.

156. Lapre, JA et al. Lytic effects of mixed micelles of fatty acids and bile acids. *Am J Physiol* 263, G333, 1992.

157. Lauterbach, F. Intestinal secretion of organic ions and drugs, in *Intestinal Permeation*, Kramer, M. et al., Eds., Excerpta Medica, Amsterdam, 1977.

158. Lebenthal, E and Duffey, ME, Eds. *Text book of Secretory Diarrhea*, Raven Press, New York, 1990.

159. Leib, MS and Matz, ME. Diseases of the large intestine, in *Textbook of Veterinary Internal Medicine*, 4th ed., Ettinger, SJ et al., Eds., W.B. Saunders, Philadelphia, 1995.

160. Leib, MS et al. Gastric emptying of liquids in the dog: serial test meal and modified emptying-time techniques. *Am J Vet Res* 46, 1876, 1985.

161. Leopold, G, Furukawa, E, Forth, W, and Rummek, W. Comparative studies of absorption of heavy metals *in vivo* and *in vitro*. *Arch Pharmacol Exp Pathol* 263, 275, 1969.

162. Levi, PE and Hodgson, E. Reactive metabolites and toxicity, in *Introduction to Biochemical Toxicology*, 3rd ed., Hodgson, E. et al., Eds., Wiley-Interscience, 2001.

163. Levi, S and Shaw-Smith, C. Non-steroidal anti-inflammatory drugs: how do they damage the gut? *Br J Rheumatol* 33, 605, 1994.

164. Levine, RR and Steinberg, GM. Intestinal absorption of pralidoxime and other aldoximes. *Nature*, 209, 269, 1966.

165. Lichtenberger LM. The hydrophobic barrier properties of gastrointestinal mucus. *Annu Rev Physiol* 57, 565, 1995.

166. Liddle RA. Cholecystokinin cells. *Annu Rev Physiol* 59, 221, 1997.

167. Lin, HC. Abnormal intestinal feedback in disorders of gastric emptying. *Dig Dis Sci* 39, 54S, 1994.

168. Lipkin, M et al. Colonic epithelial cell proliferation in responders and non-responders to supplemental dietary calcium. *Cancer Res* 49, 248, 1989.

169. Lloyd, KCK and Debas, HT. Peripheral regulation of gastric acid secretion, in *Physiology of the Gastrointestinal Tract*, 3rd ed., Johnson, LR, Ed., Raven Press, New York, 1994.

170. Macdonald IA. Physiological regulation of gastric emptying and glucose absorption. *Diabetic Med* 13, S11, 1996.

171. Macfarlane, GT and Gibson, GR. Microbiological aspects of the production of shortchain fatty acids in the large bowel, in *Physiological and Clinical Aspects of Short Chain Fatty Acids*, Cummings, JH et al., Eds., Cambridge University Press, Cambridge, 1995.

172. MacLennan, R et al. Randomized trial of intake of fat, fiber, and beta carotene to prevent colonectal adenomas. *J Natl Cancer Inst* 87, 1760, 1995.

173. Madara, L and Trier, JS. Functional morphology of the mucosa of the small intestine, in *Physiology of the Gastrointestinal Tract*, Johnson, LR, Ed., Raven Press, New York, 1994.

174. Makhlouf, GM. Neuromuscular function of the small intestine, in *Physiology of the Gastrointestinal Tract*, 3rd ed., Johnson, LR, Ed., New York, Raven Press, 1994.

175. Malcontenti-Wilson, C, Schulz, S, Penney, AG, Andrews, FJ, and O'Brien, PE. Aged gastric mucosa: mechanisms of vulnerability. *Gastroenterol Hepatol* 13, S204, 1998.

176. Marnett, LJ. Aspirin and the potential role of prostaglandins in colon cancer. *Cancer Res* 52, 5575, 1992.

177. Marve, GM. Nerves and hormones interact to control gallbladder function. *News Physiol Sci* 13, 64, 1998.

178. Mascolo, N et al. Nitric oxide and castor oil-induced diarrhea. *J Pharmacol Exp Ther* 268, 291, 1994.

179. McCallum, RW. Pharmacologic modulation of motility. *Yale J Biol Med* 72, 173, 1999.

180. McCuskey, RS and Earnest, DL. Hepatic and gastrointestinal toxicology, in *Comprehensive Toxicology*, Elsevier, New York, 1997.

181. McDonough, PL and Simpson, KW. Diagnosing emerging bacterial infections: salmonellosis, campylobacteriosis, clostridial toxicosis and helicobacteriosis. *Semin Vet Med Surg* 11, 1, 1996.

182. McHugh, PR and Moran, TH. Calories and gastric emptying: regulatory capacity with implications for feeding. *Am J Physiol* 236, R254, 1979.

183. Meade, EA, Smith, WL, and DeWitt, DL. Differential inhibition of prostaglandin endoperoxide synthase (cyclooxygenase) isozymes by aspirin and other non-steroidal anti-inflammatory drugs. *J Biol Chem* 268, 6610, 1993.

184. Mendel, JL and Walton, MS. Conversion of pp-DDT to pp-DDD by intestinal flora of the rat. *Science* 151, 1527, 1966.

185. Meyer, JH. Motility of the stomach and gastroduodenal junction, in *Physiology of the Gastrointestinal Tract*, 2nd ed., Johnson, LR, Ed., Raven Press, New York, 1987.

186. Meyer, JH et al. Effect of size and density on canine gastric emptying of nondigestible solids. *Gastroenterology* 89, 805, 1985.

187. Meyer, JH et al. Sieving of solid foods by the canine stomach and sieving after gastric surgery. *Gastroenterology* 76, 804, 1979.

188. Mezey, E and Palkovitis, M. Localization of targets for anti-ulcer drugs in cells of the immune system. *Science* 258, 1662, 1992.

189. Miller, J et al. Search for resistances controlling canine gastric emptying of liquid meals. *Am J Physiol* 241, G403, 1981.

190. Minami, H and McCallum, RW. The physiology and pathophysiology of gastric emptying in humans. *Gastroenterology* 86, 1592, 1984.

191. Misiewicz, JJ et al., in *Atlas of Clinical Gastroenterology*, Lea & Febiger, Philadelphia, 1987.

192. Mitchell, JA et al. Selectivity of nonsteroidal antiinflammatory drugs as inhibitors of constitutive and inducible cyclooxygenase. *Proc Natl Acad Sci USA* 90, 11693, 1993.

193. Moncada, S and Higgs, A. The L-arginine-nitric oxide pathway. *New Engl J Med* 329, 2002, 1993.

194. Mower, HF et al. Fecal bile acids in two Japanese populations with different colon cancer risks. *Cancer Res* 39, 328, 1979.

195. Newmark, HL and Lupton, JR. Determinants and consequences of colonic luminal pH. *Nutr Canc* 14, 161, 1990.

196. Newmark, HL, Wargovich, MJ, and Bruce, WR. Colon cancer and dietary fat, phosphate, and calcium: a hypothesis. *J Natl Cancer Inst* 72, 1323, 1984.

197. Newsholme, EA and Carrié, AL. Quantitive aspects of glucose and glutamine metabolism by intestinal cells. *Gut* 41 (Suppl. 1), S13, 1992.

198. Nickel, R, Schummer, A, and Seiferle, E. Anatomy of the domestic animals, in *The Viscera of the Domestic Mammals*, Vol. II, 2nd revised ed., Nickel, A et al., Eds., Springer-Verlag, New York, 1979.

199. O'Dorisio, MS. Neuropeptides and gastrointestinal immunity. *Am J Med* 81, 74, 1986.

200. O'Keefe, DA and Harris, CL. Toxicology of oncologic drugs. *Vet Clin North Am Small Anim Pract* 20, 483, 1990.

201. O'Reilly, WJ. Pharmacokinetics in drug metabolism and toxicology. *Can J Pharm Sc*, 7, 66, 1972.

202. Ohkohchi, N and Himukai, M. Species difference in mechanisms of D-xylose absorption by the small intestines. *Jpn J Physiol* 34, 669, 1984.

203. Otto, W and Wright, N. Trefoil peptides: coming up clover. *Curr Biol* 4, 835, 1994.

204. Owyang, C. Physiological mechanisms of cholecystokinin action on pancreatic secretion. *Am J Physiol* 271, G1, 1996.

205. Pascual, DW, Kiyono, H, and McGhee, JR. The enteric nervous and immune systems: interactions for mucosal immunity and inflammation. *Immunomethods* 5, 56, 1994.

206. Pasricha, PJ. Prokinetic agents, antiemetics, and agents used in irritable bowel syndrome, in *Goodman & Gilman's The Pharmacological Basis of Therapeutics*, 10th ed., Kunze and Furness, Eds., McGraw-Hill, New York, 1999.

207. Payne, D and Kubes, P. Nitric oxide donors reduce the rise in reperfusion-induced intestinal mucosal permeability. *Am J Physiol* 265, G189, 1993.

208. Pemberton, PW et al. An aminopeptidase N deficiency in dog and small intestine. *Res Vet Sci* 63, 195, 1997.

209. Peskar, BM et al. Gastrointestinal toxicity: role of prostaglandins and leukotrienes, *Med Toxicol* 1, Suppl .1, 39, 1986.

210. Pfeiffer, CJ. Gastroenterologic response to environmental agents-absorption and interactions, in *Handbook of Physiology*, Lee, DHK et al., Eds., American Physiological Society, Bethesda, MD, 1977, sec. 9.

211. Pohjanvirta, R and Tuomisto, J. Short-term toxicity of 2,3,7,8-tetrachlorodibenzo-p-dioxin in laboratory animals: effects, mechanisms, and animal models. *Pharmacol Rev* 46, 483, 1994.

212. Potten, CS. Role of stem cells in the regeneration of intestinal crypts after cytotoxic exposure. *Prog Clin Biol Res* 369, 155, 1991.

213. Powell, DW. Intestinal water and electrolyte transport, in *Physiology of the Gastrointestinal Tract*, Johnson, LR, Ed., Raven Press, New York, 1987.

214. Previte, JJ, in *Human Physiology*, McGraw-Hill, New York, 1983.

215. Rainsfor, KD. Mechanisms of gastrointestinal toxicity of non-steroidal anti-inflammatory drugs. *Scand J Gastroenterol Suppl* 163, 9, 1989.

216. Read, NW. Feedback regulation and sensation. *Dig Dic Sci* 39 (Suppl. 12), 37S, 1994.

217. Reddy, BS. Overview of diet and colon cancer. *Prog Clin Biol Res* 279, 111, 1988.

218. Reddy, BS. Dietary fat and colon cancer: animal models. *Prev Med* 16, 460, 1987.

219. Reddy, BS. Amount and type of dietary fat and colon cancer: animal model studies. *Prog Clin Biol Res* 222, 295, 1986.

220. Reddy, BS. Diet and excretion of bile acids. *Cancer Res* 41, 3766, 1981.

221. Renwick, AG. Toxicokinetics: pharmacokinetics in toxicology, in *Principles and Methods of Toxicology*, 4th ed., Hayes, AW, Ed., Taylor & Francis, Philadelphia, 2001, chap. 4.

222. Roderick, PJ, Wilkes, HC, and Meade, TW. The gastrointestinal toxicity of aspirin: an overview of randomised controlled trials. *Br J Clin Pharmacol* 35, 219, 1993.

223. Rodolosse, A et al. Glucose-dependent transcriptional regulation of the human sucrose-isomaltase (*SI*) gene. *Biochimie* 79, 119, 1997.

224. Rosenfield, AB and Huston, R. Infant methemoglobinemia in Minnesota due to nitrates in well water. *Minn Med* 33, 787, 1950.

225. Roussel, AJ. Intestinal motility. *Compend Contin Educ Pract Vet* 16, 1433, 1994.

226. Rowland, I R. Factors affecting metabolic activity of the intestinal microflora. *Drug Metab Rev* 19, 243, 1988.

227. Rozman, K. Fecal excretion of toxic substances, in *Gastrointestinal Toxicology*, Rosman, K et al., Eds., Elsevier, Amsterdam, 1986.

228. Rozman, K and Hanninen, O, Eds. *Gastrointestinal Toxicology*, Elsevier, Amsterdam, 1986.

229. Rozman, KK and Klaassen, CD. Absorption, distribution, and excretion of toxicants, in *Casarett and Doull's Toxicology: The Basic Science of Poisons*, 6th ed., Klaassen, CD, Ed., McGraw-Hill, New York, 2001.

230. Rutgers, HC et al, Intestinal permeability and function in dogs with small intestinal bacterial overgrowth. *J Small Anim Pract* 37, 428, 1996.

231. Rutgers, HC et al. Small intestinal bacterial overgrowth in dogs with chronic intestinal disease. *JAVMA* 206, 187, 1995.

232. Sachs, G, Zeng N, and Prinz C. Physiology of isolated gastric endocrine cells. *Annu Rev Physiol* 59, 243, 1997.

233. Sachs, G and Prinz C. Gastric enterochromaffin-like cells and the regulation of acid secretion. *News Physiol Sci* 11, 57, 1996.

234. Sachs, G. Gastric H/K ATPase: regulation and structure/function of the acid pump of the stomach, in *Physiology of the Gastrointestinal Tract*, 3rd ed., Johnson, LR, Ed., Raven Press, New York, 1994.

235. Salzman, AL. Nitric oxide in the gut. *New Horiz* 3, 33, 1995.

236. Sarna, SK and Otterson, MF. Small intestinal physiology and pathophysiology. *Gastroenterol Clin North Am* 18, 375, 1989.

237. Sarna, SK. Physiology and pathophysiology of colonic motor activity I. *Dig Dis Sci* 36, 827, 1991.

238. Sarna, SK. Physiology and pathophysiology of colonic motor activity II. *Dig Dis Sci*, 36, 998, 1991.

239. Sarosiek, J, Slomiany, A, and Slomiany, BL. Evidence for weakening of gastric mucus integrity by *Campylobacter pylori*. *Scand J Gastroenterol* 23, 585, 1988.

240. Sasser, LB and Jarboe, GE. Intestinal absorption and retention of cadmium in neonatal rat. *Toxicol Appl Pharmacol* 41, 423, 1977.

241. Sawada, M and Dickinson, CJ. The G cell. *Annu Rev Physiol* 59, 273, 1997.

242. Schanker, LS. Passage of drugs across body membranes. *Pharmacol Rev* 74, 501, 1962.

243. Schanker, LS and Jeffrey, J. Active transport of foreign pyrimidines across the intestinal epithelium. *Nature*, 190, 727, 1961.

244. Schwartze, EW. The so-called habituation to arsenic: variation in the toxicity of arsenious oxide. *J Pharmacol Exp Ther* 20, 181, 1923.

245. Sellin, JH. Intestinal electrolyte absorption and secretion, in *Sleisenger and Fordtran's Gastrointestinal and Liver Disease*, Felman, F et al., Eds., W.B. Saunders, Philadelphia, 1998.

246. Shanahan, F, in *Physiology of the Gastrointestinal Tract*, 3rd ed., Johnson, LR, Ed., Raven Press, New York, 1994.

247. Sidhu, M and Cooke, HJ. Role for 5-HT and ACh in submucosal reflexes mediating colonic secretion. *Am J Physiol* 269, G346, 1995.

248. Simanowski, UA et al. Effect of alcohol on gastrointestinal cell regeneration as a possible mechanism in alcohol-associated carcinogenesis. *Alcohol* 12, 111, 1995.

249. Simpson, KW et al. Cellular localization and hormonal regulation of pancreatic intrinsic factor secretion in dogs. *Am J Physiol* 265, 178, 1993.

250. Smith, D. Species differences in metabolism and pharmacokinetics: are we close to an understanding? *Drug Metab Rev* 23, 355, 1991.

251. Smith, GS. Gastrointestinal toxifications and detoxifications in relation to resource management, in *Gastrointestinal Toxicology*, 3d ed., Rozman, K and Hänninen, O, Eds., Elsevier, Amsterdam, 1986.

252. Smith, HW. Observations on the flora of the alimentary tract of animals and factors affecting its composition. *J Pathol Bacteriol* 89, 95, 1965.

253. Snipes, RL. *Intestinal Absorptive Surface in Mammals of Different Sizes*, Springer-Verlag, Berlin, 1997.

254. Sobel, AE, Gawson, O, and Kramer, B. Influence of vitamin D in experimental lead poisoning. *Proc Soc Exp Biol Med*, 38, 433, 1938.

255. Soll, AH and Berglindh, T. Physiology of isolated gastric glands and parietal cells: receptors and effectors regulating function, in *Physiology of the Gastrointestinal Tract*, Johnson, LR, Ed., Raven Press, New York, 1987.

256. Sorenson, AW, Slattery, MK, and Ford, MH. Calcium and colon cancer: a review. *Nutr Cancer*, 11, 135, 1988.

257. Souba, WW. Glutamine: a key substrate for the splanchnic bed. *Annu Rev Nutr* 11, 285, 1991.

258. Spinato, MT, et al. A morphometric study of the canine colon: comparison of control dogs and cases of colonic disease. *Can J Vet Res* 54, 477, 1990.

259. Stark, ME et al. Effect of nitric oxide on circular muscle of the canine small intestine. *J Physiol* (Lond) 444, 743, 1991.

260. Stark, ME and Szurszewski, JH. Role of nitric oxide in gastrointestinal and hepatic function and disease. *Gastroenterology*, 103, 1928, 1992.

261. Stefanini, E and Clement-Cormier, Y. Detection of dopamine receptors in the area postrema. *Eur J Pharmacol.* 74, 257, 1981.

262. Stein, J, Ries, J, and Barrett, KE. Disruption of intestinal barrier function associated with experimental colitis: possible role of mast cells. *Am J Physiol* 274, 203, 1998.

263. Stewart, DJ. Cancer therapy, vomiting, and antiemetics. *Can J Physiol Pharmacol* 68, 304, 1990.

264. Stewart, JJ, Burks, TF, and Weisbrodt, NW. Intestinal myoelectric activity after activation of central emetic mechanism. *Am J Physiol* 233, E131-137, 1977.

265. Strombeck, DR. Small and large intestine: normal structure and function, in *Strombeck's Small Animal Gastroenterology*, Guilford, WG et al., Eds., W.B. Saunders, Philadelphia, 1996.

266. Surprenant, A. Control of the gastrointestinal tract by enteric neurons. *Annu Rev Physiol* 56, 117, 1994.

267. Szurszewski, JH. A migrating electric complex of canine small intestine. *Am J Physiol* 217, 1757, 1969.

268. Tepperman, BL and Jacobson, ED. Circulatory factors in gastric mucosal defense and repair, in *Physiology of the Gastrointestinal Tract*, 3rd ed., Johnson, LR, Ed., Raven Press, New York, 1994.

269. Thomson, ABR, Hotke, CA, O'Brien, BD, and Weinstein, WM. Intestinal uptake of fatty acids and cholesterol in four animal species and man: role of unstirred water layer and bile salt micelle. *Comp Biochem Physiol* 75A, 221, 1983.

270. Thomson, ABR, Olatunbosun, D, and Valberg, LS. Interrelation of intestinal transport system for manganese and iron. *J Lab Clin Med* 78, 642, 1971.

271. Thomson, ABR, Valberg, LS, and Sinclair, DG. Competitive nature of the intestinal transport mechanism for cobalt and iron in the rat. *J Clin Invest* 50, 2384, 1971.

272. Thompson, RQ, Sturtevant, M, Bird, OD, and Glazko, AJ. The effect of metabolites of chloramphenicol (Chloromycetin) on the thyroid of the rat. *Endocrinology*, 55, 665, 1954.

273. Thorens, B. Facilitated glucose transporters in epithelial cells. *Annu Rev Physiol* 55, 591, 1993.

274. Thun, MJ, Namboodiri, MM, and Heath, CW, Jr. Aspirin use and reduced risk of fatal colon cancer. *New Engl J Med*, 325, 1593, 1991.

275. Thwaites, DT, Brown, CD, Hirst, BH, and Simmons, NL. H^+-coupled dipeptide (glycylsarcosine) transport across apical and basal borders of human intestinal Caco-2 cell monolayers display distinctive characteristics. *Biochem Biophys Acta* 1151, 237, 1993.

276. Toner, PG, Carr, KE, and Wyburn, GM, in *The Digestive System: An Ultrastructural Atlas Review*, Appleton-Century-Crofts, New York, 1971.

277. Tonini, M. Recent advances in the pharmacology of gastrointestinal prokinetics. *Pharmacol Res* 22, 217, 1996.

278. Triadafilopoulos, G, Pothoulakis, C, Weiss, R, Giampaolo, C, and LaMont, JT. Comparative study of *Clostridium difficile* toxin A and cholera toxin in rabbit ileum. *Gastroenterology* 97, 1186, 1989.

279. Tse, FLS and Jaffe, JM, in *Preclinical Drug Disposition,* Marcel Dekker, New York, 1991.

280. Tso, P. Intestinal lipid absorption, in *Physiology of the Gastrointestinal Tract,* 3rd ed., Johnson, LR, Ed., Raven Press, New York, 1994.

281. Tsuji, A et al. Intestinal brush border transport of the oral cephalosporin antibiotic, cefdinir, mediated by dipeptide and monocarboxylic acid transport systems in rabbits, *J Pharm Pharmacol* 45, 996, 1993.

282. Twedt, DC. Diseases of the esophagus, in *Textbook of Veterinary Internal Medicine,* 4th ed, Ettinger, SF et al., Eds., W.B. Saunders, Philadelphia, 1994.

283. Twedt, DC and Magne, ML. Diseases of the stomach, in *Textbook of Veterinary Internal Medicine,* 3rd ed, Ettinger, SJ, Ed., W.B. Saunders, Philadelphia, 1989.

284. Uchida K. and Ogami E. Intestinal microflora of dogs. *Nippon Vet Zootech Coll Bull* 17, 42, 1969.

285. Van Munster, IP et al. A new method for the determination of the cytotoxicity of bile acids and aqueous phase of stool: the effect of calcium. *Eur J Clin Invest* 23, 773, 1993.

286. Van Tilbeurgh H et al. Structure of the pancreatic lipase-protolipase complex. *Nature* 359, 159, 1992.

287. Van Tilbeurgh, H et al. Structure of the pancreatic lipase-protolipase complex. *Nature* 359, 159, 1992.

288. Vanner S and Surprenant A. Neural reflexes controlling intestinal microcirculation. *Am J Physiol* 271, G223, 1996.

289. Victor, BE et al. Protection against ethanol injury in the canine stomach: role of mucosal gluathione. *Am J Physiol* 261, G966, 1991.

290. Viluksela, M and Rozman, KK. Sources of gastrointestinal tract toxins, in *Comprehensive Toxicology,* Vol. 9, McCuskey, RS et al., Eds., Pergamon Press, Oxford, 1997.

291. Walker, MC. Physiology of the digestive system, in *Textbook of Small Animal Surgery,* 3rd ed., Slatter, D., Ed., W.B. Saunders, Philadelphia, 1993.

292. Walker, WA. Intestinal transport of macromolecules, in *Physiology of the Gastrointestinal Tract,* Johnson, LR, Ed., Raven Press, New York, 1981.

293. Wallace, JL. Cooperative modulation of gastrointestinal mucosal defense by prostaglandins and nitric oxide. *Clin Invest Med* 19, 346, 1996.

294. Walsh JH and Dockray GJ. *Gut Peptides: Biochemistry and Physiology,* Raven Press, New York, 1994.

295. Walsh, CT. Methods in gastrointestinal toxicology, in *Principles and Methods of Toxicology,* 4th ed., Hayes, AW, Ed., Taylor & Francis, London, 2001, chap. 26.

296. Walsh, JH, in *Physiology of the Gastrointestinal Tract,* 3rd ed., Johnson, LR, Ed., Raven Press, New York, 1994.

297. Walsh, CT. Anatomical, physiological, and biochemical characteristics of the gastrointestinal tract, in *Principles of Route-To-Route Extrapolation for Risk Assessment,* Gerrity, TR and Henry, CJ, Eds., Elsevier, New York, 1990.

298. Walsh, JH. Peptides as regulators of gastric acid secretion. *Annu Rev Physiol* 50, 41, 1988.

299. Wank SA. Cholecystokinin receptors. *Am J Physiol* 269, G628, 1995.

300. Wargovich, M J. Toxicants and gastrointestinal tract proliferation and cancer, in *Comprehensive Toxicology,* Vol. 9, McCuskey, RS et al., Eds., Pergamon Press, Oxford, 1997.

301. Washabau, RJ. Diseases of the esophagus, in *Textbook of Veterinary Internal Medicine Diseases of the Dog and Cat*, 5th ed., Vol. 2, Ettinger, SJ et al., Eds., W.B. Saunders, Philadelphia, 2000, chap. 135.

302. Washabau, RJ and Holt, DE. Pathophysiology of gastrointestinal disease, in *Textbook of Small Animal Surgery*, Slatter, D., Ed., W.B. Saunders, Philadelphia, 2003.

303. Watkins, PB. Drug metabolism by cytochromes P450 in the liver and small bowel. *Gastroenterol Clin N Am* 21, 511, 1992.

304. Weisburger, JH et al. Bile acids, but not neutral sterols, are tumor promoters in the colon in man and in rodents. *Environ Health Perspect* 50, 101, 1983.

305. Welsh, MJ, Smith, PL, Fromm, M and and Frizzell, RA. Crypts are the site of intestinal fluid and electrolyte secretion. *Science* 218, 1219, 1982.

306. Willard, MD. Diseases of the stomach, in *Textbook of Veterinary Internal Medicine*, 4th ed., Ettinger, SF et al., Eds., W.B. Saunders, Philadelphia, 1995.

307. Williams, RT. The influence of enterohepatic circulation on toxicity of drugs. *Ann NY Acad Sci* 123, 110, 1965.

308. Wood, D and Folb, PI. Animal tests as predictors of human response, in *Handbook of Phase I/II Clinical Drug Trials*, O'Grady, J., Ed., CRC Press, Boca Raton, 1997, chap. 4.

309. World Health Organization. *Nitrates, Nitrites and N-Nitroso Compounds*. Geneve, 1978.

310. Wright, EM. Intestinal Na+/glucose cotransporter. *Annu Rev Physiol* 55, 575, 1993.

311. Wyllie, AH. Apoptosis. *Br J Cancer*, 67, 205, 1993.

312. Wyllie, AH. Apoptosis: cell death in tissue regulations. *J Pathol*, 153, 313, 1987.

313. Zannoni, VG, in *Fundamentals of Drug Metabolism and Drug Disposition*, Williams & Wilkins, Baltimore, 1972.

7 Absorption of Macromolecules by Mammalian Intestinal Epithelium

Shayne C. Gad

CONTENTS

INTRODUCTION

Primary human oral absorption of xenobiotics is, of course, dependent on a wide range of mechanisms dictated by the structures in question. Basic patterns of metabolism are a good place to start. Consider the pattern of phase I (mainly oxidative functional group changes by cytochrome P450s), phase II (conjugating enzymes that usually add large hydrophilic molecules to the molecules in phase I metabolites), and finally phase III (elimination systems that facilitate the removal of the metabolites from cells to other places). In absorption, this pattern can be condensed from the perspective of moving things into — not out of — foods.[11]

ANATOMICAL BASIS OF ABSORPTION

The total quantity of fluid that must be absorbed each day is equal to the ingested fluid (about 1.5 liters in humans) plus that secreted in the various gastrointestinal secretions (about 7 liters). All but about 1.5 liters of the total is absorbed in the small intestine, leaving only these 1.5 liters to pass into the colon each day.

The stomach is a poor absorptive area of the gastrointestinal (GI) tract because it lacks the typical villus type of absorptive membrane and because the junctions between the epithelial cells are tight junctions. Generally only a few highly lipid-soluble substances such as alcohol and molecules like aspirin can be absorbed in small quantities. The hydrolytic process of digestion and the extreme range of pH values serve to make this entry route unattractive for many molecules such as proteins.

ABSORPTIVE SURFACE OF INTESTINAL MUCOSA: VILLI

The absorptive surface of the intestinal mucosa has many folds called valvulae conniventes that increase the surface area of the absorptive mucosa about three-fold. These folds extend circularly most of the way around the intestine and are especially well developed in the duodenum and jejunum, where they protrude markedly into the lumen.

Located over the entire surface of the small intestine, from about the point at which the common bile duct empties into the duodenum down to the ileocecal valve, are literally millions of small villi that project about 1 mm from the surface of the mucosa. These villi lie so close to one another in the upper small intestine that they touch most areas, but their distribution is less profuse in the distal small intestine. The presence of villi on the mucosal surface enhances the absorptive area an additional ten-fold.

Finally, each intestinal epithelial cell is characterized by a brush border consisting of as many as 1000 microvilli, 1 μm in length and 0.1 μm in diameter, protruding into the intestinal chyme. This increases the surface area exposed to the intestinal materials at least another 20-fold. The combination of the folds of Kerckring, the villi, and the microvilli increases the absorptive area of the mucosa perhaps 1000-fold in humans, yielding a tremendous total area of 250 or more square meters for the entire small intestine.

The general organization of the villus, emphasizing especially the advantageous arrangement of the vasculature system for absorption of fluid and dissolved material into the portal blood and the arrangement of the central lacteal for absorption into the lymphatics, which are pinched-off portions of infolded enterocyte membrane that contain inside the vesicles extracellular materials that have been entrapped. Minute amounts of substances are absorbed by this physical process of pinocytosis, although comparatively they represent a very small proportion of total absorption. Also, extending linearly into each microvillus of the brush border are multiple actin filaments that contract intermittently and cause continual movements of the microvilli, keeping them constantly exposed to new quantities of intestinal fluid.

BASIC MECHANISMS OF ABSORPTION

Absorption through the gastrointestinal mucosa occurs by active transport, diffusion, and solvent drag. Briefly, active transport imparts energy to the substance as it is transported for the purpose of concentrating it on the other side of the membrane or moving it against an electrical potential. On the other hand, transport by diffusion means simply transport through the membrane as a result of molecular movement along an electrochemical gradient. Transport by solvent drag occurs any time a solvent is absorbed because of physical absorptive forces. The movement of the solvent will "drag" dissolved substances along — the basis of many formulation approaches for pharmaceuticals.

Materials can pass from the mucosal side of the GI tract across to the serosal side via five different mechanisms: passive diffusion through a lipid membrane; diffusion through pores; active energy-dependent transport; absorption through lymphatics; and absorption of macromolecules by pinocytosis.

HYDROLYSIS AS PRIMARY STEP IN ABSORPTION OF MACROMOLECULES

Almost all carbohydrate xenobiotics are large polysaccharides or disaccharides that are combinations of monosaccharides bound to one another by condensation. The two monosaccharides then are combined with each other at these sites of removal, and the hydrogen and hydroxyl ions combine to form water. When the carbohydrates are broken down into monosaccharides, specific enzymes return the hydrogen and hydroxyl ions to the polysaccharides and thereby separate the monosaccharides from each other. This process called hydrolysis is the following (in which R-R is a disaccharide):

$$R'' - R' + H_2O \xrightarrow{\textit{digestive enzymes}} R''OH + R'H$$

Almost the entire lipid portion of the diet consists of triglycerides (neutral fats) that are combinations of three fatty acid molecules condensed with a single glycerol molecule. In condensation, three molecules of water have been removed. Digestion of the triglycerides consists of the reverse process, the fat-digesting enzymes returning molecules of water to the triglyceride molecule, thereby splitting the fatty acid molecules away from the glycerol. Here again, the digestive process is one of hydrolysis.

Finally, proteins and peptides are formed from amino acids that are bound together by peptide linkages. In this linkage, a hydroxyl ion is removed from one amino acid and a hydrogen ion is removed from the succeeding one; thus, the amino acids in the peptides or protein chain are bound together by condensation and tend to reverse the process. Proteolytic enzymes return water to the molecules to split them into their constituent amino acids. The chemistry of digestion and the break-down of xenobiotics for absorption in the GI tract is simple because in the case of all three major types of primary organic structures, the basic process of hydrolysis is involved. The only difference lies in the enzymes required to promote the reactions for each type of molecule.

ABSORPTION OF WATER

Water is transported through the intestinal membrane entirely by diffusion, obeying the usual laws of osmosis. Therefore, when the stomach contents are dilute, water is absorbed through the intestinal mucosa into the blood of the villi by osmosis. At the same time, water can also be transported in the opposite direction, from the plasma into the contents. This occurs especially when hyperosmotic solutions are discharged from the stomach into the duodenum. Sufficient water usually is rapidly transferred by osmosis to make the chyme isosmotic with the plasma. Generally, nature abhors a vacuum.

As dissolved substances are absorbed from the lumen of the gut into the blood, absorption tends to decrease the osmotic pressure of the GI tract contents (chyme). However, water diffuses so readily through the intestinal membrane (because of large 0.7- to 1.5-nm paracellular pores through the so-called tight junctions between the epithelial cells) that it almost instantaneously "follows" the absorbed substances into the blood. Therefore, as molecules are absorbed, so also is an isosmotic equivalent of water absorbed.

ABSORPTION OF IONS

Twenty to thirty grams of sodium are secreted into the intestinal secretions each day. In addition, a normal person eats 5 to 8 g of sodium each day. Combining these, the small intestine must absorb 25 to 35 g of sodium each day, which is equal to about one-seventh of all the sodium present in the body. Therefore, one can well understand that whenever intestinal secretions are lost to the exterior as in extreme diarrhea, the body's sodium reserves can be depleted to a lethal level within hours. Normally, however, less than 0.5% of the intestinal sodium is lost in the feces each day because of its rapid absorption through the intestinal mucosa. Sodium also plays an important role in the absorption of sugars and amino acids.

The motive power for the sodium absorption is provided by active transport of sodium from inside the epithelial cells through the basal and side walls of these cells into the paracellular spaces. This active transport obeys the usual laws of active transport: it requires energy, and the energy process is catalyzed by appropriate adenosine triphosphatase enzymes in the cell membranes. Part of the sodium is absorbed simultaneously with chloride ions; the chloride ions are passively dragged along by the positive electrical charges of the sodium ion. Additional sodium ions are absorbed while either potassium or hydrogen ions are transported in the opposite direction in exchange for the sodium ions.

ABSORPTION IN LARGE INTESTINE: FORMATION OF FECES

About 1500 mL of chyme normally pass into the large intestine each day. Most of the water and electrolytes in the chyme are absorbed in the colon, usually leaving less than 100 mL of fluid to be excreted in the feces. Essentially all the ions are absorbed, leaving only 1 to 5 meq each of sodium and chloride ions to be lost in the feces. Most of the absorption in the large intestine occurs in the proximal one half of the colon, whereas the distal colon functions principally for storage.

The mucosa of the large intestine also has a high capability for active absorption of sodium, and the electrical potential created by the absorption of the sodium causes chloride absorption as well. The tight junctions between epithelial cells of the large intestinal epithelium are much tighter than those of the small intestine. This prevents significant amounts of back-diffusion of ions through these junctions, thus allowing the large intestinal mucosa to absorb sodium ions far more completely than can occur in the small intestine. This is especially true when large quantities of aldosterone are available to enhance sodium transport capability.

In addition, as in the distal portion of the small intestine, the mucosa of the large intestine secretes bicarbonate ions while it simultaneously absorbs an equal number of chloride ions in an exchange transport process. The bicarbonate helps neutralize the acidic end products of bacterial action in the colon. The absorption of sodium and chloride ions creates an osmotic gradient across the large intestinal mucosa, which in turn enhances absorption of water.

A human large intestine can absorb up to 5 to 7 liters of fluid and electrolytes each day. When the total quantity entering the large intestine exceeds this amount, the excess appears in the feces as diarrhea. As noted earlier, toxins from cholera, other bacterial infections, and certain other xenobiotics can often cause the crypts of Lieberkühn in the terminal ileum and the large intestine to secrete more liters of fluid each day, leading to severe and sometimes lethal diarrhea.

Numerous bacteria, especially colon bacilli, are normally present in the absorbing colon. They are capable of digesting small amounts of cellulose, in this way providing a few calories of nutrition to the body each day. In herbivorous animals, this source of energy is significant, although it is of negligible importance in human beings. Other substances formed as a result of bacterial activity are vitamin K, vitamin B_{12}, thiamin, riboflavin, and various gases that contribute to flatus in the colon, especially carbon dioxide, hydrogen gas, and methane. Vitamin K is especially important because the amount of this vitamin ingested in foods is normally insufficient to maintain proper blood coagulation.

The feces normally are about three-fourths water and one-fourth solid matter which is composed of about 30% inorganic matter, 2 to 3% protein, and 30% undigested roughage of the food and dried constituents of digestive juices such as bile pigment and sloughed epithelial cells. The large amount of fat derives mainly from fat formed by bacteria and fat in the sloughed epithelial cells. The brown color of feces is caused by stercobilin and urobilin, derivatives of bilirubin. The odor is caused principally by the products of bacterial action; these products vary from one individual or species to another, depending on colonic bacterial flora and on the type of food eaten.

EFFECTS OF pH AND VOLUME

A number of barriers are present to impede the simple diffusion of molecules across the membranes of the epithelial cells lining the tract. First, the molecules must transverse the unstirred layers of fluid lying immediately adjacent to the membrane, then cross the mucus layer coating the membrane, and finally cross the bilipid membrane into the cell. Once within the cytoplasm of the cell, the molecule must pass through the cytoplasm and then through the basement membrane and the capillary or lymphatic wall membranes. The bilipid structure of the cell membrane greatly favors the absorption of hydrophobic structures over hydrophilic ones. The fact that ionized forms are marginally absorbed may be the result of microenvironments of lower pH in the unstirred layers immediately adjacent to the membrane or the acidity of the membrane.

The process of diffusion is driven by the concentration gradient across the membrane, and thus the fluid volume in the tract can have a major influence on the rate at which an ingested material may appear in the bloodstream. The active transport of sodium through the basolateral membranes of the cell reduces the sodium concentration inside the cell to a low value. Sodium moves down a steep electrochemical gradient from the chyme through the brush border of the epithelial cell into the epithelial cell cytoplasm, replacing the sodium that is actively transported out of the epithelial cells into the paracellular spaces.

Next, water moves by osmosis into the paracellular spaces. This is caused by the gradient created by the elevated concentration of ions in the paracellular space. Most of this osmosis occurs through the tight junctions between the apical borders of the epithelial cells, but a smaller proportion occurs through the cells themselves. The osmotic movement of water creates a flow of fluid into and through the paracellular space and from there to the circulating blood of the villus.

When a person or animal becomes dehydrated, large amounts of aldosterone are almost always secreted by the adrenal glands. Within 1 to 3 hours the excess aldosterone greatly enhances all the enzyme and transport mechanisms for all aspects of sodium absorption by the intestinal epithelial cells. The increased sodium absorption then causes secondary increases in absorption of chloride ions, water, and some other substances. Aldosterone in the intestinal tract acts the same as that activated by aldosterone in the renal tubules, which also serves to conserve salt and water in the body when an organism becomes dehydrated.

In the upper part of the small intestine, chloride absorption is rapid and mainly by passive diffusion. The absorption of sodium ions through the epithelium creates slight electronegativity in intestinal chyme and electropositivity on the basal sides of the epithelial cells. Chloride ions move along this electrical gradient to follow the sodium ions.

Often large quantities of bicarbonate ions must be reabsorbed from the upper small intestine because of the large amounts of bicarbonate ions in both the pancreatic secretion and the bile. The bicarbonate ion is absorbed individually as follows. When sodium ions are absorbed, moderate amounts of hydrogen ions are secreted into the gut in exchange for some of the sodium. Such hydrogen ions combine with the bicarbonate ions to form carbonic acid (H_2CO_3), which then dissociates to form water and carbon dioxide. The water remains in the intestines, but the carbon dioxide is readily absorbed into the blood and subsequently expired through the lungs. This is a so-called active absorption of bicarbonate ions. It is the same mechanism that occurs in some of the tubules of the kidneys.

SECRETION OF BICARBONATE IONS IN ILEUM AND LARGE INTESTINE: SIMULTANEOUS ABSORPTION OF CHLORIDE IONS

The epithelial cells on the surfaces of the villi in the ileum and on all surfaces of the large intestine have a special capability of secreting bicarbonate ions in exchange for absorption of chloride ions. This provides alkaline bicarbonate ions that are used to neutralize acid products formed by bacteria, especially in the large intestine. The exact mechanism of this exchange is unclear, but depends on the exchange of protein in the luminal membrane of the epithelial cell that forcibly exchanges bicarbonate ions formed inside the cell for chloride ions in the intestinal lumen. The excess chloride in the cell is then transported by facilitated diffusion through the basolateral membrane of the epithelial cell, completing the chloride absorption.

Immature epithelial cells in the crypts of Lieberkühn continually divide to form new epithelial cells that then spread outward over the luminal surfaces of the intestines. These new cells have properties different from those of the mature cells already on the outer luminal surfaces. Normally, they secrete small quantities of sodium chloride and water into the intestinal lumen, but this secretion is immediately reabsorbed by the older epithelial cells outside the crypts, providing a watery solution for absorbing intestinal digestates.

Extreme secretion is initiated by entry of a subunit of the cholera toxin into a cell. This stimulates the formation of excess cyclic adenosine monophosphate, which then opens tremendous numbers of chloride channels, allowing chloride ions to flow rapidly from inside the cell into the crypts. In turn, this is believed to activate a sodium pump that pumps sodium ions into the crypts to go along with the chloride ions. Finally, all this extra sodium chloride causes extreme osmosis of water into the crypts as well, thus providing the rapid flow of fluid along with the salt. Initially, all this excess fluid washes away the bacteria and is of value in combating the disease, but ultimately can be lethal because of the serious dehydration of the body that may ensue.

The transport of an absorbed molecule into the bloodstream is driven by a large concentration gradient between the luminal side and the serosal side of the intestine. Because of the rapid blood flow and concomitant rapid removal of absorbed solutes into the general systemic circulation, concentration gradients are invariably favorable for movement from the gut into the circulatory system. The major impediment to absorption of nutrients and exogenous chemicals is the initial movement across the mucosal cell membrane.

It is believed that a major portion of the water present in the GI tract is reabsorbed through pores present in the apical junctions of the epithelial cell lining. These pores are large enough to allow penetration of small molecules, particularly small ionized species. The net direction of flow of water is either from the GI tract into the serosal fluid, as is generally the case when the contents are either iso-osmotic or hypotonic, or into the GI tract, as might occur when the gastrointestinal contents are hyper-osmotic or in certain pathological states.

Vogel et al.[70] studied the effect of water flow on the toxicity of atropine, an azoniaspiro compound, phenobarbitol, and nicotine by infusing solutions of these substances into the duodenum of rats. Mannitol was concomitantly infused to adjust the osmotic concentration of the contents and thus the flow of water from the serosal side to the mucosal side of the GI tract. Toxic effects were increased by a factor of two to four, with a decrease in osmotic concentration from triple isotonicity to isotonicity for three of the four materials; the only exception was the azoniaspiro compound. The depression of absorption of solutes resulting from the flow of water from the serosa into the lumen of the intestine is termed solvent drag. This process can play an important role in evoking toxic responses of certain compounds, primarily small water-soluble ions.

ACTIVE TRANSPORT

Active energy-dependent transport mechanisms of absorption are primarily for molecules resembling nutrients, i.e., amino acids, sugars, essential vitamins, and minerals, etc. Specific exogenous substances can also be absorbed from the GI tract using these same transport systems. For instance, pyrimidines and amino acids are absorbed by active transport systems. 5-Fluorouracil and 5-bromouracil are actively transported across the rat intestinal epithelium by the process that transports natural pyrimidines.[65] Penicillamine and levodopa utilize an active transport mechanism for natural amino acids. Processes designed for the transport of essential metals are also responsible for the absorption of such toxic metals as lead and aluminum. Chlorothiazide has been demonstrated to be absorbed by a non-saturable active absorption process.[79]

MAMMALIAN ABSORPTION TRANSPORTERS

Absorption is not purely a matter of passive mechanisms based on physiochemical characteristics of a xenobiotic. Molecules are taken into the body via a number of active mechanisms. The GI tract contains a whole family of active "transporter" mechanisms. All the transporters listed below are present to varying extents in humans and most common laboratory species.

PEPTIDE TRANSPORTERS

- Located in the brush border membrane of the intestine.
- Broad substrate specificity of various peptidomimetic drugs and small peptides.
- Many -lactam antibiotics and some other drugs can be transported via this system, e.g., cephalexin, ampicillin, amoxicillin, captopril (and other ACE inhibitors), and the amino acid prodrug of acyclovir (has no peptide bond, suggesting a broader spectrum than just peptides).

NUCLEOSIDE TRANSPORTERS

- One type involved in facilitated diffusion (carrier attachment without energy input).
- Another type involved in active transport (requires input of energy).
- Probably affect absorption of nucleoside analogues used in antiviral and anticancer therapies.

SUGAR TRANSPORTERS

- There are at least two types with high affinities for D-glucose and D-fructose and low affinities for D-galactose and mannose. At least one type is facilitated transport.
- L sugars have affinities about 1000 times lower than D sugars.

BILE ACID TRANSPORTERS

- Preserve bile salts via absorption from the ileum (enterohepatic recirculation).

AMINO ACID TRANSPORTERS

- Many different types exist in the intestine.
- Some drugs absorbed with these transporters include α-methyldopa, baclofen and D-cyclosporin.

ORGANIC ANION TRANSPORTERS

- Anions are generally negatively charged moieties, such as produced by carboxylic acids in neutral or basic media, e.g., acetate.

VITAMIN TRANSPORTERS

- The following have specific transporters: thiamine, vitamin C, folic acid, vitamin B_{12}.
- Methotrexate (analogue of folic acid) is absorbed by the intestine in a manner similar to folic acid.
- The nicotinic acid transporter also has affinity for valproic acid, salicylic acid, and penicillins.

PHOSPHATE TRANSPORTERS

- Foscarnet (antiviral drug) and fosfomycin (water soluble antibiotic) utilize this transporter.

BICARBONATE TRANSPORTERS

- These are the principal regulators of pH in cells and play a vital role in acid–base movement.
- These transporters help exchange bicarbonate, sodium, and chloride.

ORGANIC CATION TRANSPORTERS

- Choline is a substrate.

FATTY ACID TRANSPORTERS

- Long chain fatty acids such as palmitate and oleate, but not short chain fatty acids, can saturate the transporter.
- A protein may assist in directing fatty acids to transporter sites.

Human Efflux Transporters (P-Glycoprotein)

- Exists on the brush border.
- Pumps out (exorbs) a large number of drugs (broad substrate specificity).
- Substrates include vincristine, taxol, digoxin, some fluoroquinolone antibacterials, quinidine, etoposide, cyclosporine, varapamil, and nifedipine.

ABSORPTION BY LYMPHATICS

Absorption by way of the lymphatics is limited to nonpolar materials and operates by mechanisms analogous to the mechanism that absorbs fatty acids. Bile salts play an important role in dispersing triglycerides and other fat-soluble molecules and are critical in the formation of micelles that allow dissolution of fatty materials within the chyme. The fact that rats do not possess gallbladders may lead to differences in their ability to absorb materials efficiently by way of the lymphatics.

Fatty acids derived from the hydrolysis of triglycerides by various lipases migrate to the brush borders of the mucosal cells and readily diffuse through the mucosal membrane into the cytosol of the cell. Once in the cell, the fatty acids are reincorporated into triglycerides within the endoplasmic reticulum and packaged into chylomicrons — conglomerates of triglycerides, cholesterol, and phospholipids encased in a protein coat. These provide an ideal environment to entrain other lipid-soluble molecules. The protein coat provides a hydrophilic exterior to the conglomerate that is extruded from the cell into the serosal fluid and into the central lacteals of the villi.

The chylomicrons are pumped through the lymphatic system and empty into the systemic circulatory system at the entrance of the thoracic duct in the veins of the neck. In this manner, fatty lipophilic materials avoid entering the hepatic portal circulatory system and first-pass effects of metabolism by liver enzymes. Sieber[67] has shown that p,p'-DDT and structurally related analogues are absorbed through the lymphatics. The extent of lymphatic absorption is limited, however, presumably because of the relatively slow rate of movement of lymph through the lymphatics as compared with movement of blood through the general circulatory system. The extent of absorption may vary greatly, depending on the vehicle in which a test substance is administered. Thus, Sieber[67] recovered only 15% of a dose of p,p'-DDT in the lymph when administered in ethanol compared with 34% when administered in corn oil.

P-aminosalicylic acid (PAS) and tetracycline have also been demonstrated to be absorbed by way of the lymphatics. Both these drugs and silicone oils are also rapidly distributed throughout the extracellular fluid, including lymph, when administered by the intravenous route.[19] Thus, care must be taken in interpretation of data in which accountability of a substance in lymph is used to determine absorption through lymphatics after peroral dosing. Other materials shown to be absorbed by way of the lymphatics include 3-methylcholanthrene, polychlorinated biphenyls, and benzpyrene.

MACROMOLECULES

The direct absorption of macromolecules from the GI tract is well established and has both wide application in pharmacotherapeutics and grave toxicological implications in some instances, e.g., the absorption of botulinum toxins, which are proteins of molecular weights ranging from 200,000 to 400,000. Macromolecules are believed to be absorbed by pinocytosis. Intestinal mucosas in the area of the Peyer's patches and lymphoid follicle aggregates are believed to be particularly active in this respect.[1] Peyer's patches are the sites of lymphoid follicle-associated epithelium that contain cells capable of transporting antigens and microorganisms.[26] Mucosa-associated lymphoid tissue is separated from the lumen of the intestine by lymphoid follicle-associated epithelium.

The ability of macrostructures to cross the epithelium lining, particularly in the area of Peyer's patches, has been explored for use in the delivery of pharmaceutical and molecular biological preparations. Polyanhydride copolymers of fumaric and sebacic acid have demonstrated high biological adhesive properties.[45] Microspheres of the polyanhydride copolymer with diameters ranging from 0.1 to 10 μm have been fed to rats and observed by histological procedures to transverse both the mucosal epithelium through and between individual cells and the follicle-associated epithelium covering the lymphatic elements of Peyer's patches. Once taken into mucosal cells, the macromolecules are transported to the general circulation by way of the lymphatics. The process is age dependent, decreasing with age.

ACQUISITION OF PASSIVE POSTNATAL
HUMORAL IMMUNITY

We should at this point recall that the GI tract serves as one of the three principal routes for entry of xenobiotics into the body for mammals and also as one of the major routes for immune system interaction with the environment. Two major avenues are available for absorption of macromolecules such as immunoglobulin G (IgG) by the intestine. One is receptor-mediated endocytosis and the other is nonreceptor-mediated endocytosis.

Coated pits and vesicles are involved in receptor-mediated endocytosis.[17,50] Clathrin, with a molecular weight 180,000, is the major structural protein of coated pits and vesicles.[50,54] Clathrin defines the cytoplasmic sides of endocytotic organelles by enclosing them in a lattice of pentamers and hexamers. Finally a polyhedral vesicle is produced. In receptor-mediated endocytosis, it is believed that specific protein receptors are randomly dispersed in the lipid bilayer of the plasmalemma.[49] To initiate internalization, the macromolecule or ligand binds to its receptor. This in turn promotes the binding of clathrin to the other end of the receptor. Ligand–receptor–clathrin complexes cluster at the base of the microvilli, causing the plasmalemma to invaginate or pit. The coated pit pinches off, forming a coated submicroscopic vesicle that then traverses the cell and fuses with the basal lateral membrane. Finally, the microvesicle undergoes reverse pinocytosis (exocytosis), resulting in the discharge of the ligand into extracellular space.[70,72]

In nonreceptor-mediated endocytosis, macromolecules are trapped within a submicroscopic apical tubular system, which is contiguous with the plasmalemma.[70,72] The trapped macromolecules flow down the tubule, eventually reaching the apical cytoplasm. The blind end pinches off and forms a microvesicle, visible by light microscopy. These microvesicles join lysosomes, becoming phagolysosomes. Intracellular digestion is the most probable fate of macromolecules internalized by this nonselective route.

Another mechanism exists for transporting macromolecules (soluble antigens, bacteria, viruses, etc.) through endocytosis.[10,52,53,75] M cells (specialized cells sandwiched between enterocytes overlying Peyer's patches) may be responsible for initiating a local immune response by transferring g antigens from the gut lumen to the lymphoid tissue in the Peyer's patches.

WHEN DO MAMMALS ACQUIRE PASSIVE HUMORAL IMMUNITY?

Mammals can be divided into three groups based on when they acquire passive humoral immunity.[8,28] Group I mammals acquire passive immunity exclusively postpartum; some examples are pigs, horses, and ruminants. Group II mammals acquire passive immunity both pre- and postpartum; examples are mice, rats, hamsters, dogs, and cats. Group III mammals acquire passive immunity exclusively prepartum and include humans, other primates, and guinea pigs.

Neonates in Group I nonselectively absorb macromolecules for a short period postpartum. Enterocytes on the intestinal epithelium of neonates in Group I nonselectively transport macromolecules from the lumen of the gut into the blood for about 2 days postpartum.[2,8,9,28,31,35] However, enterocytes continue to internalize (but do not transport) macromolecules nonselectively for a much longer period. Because of the dichotomy between internalization and transport, the absorption of macromolecules is divided into two phases: (1) uptake or internalization within the enterocyte and (2) transport through the enterocyte. The period after which enterocytes can no longer internalize macromolecules is called *closure*.[9,31,32,36]

In neonatal pigs, dietary regimens influence both cessation of transport and closure.[25,27,31,32,36,37] Piglets denied food from birth transport macromolecules from the gut into the blood as long as they live (about 3.5 days), while nursing pigs eating about 300 mL of colostrum or milk cease transporting within 24 hours postpartum.[37] It appears that eating stimulates the release of a humoral signal (hormone) that turns off transport. Although transport is qualitatively nonselective, the process is energy-dependent [29] and preferential, i.e., more immunoglobulin is transported than albumin when ligated segments of neonatal gut are injected with a solution containing both albumin and IgG. Also, the upper half of the small intestine transports more efficiently than the lower half. Enterocytes in the lower half have more lysosmal-like proteolytic activity.[27]

By the time a pig has nursed for 2 days, the intestine can no longer transport macromolecules, but the lower half of the small intestine can still internalize them. As the pig ages, more and more of the small intestine (proceeding toward the ileum) ceases internalizing macromolecules. Finally, by 2 to 3 weeks of age all enterocytes throughout the length of the small intestine are closed and the pig cannot internalize macromolecules.[31] As with transport, dietary regimens affect the time of closure and the signal for closure seems to be humoral, since an intestinal segment surgically removed from the digestive pathway closes at the same time as its counterpart in the digestive pathway.[24]

Histological studies show that enterocytes capable of transporting macromolecules have a submicroscopic noncoated interconnecting tubule system that traverse enterocytes from the plasmalemma to the basal lateral membrane.[22] These kinds of enterocytes are found mainly in the upper thirds of the small intestines of newborn pigs. In the lower thirds, enterocytes mainly internalize macromolecules for digestion. These enterocytes have a few apical tubules and many small vacuoles that appear to fuse, eventually producing large macroscopic vacuoles. Enterocytes in the mid small intestines of newborn pigs contain numerous apical tubules and vacuoles, indicating that they are both internalizing and transporting macromolecules.

Thus, the neonatal pig has enterocytes that transport macromolecules (mainly upper small intestines), enterocytes that internalize and digest macromolecules (mainly lower small intestines), and enterocytes that do both (mainly mid small intestines).

At about 2 days of age, neonatal pigs cease transporting macromolecules from the gut lumen to the blood. They cease internalizing macromolecules in the upper half of the small intestines. They continue to internalize nonselectively macromolecules in the ileal area for 2 more weeks. Time of cessation of transport and closure are both influenced by a humoral signal induced by eating. The separation of transport from digestion would be of value to a neonate requiring intact protein for transport (IgG) and digested protein for amino acid building blocks.

Animals in Group II selectively absorb macromolecules for extended periods, e.g., rats for 21 days, mice for 17 days, and hamsters for 7 days postpartum.[8,30,32]

Rats, mice, and hamsters have been extensively studied regarding this phenomenon. Absorption can be divided into a transport in rats and mice that occurs exclusively in the upper third of the small intestines and is selective for IgG.[30,42,57] The lower third of the small intestine nonselectively internalizes macromolecules and the mid third does both absorption and transport.

Clathrin-like coated pits, coated vesicles, and Fc-receptors for IgG have been associated with apical tubular systems in enterocytes located in the upper part of the small intestines but not with the apical tubular systems of enterocytes in the ileal area.[40,57,70,72,73] Thus, it seems that IgG is routed through the enterocyte of the upper gut in coated submicroscopic vesicles[70,72] and tubules to the basal lateral membrane, a process not too different from that of the pig except that neonatal rat enterocytes absorb selectively via clathrin-coated organelles.

Enterocytes in the lower part of the small intestine internalize macromolecules nonselectively in uncoated submicroscopic vesicles that fuse with others. Eventually, as with the ileal area in the pig, these fusing vesicles produce a macroscopic vesicle that appears to join the supranuclear vacuole.[70] Thus, the internalization of macromolecules in the ileal area leads to the digestion or storage of the macromolecules rather than transport. Compartmentation is an elegant way to reconcile the neonate's distinct needs for intact immunoglobulin for transport into the blood and digested proteins for building blocks. Cessation of transport and closure occur at the same time, coincident with weaning. These phenomena may be under adrenal hormone control in that glucocorticoids (at unphysiologically high levels) can precociously initiate closure, provided the neonate's adrenals have reached the proper maturational state.[21,43,44]

Neonates in Group III lack the capacity to transport macromolecules postnatally in appreciable amounts.[8] Even though they do not transport appreciable amounts of macromolecules, perhaps they can internalize and digest macromolecules for a short period. This notion is supported by evidence from guinea pigs.

Guinea pigs can nonselectively internalize macromolecules for about 2 days postnatally.[32,58] Pinocytotic macrovesicles are present in enterocytes during the internalization phase and probably contribute to the digestion of soluble protein in this early neonatal period.[32] Thus, enterocytes in neonatal guinea pigs have internalizing and digesting organelles that are similar to those seen in the neonates in Groups I and II.

Reports have noted small amounts of antibody transported by the nursing human infant gut.[5,20] Interestingly, the human infant gut during fetal development undergoes maturational changes analogous to those seen postnatally in pigs and rats.[3,39,46–48] These structural changes are apical tubules that appear in enterocytes throughout the entire length of the small intestine at the time villi are formed, around 10 weeks of gestation. (This same kind of structure is seen in suckling rats and newborn pigs as noted above.) Apical tubules and lysosomal elements are more numerous in the lower third of the intestine (again, like suckling rats and pigs). By 22 weeks of gestation, apical tubules disappear, and enterocytes in the upper area of the small intestine resemble adult-type enterocytes (a pattern seen in 2- to 8-day old pigs). At term or shortly thereafter, the infant's gut is replete with adult-type enterocytes. Although fetal enterocytes in humans seem capable of internalizing macromolecules, some doubt surrounds the capacity of these enterocytes to transport macromolecules through cells in appreciable amounts.[48]

NORMAL ADULTS

Investigators using a highly sensitive enzymatic macromolecular marker (horseradish peroxidase) found evidence for transport of this macromolecule through adult rat and rabbit enterocytes.[12,18,61,69] Horseradish peroxidase injected into ligated segments of adult jejunum was visualized histochemically within enterocytes in an apical tubular system. Further, this marker was transmitted into the extracellular space of the lamina propria. Others, using horseradish peroxidase and lactoperoxidase, detected apical tubular systems in enterocytes on villi in organ-cultured adult human small intestine.[5-7] Adult enterocytes internalize macromolecules in a manner analogous to that described for neonatal rats except that the apical tubular system is less well developed in the adult.[12,61,69]

Thus, evidence indicates that low levels of macromolecules (antigens) can break the adult mucosal barrier. They can be absorbed nonselectively by enterocytes via an apical tubular system (that may be a vestige of the neonatal system) or they can be absorbed by M cells.

ABNORMAL ADULTS

In the normal adult, low-level absorption of macromolecules does not seem to be a threat to health.[60,62] However, disease could result if increased quantities of antigens or toxic substances were absorbed. For example, in adults with gastric and pancreatic insufficiency, macromolecules are less efficiently digested. Thus, higher concentrations of macromolecules would be presented to the enterocytes and more macromolecules would likely be absorbed.[23,59,60,62,68] Also, an increase in absorption would occur if intracellular digestion was decreased because of faulty lysosomes.

Mucosa that no longer functions as a viable structure (radiation damage) could serve as a source of passively transmitted macromolecules. Increased absorption of macromolecules could result from an immune deficiency. In this case, secretory antibodies capable of reacting with antigens and thereby blocking their absorption would be lacking.[14,16,63,64] Certain diseases, e.g., celiac disease, allergic gastroenteropathies, inflammatory bowel disease, viral and bacterial enteritis, parasitic infestations of the gut, and radiation enteritis may be associated with increased absorption and transport of macromolecules.[4,60,62]

CONCLUSION

Neonatal mammals have mechanisms for absorbing macromolecules. The normal function of the mechanism is to absorb physiologically useful macromolecules such as immunoglobulins. However, if the neonate is ill managed and placed in an environment replete with toxic macromolecules, the potential exists for absorbing these toxins. In the neonatal period when pigs and mice have immature intestinal epithelium, they are more susceptible to enteric pathogens like *Escherichia coli* and rotaviruses and they can internalize toxins like endotoxins from Gram-negative rods.[13,33,34,38,55,74] As the intestine matures and can no longer absorb macromolecules, these animals become less susceptible to these enteropathogens.

A remnant of the neonatal system for absorbing macromolecules continues to exist in mature mammals. Thus, adults can absorb macromolecules at a low level. In a normal adult, the absorption of insignificant quantities of macromolecules produces no ill effects. However, if alteration in the intraluminal digestive process occurs or if the mucosal barrier becomes defective, increased quantities of antigenic or toxic substances could gain entrance to the body, resulting in local intestinal or systemic disorders.

REFERENCES

1. Aungst, B. and Shen, D.D., Gastrointestinal absorption of toxic agents, in *Gastrointestinal Toxicology*, Rozman, K. and Hänninen, O., Eds., Elsevier, New York, 1986, p. 35.
2. Balconi, I.R. and Lecce, J.G., Intestinal absorption of homologous lactic dehydrogenase isoenzyme by the neonatal pig, *J. Nutr.*, 88, 233, 1966.
3. Bierring, F. et al., On the nature of the meconium corpuscles in human foetal intestinal epithlium I. Electron microscopic studies, *Acta Pathol. Micromiol. Scand.*, 61, 365, 1964.
4. Bloch, K.J. et al., Intestinal uptake of macromolecules VI. Uptake of protein antigen *in vivo* in normal rats and rats infected with *Nippostrongylus brasiliensis* or subjected to mild systemic anaphylaxis, *Gastroenterology*, 77, 1039, 1979.
5. Blok, J. et al., The effect of chloroquine on lysomal function and cell-coat glycoprotein transport in the absorptive cells of cultured human small intestinal tissue, *Cell Tissue Res.*, 218, 227, 1981.
6. Blok, J. et al., Endocytosis in absorptive cells of cultured human small-intestinal tissue: horseradish peroxidase, lactoperoxidase and ferritin as markers, *Cell Tissue Res.*, 216, 1, 1981.
7. Blok, J. et al., Endocytosis in absorptive cells of cultured human small-intestinal tissue: effect of cytochalasin B and D, *Cell Tissue Res.*, 222, 113, 1982.
8. Brambell, F.W.R., The passive immunity of the young mammal, *Biol Rev.*, 33, 488, 1958.
9. Broughton, C.W. and Lecce, J.G., Electron-microscopic studies of the jejunal epithelium from neonatal pigs fed different diets, *J. Nutr.*, 100, 445, 1970.
10. Bukinskaya, A.G., Penetration of viral genetic material into host cell, *Adv. Virus Res.*, 27, 141, 1982.
11. Coleman, M.D., *Human Drug Metabolism: An Introduction*, John Wiley & Sons, Chichester, 2005.
12. Conning, D.M., Toxicology of food and food additives, in *General and Applied Toxicology*, 2nd ed., Macmillan, New York, 1999, p. 93.
13. Cornell, R., Walker, W.A., and Esselbacher, K.J., Small intestinal absorption of horseradish peroxidase: a cytochemical study, *Lab. Invest.*, 25, 42, 1971.
14. Crawford, P.C. and Lecce, J.G., Internalization of endotoxin (LPS) by enterocytes of neonatal pigs inoculated with *Escherichia coli* (abstr.), *Proc. 79th Ann. Mtg. A. Soc. Microbiol.*, 24, 1979.
15. Crouthamel, W.G. et al, Drug absorption IV. Influence of pH on absorption kinetics of weakly acidic drugs, *J. Pharm. Sci.*, 60, 1160, 1971.
16. Cunningham-Rundles, C. et al., Milk precipitins, circulating immune complexes and IgA deficiency, *Proc. Natl. Acad. Sci. USA*, 75, 3387, 1978.
17. Cunningham-Rundles, C. et al, Bovine antigens and the formation of circulating immune complexes in selective immunoglobulin A deficiency, *J. Clin. Invest.*, 64, 272, 1979.

18. Dayton, A.C. and Hall, J.E., *Textbook of Medical Physiology*, W.B. Saunders, Philadelphia, 1996.

19. DeMarco, T.J. and Levine, R.R., Role of the lymphatics in the intestinal absorption and distribution of drugs, *J. Pharmacol. Exp. Ther.*, 169, 142, 1969.

20. Engel, E. et al, Barrier function of the gastric mucus gel, *Am. J. Physiol.*, G994, 1995.

21. Goldstein, J.L. and Anderson, F.G.W., and Brown, M.S., Coated vesicles and receptor-mediated endocytosis, *Nature*, 279, 679, 1979.

22. Guyton, A.C. and Hall, J.E., Digestion and absorption in the gastrointestinal tract, in *Textbook of Medical Physiology*, 9th ed., W.B. Saunders, Philadelphia, 1996.

23. Haliday, R., The effect of steroid hormones on the absorption of antibodies by the young rat, *J. Endocr.*, 18, 56, 1959.

24. Heyman, M. et al., Horseradish peroxidase transport across adult rabbit jejunum *in vitro*, *Am. J. Physiol.*, 242, G558, 1982.

25. Iyengar, L. and Selvaraj, R.J., Intestinal absorption of immunoglobulins by newborn infants, *Arch. Dis. Child.*, 47, 411, 1972.

26. Kerneis, S. et al., Conversion by Peyer's patch lymphocytes of human enterocytes into M cells that transport bacteria, *Science,* 277, 949, 1997.

27. King, M.W. and Lecce, J.G., Transport of macromolecules through enterocytes of the neonatal piglet intestine, 1983.

28. Kraft, S.C. et al., Gastric acid output and circulating antibovine serum albumin in adults, *Clin Exp. Immunol.*, 2, 321, 1967.

29. Leary, H.L. and Lecce, J.G., Uptake of macromolecules by enterocytes on transposed and isolated piglet small intestine, *J. Nutr.*, 106, 419, 1976.

30. Leary, H.L. and Lecce, J.G., The effect of feeding on the cessation of transport and macromolecules by enterocytes of neonatal piglet intestine, *Biol. Neonat.,* 34, 174, 1978.

31. Leary, H.L. and Lecce, J.G., The preferential transport of immunoglobulin G by the small intestine of the neonatal pig, *J. Nutr.*, 109, 458, 1979.

32. Lecce, J.G., Absorption of macromolecules by neonatal intestine, *Bio. Neonat.*, 9, 50, 1966.

33. Lecce, J.G., *In vitro* absorption of γ-globulin by neonatal intestinal epithelium of the pig, *J. Physiol.*, 184, 594, 1966.

34. Lecce, J.G., Selective absorption of macromolecules into intestinal epithelium and blood by neonatal mice, *J. Nutr.*, 102, 69, 1972.

35. Lecce, J.G., Effect of dietary regimen on cessation of uptake of macromolecules by piglets intestinal epithelium (closure) and transport to the blood, *J. Nutr.*, 103, 751, 1973.

36. Lecce, J.G. and Broughton, C.W., Cessation of uptake of macromolecules by neonatal guinea pig, hamster and rabbit intestinal epithelium (closure), *J. Nutr.*, 103, 744, 1973.

37. Lecce J.G. and King, M.W., Role of reovirus-like agent associated with fatal diarrhea in neonatal pigs, *Infect. Immunol.*, 14, 816, 1978.

38. Lecce, J.G., King, M.W., and Mock, R., Reovirus-like agent associated with fatal diarrhea in neonatal pigs, *Infect. Immunol.*, 14, 816, 1976.

39. Lecce, J.G., Matrone, G., and Morgan, D.O., Porcine neonatal nutrition: absorption of unsaltered non-porcine proteins and polyvinylpyrrolidone from the gut of piglets and the subsequent effect of the maturation of the serum protein profile, *J. Nutr.*, 73, 158, 1961.

40. Lecce, J.G., and Morgan, D.O., The effect of dietary regimen on the cessation f absorption of large molecules (closure) in the neonatal piglet and lamb, *J. Nutr.* 73, 158, 1962.

41. Lecce, J.G., Morgan, D.O., and Matrone, G., Effect of feeding colostral and milk components on the cessation of intestinal absorption of large molecules (closure) in neonatal pigs, *J. Nutr.*, 84, 43, 1964.

42. Lecce, J.G. and Reep, B.R., *Escherichia coli* associated with colostrum-free neonatal pigs raised in isolation, *J. Exp. Med.*, 115, 491, 1962.

43. Lev, R., Siegel, H.I., and Bartman, J., Histochemical studies of developing human fetal small intestine, *Histochemie*, 29, 103, 1972.

44. Mackenzie, N.M., Morris, B., and Morris, R., Protein binding to brush borders of entrocytes from the jejunum of the neonatal rat, *Biochim. Biophys. Acta*, 755, 204, 1983.

45. Mathiowitz, E. et al., Biologically erodable microspheres as potential oral drug delivery systems, *Nature*, 386, 410, 1997.

46. McNabb, P.C. and Tomasi, T.B., Host defense mechanisms at mucosal surfaces, *Annu. Rev. Microbiol.*, 35, 477, 1981.

47. Morris, B. and Morris, R., The absorption of ^{125}I -labeled immunoglobulin G by different regions of the gut in young rats, *J. Physiol.*, 241, 761, 1974.

48. Morris, B. and Morris, R., The effect of corticosterone and cortisone on the transmission of IgG and the uptake of polyvinyl pyrrolidone by the small intestine in young rats, *J. Physiol.*, 255, 619, 1976.

49. Morris, B., Morris, R., and Kenyon, C.J., Effect of adrenalectomy on the transmission of IgG in young rats, *Biol. Neonat.*, 39, 239, 1981.

50. Moxey, P.C., Specialized cell types in the human fetal small intestine, *Anat. Rec.*, 191, 269, 1978.

51. Moxey, P.C. and Trier, J.S., Structural features of the mucosa of human fetal intestine, *Gastroenterology*, 68, 102, 1975.

52. Moxey, P.C. and Treir, J.S., Development of villus absorptive cells in the human fetal small intestine: a morphological and morphometric study, *Anat. Rec.*, 195, 463, 1979.

53. Ockleford, C.D. and Munn, E.A., Dynamic aspects of coated vesicle function, in *Coated Vesicles*, Ockleford, C.D. and Whyte, A., Eds., Cambridge University Press, Cambridge, 1980, p. 265.

54. Ockleford, C.D. and Whyte, A., Eds., *Coated Vesicles*. Cambridge University Press, Cambridge, 1980.

55. Ogra, S.S., Weintraub, D., and Ogra, P.L., Immunologic aspects of human colostrums and milk III. Fate and absorption of cellular and soluble components in the gastrointestinal tract of the newborn, *J. Immunol.*, 119, 245, 1977.

56. Oh, D.M., Han, H. K., and Amidon G.L., Drug transport and targeting: intestinal transport, in *Membrane Transporters as Drug Targets*, Amidon, G.L. and Sadee, W., Eds., Kluwer Academic, New York, 1999, chap. 3.

57. Owen, R.L., Sequential uptake of horseradish peroxidase by lymphoid follicle epithelium of Peyer's patches in the normal unobstructed mouse intestine: an ultrastructure study, *Gastroenterology*, 72, 440, 1977.

58. Owen, R.L. and Jones, A.L., Epithelial cell specialization within human Peyer's patches: An ultrastructural study of intestinal lymphoid follicles, *Gastroenterology*, 66, 189, 1974.

59. Pearse, B.M.F., On the structural and functional components of coated vesicles, *J. Mol. Biol.*, 126, 803, 1978.

60. Riepenhoff-Talty, M. et al., Age-dependent rotavirus-enterocyte interactions, *Proc. Soc. Exp. Biol. Med.*, 170, 146, 1982.

61. Rodewald, R., Selective antibody transport in the proximal small intestine of the neonatal rat, *J. Cell Biol.*, 45, 635, 1970.

62. Rozman, K.K. and Klaassen, C.D., Absorption distribution and excretion of toxicants, in *Casarett and Doulls Toxicology*, 6th ed., McGraw Hill, New York., 2001, chap. 5.

63. Rundell, J.O. and Lecce, J.G., Relationship of incorporation of radioprecursors into protein and phospholipids of the plasmalemma of guinea pig (neonate) intestinal epithelium and the cessation of uptake of macromolecules (closure), *Biol. Neonat.*, 34, 278, 1978.

64. Saffran, M. et al., A model for the study of the oral administration of peptide hormones, *Can. J. Biochem.*, 57, 548, 1979.

65. Schanker, L.S. and Jeffery, J.J., Active transport of foreign pyrimidines across the intestinal epithelium, *Nature*, 190, 727, 1961.

66. Schanker, L.S. et al., Absorption of drugs from the stomach I. The rat, *Pharmacol. Exp. Ther.*, 120, 528, 1957.

67. Sieber, S.M., The lymphatic absorption of p,p´-DDT and some structurally related compounds in the rat, *Pharmacology*, 14, 443, 1976.

68. Tyler, T.R., Peroral toxicity, in *General and Applied Toxicology*, 2nd ed., Macmillan, Oxford, 2000, p. 543.

69. Udall, J.N. and Walker, W.A., The physiologic and pathologic basis for the transport of macromolecules across the intestinal tract, *J. Pediatr. Gastroenterol. Nutr.*, 1, 295, 1982.

70. Vogel, G., Becker, U., and Ulbrich, M., The relevance of the osmolarity of the intestinal fluid to the effectiveness and toxicity of drugs given by the intraduodenal route-solvent drug influence on the intestinal absorption of drugs, *Arzneim. Forsch.*, 25, 1037, 1975.

71. Walker, W.A. et al., Macromolecular absorption: mechanism of horseradish peroxidase uptake and transport in adult and neonatal rat intestine, *J. Cell Biol.*, 54, 195, 1972.

72. Walker, W.A. and Isselbacher, K.J., Uptake and transport of macromolecules by the intestine: possible role in clinical disorders, *Gastroenterology*, 67, 531, 1974.

73. Walker, W.A. and Isselbacher, K.J., Intestinal antibodies, *New Engl. J. Med.*, 297, 767, 1977.

74. Walker, W.A., Isselbacher, K.J., and Bloch, K.J., Intestinal uptake of macromolecules: effect of oral immunization, *Science*, 177, 608, 1972.

75. Walker, W.A. et al., Intestinal uptake of macromolecules IV. The effect of pancreatic duct ligation on the breakdown of antigen and antigen-antibodycomplexes on the intestinal surface, *Gastroenterology*, 69, 1223, 1975.

76. Warshaw, A.L., Walker, W.A., and Isselbacher, K.J., Protein uptake by the intestine: evidence for absorption of intact macrocoleules, *Gastroenterology*, 66, 987, 1974.

77. Welling, P.G., Interactions affecting drug absorptions, *Clin. Pharmacokinet.*, 9, 404, 1984.

78. Wild, A.E., Role of the cell surface in selection during transport of proteins from mother to fetus and newly born, *Philos. Trans. R. Soc.*, London B, 271, 495, 1975.

79. Wild, A.E., Coated vesicles: a morphologically distinct subclass of endocytic vesicles, in *Coated Vesicles*, Ockleford, C.D. and Whyte, A., Eds., Cambridge University Press, Cambridge, 1980, p. 14.

80. Wild, A.E., Distribution of FC receptors on isolated gut enterocytes of the suckling rat, *J. Reprod. Immunol.*, 3, 283, 1981.

81. Wolf, J.L. et al., Suceptibility of mice to roavirus infection: effects of age and administration of corticosteroids, *Infect. Immun.*, 33, 565, 1981.

82. Wolf, J.L. et al., Intestinal M cells: a pathway for entry of retrovirus into the host, *Science*, 212, 471, 1981.

8 Peyer's Patch Epithelium: An Imperfect Barrier

Gary R. Burleson and Florence G. Burleson

CONTENTS

GASTROINTESTINAL TRACT: DESCRIPTION

Morphologically, the gastrointestinal (GI) tract can be described as a tube extending from the oral cavity to the anus. The longest section is the small intestine that connects the pylorus of the stomach to the large intestine or colon. The small intestine is divided into three sections: the duodenum, the jejunum, and the ileum. The GI tract consists of four distinct layers extending from the mucosa (ablumina or innermost layer closest to the lumen) to the adventitia or serosa or most ablumina or outermost layer from the lumen. These four layers include: (1) the mucosa which includes the epithelium, lamina propria, and muscularis mucosae, (2) the submucosa which includes the connective tissue, (3) the muscularis externa which is the muscular wall, and (4) the adventitia or serosa layer (see Figure 8.1).

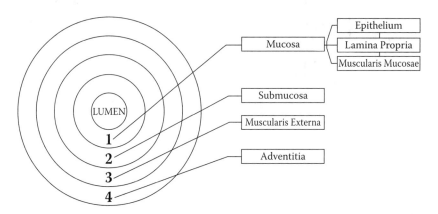

FIGURE 8.1 Four layers of gastrointestinal tract.

The mucosal epithelium lines the entire GI tract and is characterized by folds resulting in crypts and villi that increase the surface area for nutrient absorption — one of the major functions of the GI tract — performed by enterocytes. The crypts or invaginations also provide sites for stem cells and are the locations of Paneth's cells. The mucosa is the most highly differentiated layer of the GI tract. The mucosal epithelium includes the apical surface (gut luminal side) and the basal or connective tissue side. The gastrointestinal differentiation is related to function along the GI tract and includes protective aspects of the epithelium, production of digestive acid and enzymes, mucus-secreting cells, absorption of nutrients, secretory epithelium, stem cells for replenishment, smooth muscle fibers, and lymphoid cells. Specialized functions include sensory discrimination, mechanical processing, enzymatic and chemical digestion, and immunological surveillance.

MUCOSAL EPITHELIUM BARRIER FUNCTION

The mucosal epithelium with its tight junctions forms an effective physical barrier that normally functions as a perfect barrier. The cells of the mucosal epithelium form a continuous intact physical barrier with tight junctions formed with each neighboring cell. This tight physical barrier separates the inside of the human body from the outside. Cells of the mucosal epithelium have three important functions: (1) nutritional function (see Chapters 1 and 7), (2) barrier function (see Chapters 1 and 7), and (3) immunological function.

The mucosal epithelium thus acts as a watchdog, sentinel, or security guard to allow essential nutrients and electrolytes to enter, to deny passage of pathogenic microorganisms, to generate immune responses against pathogenic microorganisms, and to prevent immune responses against non-pathogenic or commensal microorganisms and foods that provide nourishment. However, the complexity of the mucosal epithelium which includes the multitude of tissue layers, cell types, cell functions, cellular control mechanisms, and messenger molecules such as hormones, neurotransmitters, cytokines, and chemokines makes providing the perfect barrier a difficult balancing act to maintain. The mucosal epithelium must perform disparate functions: serve as a barrier to protect the body from the outside world while serving as a mechanism to allow entry of nutrients, electrolytes, water, and antigens in order to allow initiation of an immune response.

The mucosal epithelium of the small intestine is folded into repeated villus and crypt structures and has a surface area of 400 m^2 (MacDonald and Monteleone, 2005). While this large surface area is beneficial for the absorption of nutrients, water, and electrolytes, the large access area is not beneficial and in fact complicates the immunological function.

MUCOSAL IMMUNITY

The perfect immunological GI barrier would prevent disease from infectious pathogenic microorganisms. Protection from infectious disease would be mediated by (1) a physical barrier to infection, (2) innate immunity, and (3) adaptive immunity. The perfect barrier would prevent an inappropriate immune response including responses to commensal microorganisms, food hypersensitivity, Crohn's disease, and IBD. The perfect barrier would allow commensal microorganisms of the normal GI flora to co-exist.

Control mechanisms must not allow immune responses to food antigens or against the commensal microorganisms residing in the intestines as part of the normal flora or allow entry of infectious agents that may result in serious local or systemic infection. The entry must allow antigenic sampling in order that an immunological response can be initiated and produced in defense against pathogenic microorganisms, but not against commensal microorganisms, nutrients, or food antigens. While the mucosal epithelium with its tight junctions performs as a barrier, the selective entry or antigenic sampling is performed by specialized immune cells in the Peyer's patches.

MALT AND MUCOSAL IMMUNITY OF GI TRACT

The mucosa-associated lymphoid tissue (MALT) term is used to describe all the mucosal lymphoid tissues in the body. One component of the MALT is the mucosal intestinal immune system that provides immunological surveillance and includes the GALT or gut-associated lymphoid tissue. Resistance to infectious and neoplastic disease is the raison d'être of the immunological armamentarium (Burleson, 2000). The total immune system of the body consists of a vast network of lymphoid and non-lymphoid cells communicating via messenger molecules to create a functional immune system to protect against disease. This network, while interconnected via mediator molecules, contains compartmentalized units especially equipped to defend against insults to the integrity of the immune system (Burleson, 2000). The intestinal immune system, like the pulmonary immune system, is specialized and compartmentalized. It is capable of performing all immunological functions locally and is also capable of interacting with the systemic immune system (reviewed by Burleson, 1987, 1995, 1996, 2000; and Lebrec and Burleson, 1994).

Mucosal immunity in the GI tract is composed of physical factors and non-immune molecules, plus non-immune (non-lymphoid cells) and immune (lymphoid) cells of the mucosal epithelium and Peyer's patches.

PHYSICAL FACTORS AND NON-IMMUNE MOLECULES

The physical barrier is provided by a continuous line of epithelial cells to protect against infection, exclude unwanted macromolecules, and minimize fluid and electrolyte loss into the intestinal lumen (Figure 8.2). Several components of the physical barrier are designed to keep potential pathogens from reaching the epithelium. Pathogenic microorganisms must compete with microorganisms of the normal flora for nutrients and space. Mucus secreted by goblet cells not only binds and immobilizes potential pathogens but also contains antimicrobial substances including lysozyme, hydrolytic enzymes, lactoferrin, and secretory antibodies.

The brush border with its glycocalyx containing mucin-like molecules provides a protective shield over the epithelial cells and also immobilizes potential threats to the epithelium (MacDonald and Monteleone, 2005). Peristalsis is another physical mechanism that moves infectious agents along unless they attach to susceptible epithelial cells.

Nevertheless, the gut epithelial barrier does not completely prevent luminal antigens from entering the tissues. Thus, intact food proteins can be detected in plasma (Husby et al., 1985) and a few gut bacteria can be detected in the mesenteric lymph nodes draining the guts of healthy animals (Berg, 1995). Antigens can cross the epithelial surfaces through breaks in tight junctions,

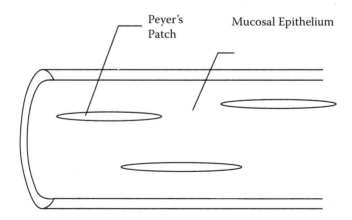

FIGURE 8.2 Gastrointestinal tract with mucosal epithelium and Peyer's patches.

perhaps at villus tips where epithelial cells are shed or through the follicle-associated epithelium (FAE) that overlies the organized lymphoid tissues of the intestinal wall (Neutra et al., 2001).

Non-Lymphoid Cells

Non-lymphoid cells include the intestinal epithelial cells (IECs) that form a continuous monolayer separating the outside world from the human body (Christ and Blumberg, 1997). IECs are capable of producing defensins such as cryptdins and numerous cytokines as messenger molecules that call in and activate the effector cells of the immune system. IECs are also involved in IgA transport as well as antigen uptake and presentation (Christ and Blumberg, 1997). IECs, enterocytes (absorptive intestinal cells), goblet cells, Paneth's cells (located at the bottoms of intestinal crypts), and enteroendocrine cells that produce neuroendocrine molecules with autocrine and paracrine effects on intestinal cells are all important non-lymphoid cell contributors to immunological protection.

Lymphoid Cells: Mucosal Epithelium

Lymphoid cells residing in the mucosal epithelium consist predominantly of the following types: intestinal intraepithelial lymphocytes (IELs) including IELαB and IELγδ, natural killer (NK) cells, T lymphocytes including Tαβ and Tγδ and macrophages (Figure 8.3). These cells are capable of providing both innate (non-specific) and specific (acquired) immunity.

Peyer's Patches: Description and Function

Peyer's patches are lymphoid aggregates or nodules that were first described by Johanni Conradi Peyeri in 1677 in his thesis titled "De glandulis Intestinorum

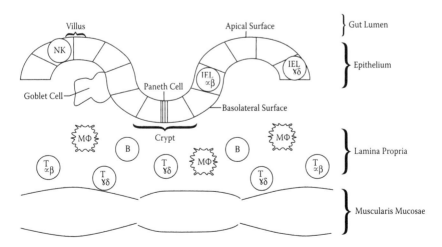

FIGURE 8.3 Non-immune and immune cells of mucosal epithelium and lamina propria.

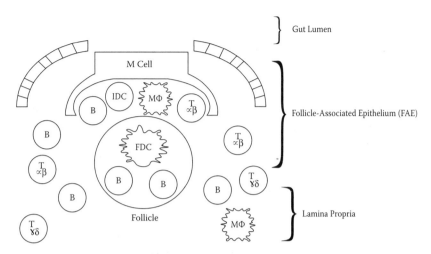

FIGURE 8.4 M cell, Peyer's patches, and immune cells.

Earumque Usu et Affectionibus Cui Fubjungitur Anatome Ventriculi Gallinacei"
(Croitoru and Bienenstock, 1994). Peyer's patches are located in the distal ileum
of the small intestine. In addition to increased numbers of Peyer's patches or
mucosal lymphoid tissue, the ileum also has more goblet cells than proximal
sections of the small intestine.

Immunological surveillance within the mucosal epithelium is primarily provided by Peyer's patches (Figure 8.2 and Figure 8.4). The mucosal lymphoid
aggregates comprising Peyer's patches functionally perform the important role
of initiating the local immune system. Peyer's patches are collections of lymphoid
tissue underneath the follicle-associated epithelium (FAE) consisting of cells with
microvilli. These lymphoid follicles differ from lymph nodes in that they lack
capsules, medullae, afferent lymphatic ducts, and clear borders. M cells are
situated within this epithelium among the microvilli-covered cells. Also present
are B lymphocytes, macrophages, follicular dendritic cells, and NK cells.

M CELLS

Specialized epithelial cells designated membranous or microfold (M) cells provide access to Peyer's patches (Figure 8.4). Antigen attaches and enters M cells
that contain a specialized epithelium and are located above the lymphoid follicles.
M cells continuously transport intestinal bacteria and antigens from the lumen
into lymphoid tissues. These specialized M cells in the FAE sample foreign
material and deliver it to the organized mucosal lymphoid tissue. The purpose is
to initiate the specific immune response. While induction of the immune response
occurs in M cells of the Peyer's patches, the effector region is the lamina propria.

Follicular dendritic cells (DCs) are numerous in the subepithelial dome (SED)
region located beneath the FAE. DCs are professional antigen-presenting cells
(APCs); they are able to engulf, process, and present the antigen that has been

sampled from the intestinal lumen by the M cell. While normally maturing and migrating through the lymphatics or blood vessels to T cell areas in secondary lymphoid organs, the DCs in the SED region are in close proximity to T and B cell zones and thus present antigen locally.

PEYER'S PATCHES: LYMPHOID CELLS

Lymphoid cells include dendritic cells, macrophages, mast cells, polymorphonu- clear (PMN) leukocytes, NK cells, T lymphocytes (CD4+ helper T lymphocytes and CD8+ cytotoxic T lymphocytes), and B lymphocytes. More than 80% of the body's activated B cells are located in the intestines and 80 to 90% of the terminally differentiated B cells are found in the lamina propria IgA blasts and plasma cells (Brandtzaeg et al., 2001; Campbell, et al., 2003).

BARRIER DYSFUNCTION

As noted above, the mucosal epithelium performs numerous specialized functions required for health, nutrition, and protection of the body from the outside envi- ronment. Perturbation of this finely balanced homeostasis may result in altered function such as altered barrier function. Furthermore, the immunological mech- anisms designed to prevent infection with enteric pathogens may be circumvented by the M cells to actually transport pathogenic microorganisms into the body.

IMMUNE-INDUCED BARRIER DYSFUNCTION

Immunological defense against infection results in the production of various cytokines and chemokines that have a multitude of autocrine and paracrine effects. While immunological defense is the designated and desired role of the mucosal immune system, infectious disease may regulate in a positive or negative fashion the delicate and tightly controlled homeostatic balance required in the GI tract. Infection by microorganisms results in the production of cytokines by T helper or CD4+ cells that is termed either a TH_1 or TH_2 response. TH_1 cells produce IFNγ and IL-2, are active against intracellular bacteria and viruses, and induce isotype switching in humans to IgG1 and IgG3. TH_2 cells produce IL-4, IL-5, and IL-10, are active against extracellular bacteria and parasites, and induce isotype switching to IgA, IgE, and IgG4.

Lymphocytes in the intestines include CD8+ IELs or submucosal popula- tions of CD4+ lamina propria lymphocytes (LPLs). While CD4+ TH_2 T cells are known to produce IL-4, evidence now demonstrates that subsets of IEL also produce IL-4 (Fujihashi et al., 1993a and 1993b). Thus, infection by intracellular bacteria or viruses results in the production of IFNγ while infection by extra- cellular bacteria or parasites results in the production of IL-4.

Either IL-4 or IFNγ can act directly on epithelial cells to alter the barrier function of the mucosal epithelium and modulate the effect of electrolyte and water loss through the intestinal barrier as a result of a derangement or pertur- bation of epithelial tight junctions (Watson et al., 2004).

Trojan Horse Barrier Dysfunction: Reovirus, Local, and Systemic Infection through Peyer's Patches Epithelium

Reoviruses (respiratory, enteric, orphan viruses) have been studied in the respiratory and GI tracts. Reovirus serotype 1 (Lang) and serotype 3 (Dearing) strains have been most thoroughly characterized. Reovirus type 1 (Lang) replicates to high titers after oral infection in suckling mice while reovirus type 3 (Dearing) does not. The molecular basis for this differential replication and subsequent viral shedding from the GI tract resides in the L2 and S1 genes. The S1 gene that codes for the outer capsid protein -1 and the L2 gene that codes for the -2 core spike protein are responsible for the difference in allowing the Lang strain (but not the Dearing strain) to replicate in intestinal tissue (Keroack and Fields, 1986; Bodkin and Fields, 1989).

Reoviruses enter the body through the very mechanism that protects and initiates an immune response against infections agents – demonstrating the imperfect barrier function of Peyer's patches. Reoviruses (respiratory, enteric, orphan viruses) were named by Sabin in 1959 because they were typically isolated from the respiratory and GI tracts and were not associated with any known disease. Infection in the GI tract occurs when intestinal M cells are used as portals of entry.

Studies in mice demonstrated that reovirus type 1 was detected adhering to the surfaces of intestinal M cells (but not other epithelial cells) 30 min after administration into the intestinal lumen. Viruses were detected in the M cell cytoplasm within 1 hr (Wolf et al., 1981). Thus, reoviruses attach to the surfaces of specialized epithelial M cells that overlie the domes of Peyer's patches. M cells transport macromolecules from the intestinal lumen to the intercellular space. Following facilitated access through M cells, a reovirus is spread and is sequentially detected in Peyer's patches, mesenteric lymph nodes, spleen, and the CNS (Kauffman et al., 1983).

Numerous other bacteria, viruses, protozoa, and helminths are capable of causing intestinal infections with clinical illness (Table 8.1). The majority of these infectious agents cause diseases ranging from mild to severe, including diarrheal illnesses, dysenteries, enteric fevers, and malabsorptive states. Virulence properties typically include cytotoxic enterotoxins, fimbrial attachment factors, expression of proteins leading to effacement of outer membrane proteins that allow bacteria to be internalized by epithelial cells, cytotoxins that suppress protein synthesis and lead to cell death, and expression of proteins that allows survival within macrophage phagolysosomes. Two recurrent bacterial properties of enteric bacterial pathogens include: (1) mechanisms allowing adherence to mucosal epithelial cells, and (2) elaboration of toxins (reviewed by Levine and Nataro, 1994).

In cholera, the cholera toxin is capable of killing epithelial cells so that cell-to-cell junctions no longer maintain the integrity of the fluid barrier between lumen and lamina propria. Body fluid thus accumulates in the lumen and passes through the intestine as watery diarrhea, leading to rapid dehydration and may even lead to death. Treatment involves antibiotics and hydration therapy, with an

TABLE 8.1
Infectious Microorganisms, M Cells, and the GI Tract

Pathogenic Microorganisms	References
Viruses	
Adenovirus	Buller and Moxley, 1988
Astrovirus	Woode et al., 1984
Breda virus	Woode et al., 1984
Coxsackievirus	Heinz and Cliver, 1988
Human immunodeficiency virus Type 1 (HIV-1)	Amerongen et al., 1991; Fotopoulos et al., 2002
Mouse mammary tumor virus	Neutra and Kraehenbuhl, 1992
Poliovirus type 1	Ouzilou et al., 2002
Reovirus Type 1	Bass et al., 1988; London et al., 1987; Wolf et al., 1987; Helander et al., 2003
Reovirus Type 3	Wolf et al., 1983
Rotovirus	Buller and Moxley, 1988
Transmissible gastroenteritis virus	Chu et al., 1982
Bacteria	
Calmette–Guerin bacillus	Van der Brugge-Gamelkoorn et al., 1985; Fujimura, 1986
Brucella abortus	Ackermann et al., 1988
Campylobacter jejuni	Walker et al., 1988
Chlamydia	Landsverk, 1981
Escherichia coli RDEC-1 strain	Inman and Cantey, 1983; Inman et al., 1986
Escherichia coli O:124 K:72	Uchida, 1987
Listeria monocytogenes	Jenson et al., 1998
Mycobacterium paratuberculosis	Momotani et al., 1988
Rhodococcus equi	Johnson et al., 1983
Shigella flexneri	Wassef et al., 1989; Jenson et al., 1998
Salmonella choleraesuis	Pospischil et al., 1990
Salmonella enteritidis	Kanoi, 1991
Salmonella gallinarium	Pascopella et al., 1995
Salmonella typhi	Kohbata et al., 1986; Pascopella et al., 1995
Salmonella typhimurium	Hohman et al., 1978; Jenson et al., 1998
Streptococcus pyogenes	Nagasaki et al., 1988
Yersinia enterocolitica	Grutzkau et al., 1990
Yersinia pseudotuberculosis	Fujimura et al., 1989; Fujimura et al., 1992; Clark et al., 1998
Vibrio cholerae	Owen et al., 1986; Pearch et al., 1987
Vibrio parahemolyticus	Yamamoto and Yokota, 1989
Protozoa	
Cryptosporidium	Marcial and Madara, 1986
Prions	
Scrapie prion protein (PrP)	Heggebo et al., 2000

intravenous plasma substitute or a properly balanced solution of salt delivered orally. The cholera bacteria will clear and the epithelium will be replaced by stem cells dividing in the crypts.

Enterotoxigenic *Escherichia coli*, enteropathogenic *E. coli*, Shigella, rotaviruses, *Vibrio cholera* 01 and *Shigella dysenteriae* 1, *Salmonella typhi*, *Campylobacter jejuni*, enteric adenoviruses and *Entamoeba histolytica* are among the most important pathogens from a public health view that cause intestinal disease (reviewed by Levine and Nataro, 1994).

REFERENCES

Ackermann, M.R., N.F. Cheville, and B.L. Deyoe. 1988. Bovine ileal dome lymphoepithelial cells: endocytosis and transport of *Brucella abortus* strain 19. *Vet. Pathol.* 25: 28–35.

Amerongen, H.M., R. Weltzin, C.M. Farnet, P. Michetti, W.A. Haseltine, and M.R. Neutra. 1991. Transepithelial transport of HIV-1 by intestinal M cells: a mechanism for transmission of AIDS. *J. Acquir. Immun. Defic. Syndr.* 4: 760–765.

Bass, D.M., J.S. Trier, R. Dambrauskas, and J.L. Wolf. 1988. Reovirus type 1 infection of small intestinal epithelium in suckling mice and its effect on M cells. *Lab. Invest.* 58: 226–235.

Berg, R.D. 1995. Bacterial translocation from the gastrointestinal tract. *Trends Microbiol.* 3: 149–154.

Bodkin, D.K. and B.N. Fields. 1989. Growth and survival of reovirus in intestinal tissue: role of the L2 and S1 genes. *J. Virol.* 63: 1183–1193.

Brandtzaeg, P., E.S. Baekkevold, and H.C. Morton. 2001. From B to A the mucosal way. *Nature Immunol.* 2: 1093–1094.

Buller, C.R. and R.A. Moxley. 1988. Natural infection of porcine ileal dome M cells with rotavirus and enteric adenovirus. *Vet. Pathol.* 25: 516–517.

Burleson, G.R. 1987. Alteration of cellular interactions in the immune system: natural killer activity and N lymphocytes, in H.A. Milman and E. Elmore, Eds., *Biochemical Mechanisms and Regulation of Intercellular Communication*. Princeton Scientific Publishing, Princeton, NJ, pp. 51–96.

Burleson, G.R. 1995. Influenza virus host resistance model for assessment of immunotoxicity, immunostimulation, and antiviral compounds, in G.R. Burleson et al., Eds., *Methods in Immunotoxicology*, Vol. 2, Wiley-Liss, New York, pp. 181–202.

Burleson, G.R. 1996. Pulmonary immunocompetence and pulmonary immunotoxicology, in R.J. Smialowicz, and M.P. Holsapple, Eds., *Experimental Immunotoxicology*. CRC Press, Boca Raton, FL, pp. 119–141.

Burleson, G.R. 2000. Models of respiratory immunotoxicology and host resistance. *Immunopharmacology* 48: 315–318.

Campbell, D.J., C.H. Kim, and E.C. Butcher. 2003. T and B cells express $\alpha 4 B7$ integrin and migrate to the blood after being activated in the Peyer's patches. *Immunol. Rev.* 195: 58–71 .

Christ, A.D. and R.S. Blumberg. 1997. The intestinal epithelial cell: immunological aspects. *Springer Semin. Immunopathol.* 18: 449–461.

Chu, R.M., R.D. Glock, and R.F. Ross. 1982. Changes in gut-associated lymphoid tissues of the small intestine of eight-week-old pigs infected with transmissible gastroenteritis virus. *Am. J. Vet. Res.* 43: 67–76.

Clark, M.A., B.H. Hirst, and M.A. Jepson. 1998. M-cell surface beta-1 integrin expression and invasin-mediated targeting of *Yersinia pseudotuberculosis* to mouse Peyer's patch M cells. *Infect. Immun.* 66: 1237–1243.

Croitoru, K. and J. Bienenstock. 1994. Characteristics and functions of mucosa-associated lymphoid tissue, in P.L. Ogra et al., Eds., *Handbook of Mucosal Immunology*, Academic Press, New York, chap. 12.

Fotopoulos, G., A. Haran, P. Michetti, D. Trono, G. Pantaleo, and J.P. Kraehenbuhl. 2002. Transepithelial transport of HIV-1 by M cells is receptor mediated. *Proc. Natl. Acad. Sci. USA* 99: 9410–9414.

Fujihashi, K., M. Yamamota, J.R. McGhee, and H. Kiyono. 1993a. TCR-αB-positive intraepithelial lymphocytes with CD4+CD8- and CD4+CD8+ phenotypes from orally immunized mice provide Th2-like function for B cell responses. *J. Immunol.* 151: 6681–6691.

Fujihashi, K., M. Yamamoto, J.R. McGhee, K.W. Beagley, and H. Kiyono. 1993b. Function of αB T cell receptor-positive intraepithelial lymphocytes: Th1 and Th2-type cytokine production by CD4+ CD8- and CD4+CD8+ T cells for helper activity. *Int. Immunol.* 5: 1473–1481.

Fujimura, Y. 1986. Functional morphology of microfold cells (M cells) in Peyer's patches: phagocytosis and transport of BCG by M cells into rabbit Peyer's patches. *Gastroenterol. Jpn.* 21: 325–335.

Fujimura, Y., K. Ohtani, R. Kamoi, T. Kato, K. Kozuka, N. Miyashima, J. Uchida, T. Kihara, and H. Mine. 1989. An ultrastructural study of ileal invasion process of *Yersinia pseudotuberculosis* in rabbits. *J. Clin. Electron Microsc.* 22: 712–716.

Fujimura, Y., T. Kihara, and H. Mine. 1992. Membranous cells as a portal of *Yersinia pseudotuberculosis* entry into rabbit ileum. *J. Clin. Electron Microsc.* 25: 35–42.

Grutzkau, A., C. Hanski, H. Hahn, and E.O. Riecken. 1990. Involvement of M cells in the bacterial invasion of Peyer's patches: a common mechanism shared by *Yersinia enterocolitica* and other enteroinvasive bacteria. *Gut* 31: 1011–1015.

Heggebo, R., C.M. Press, G. Gunnes, K.I. Lie, M.A. Tranulis, M. Ulvund, M.H. Groschup, and T. Landsverk. 2000. Distribution of prion proteins in the ileal Peyer's patch of scrapie-free lambs and lambs naturally and experimentally exposed to scrapie agent. *J. Gen. Virol.* 81: 2327–2337.

Heinz, B.A. and D.O. Cliver. 1988. Coxsackievirus–cell interactions that initiate infection in porcine ileal explants. *Arch. Virol.* 101: 35–47.

Helander, A., K.J. Silvey, N.J. Mantis, A.B. Hutchings, K. Chandran, W.T. Lucas, M.L. Nibert, and M.R. Neutra. 2003. The viral sigma-1 protein and glycoconjugates containing alpha 2-3-linked sialic acid are involved in type 1 reovirus adherence to M cell apical surfaces. *J. Virol.* 77: 7964–7977.

Hohman, A.W., G. Schmidt, and D. Rowley. 1978. Intestinal colonization and virulence of Salmonella in mice. *Infect. Immun.* 22: 763–770.

Husby, S., J.C. Jensenius, and S.E. Svehag. 1985. Passage of undegraded dietary antigen into the blood of healthy adults: quantification, estimation of size distribution, and relation of uptake in levels of specific antibodies. *Scand. J. Immunol.* 22: 83–92

Inman, L.R. and J.R. Cantey. 1983. Specific adherence of *Escherichia coli* (strain RDEC-1) to membranous M cells of the Peyer's patch in *Escherichia coli* diarrhea in the rabbit. *J. Clin. Invest.* 71: 1– 8.

Inman, L.R., J.R. Cantey, and S.B. Formal. 1986. Colonization, virulence, and mucosal interaction of an enteropathogenic *Escherichi coli* (strain RDEC-1) expressing Shigella somatic antigen in the rabbit intestine. *J. Infect. Dis.* 154: 742–751.

Jenson, V.B., J.T. Harty, and B.D. Jones. 1998. Interactions of the invasive pathogens *Salmonella typhimurium*, *Listeria monocytogenes*, and *Shigella flexneri* with M cells and murine Peyer's patches. *Infect. Immun.* 66: 3758–3766.

Johnson, J.A., J.F. Prescott, and R.J. Markham. 1983. The pathology of experimental *Corynebacterium equi* infection in foals following intragastric challenge. *Vet. Pathol.* 20: 450–459.

Kanoi, R. 1991. Morphological studies of *Salmonella enteritidis* uptake by microfold cells (M cells) of the Peyer's patch. *Kaw. Igak.* 17: 225–231.

Kauffman, J.L. Wolf, R. Finberg, J.S. Trier, and B.N. Fields. 1983. The sigma-1 protein determines the extent of spread of reovirus from the gastrointestinal tract of mice. *Virology* 124: 403–410.

Keroack, M. and B.N. Fields. 1986. Viral shedding and transmission between hosts determined by reovirus L2 gene. *Science* 232: 1635–1638.

Kohbata, S., H. Yokoyama, and E. Yabuuchi. 1986. Cytopathogenic effect of *Salmonella typhi* GIFU 10007 on M cells of murine ileal Peyer's patches in ligated ileal loops: an ultrastructural study. *Microbiol. Immunol.* 30: 1225–1237.

Landsverk, T. 1981. Peyer's patches and the follicle-associated epithelium in diarrheic calves: pathomorphology, morphometry and acid phosphatase histochemistry. *Acta Vet. Scand.* 22: 459–471.

Lebrec, H. and G.R. Burleson. 1994. Influenza virus host resistance models in mice and rats: utilization for immune function assessment and immunotoxicology. *Toxicology* 91: 179–188.

Levine, M.M. and J.P. Nataro. 1994. Intestinal infections, in P.L. Ogra et al., Eds., *Handbook of Mucosal Immunology*, Academic Press, New York.

London, S.D., D.H. Rubin, and J.J. Cebra. 1987. Gut mucosal immunization with reovirus serotype 1/L stimulates virus-specific cytotoxic T cell precursors as well as IgA memory cells in Peyer's patches. *J. Exp. Med.* 165: 830–847.

MacDonald, T.T. and G. Monteleone. 2005. Immunity, inflammation, and allergy in the gut. *Science* 307: 1920–1925.

Marcial, M.A. and J.L. Madara. 1986. Cryptosporidium: cellular localization, structural analysis of absorptive cell-parasite membrane-membrane interactions in guinea pigs, and suggestion of protozoan transport by M cells. *Gastroenterology* 90: 583–594.

Momotani, E., D.L. Whipple, A.B. Thiermann, and N.F. Cheville. 1988. Role of M cells and macrophages in the entrance of *Mycobacterium paratuberculosis* into domes of ileal Peyer's patches in calves. *Vet. Pathol.* 25: 131–137.

Nagasaki, S., R. Kamoi, T. Kato, K. Kozuka, N. Miyashima, Y. Fujimura, J. Uchida, and T. Kihara. 1988. M cell transport of *Streptococcus pyogenes* Su strains ATCC 2106 and OK-432 from the intestinal lumen into rabbit Peyer's patches. *J. Clin. Electron Microsc.* 21: 588–594.

Neutra, M.R. and J.P. Kraehenbuhl. 1992. M cell-mediated antigen transport and monoclonal IgA antibodies for mucosal immune protection. *Adv. Exp. Med. Biol.* 327: 143–150.

Neutra, M.R., N.J. Mantis, and J.P. Kraehenbuhl. 2001. Collaboration of epithelial cells with organized lymphoid tissues. *Nature Immunol.* 2: 1004–1009.

Owen, R.L., N.F. Pierce, R.T. Apple, and W.C. Cray Jr. 1986. M cell transport of *Vibrio cholerae* from the intestinal lumen into Peyer's patches: a mechanism for antigen sampling and for microbial transepithelial migration. *J. Infect. Dis.* 153: 1108–1118.

Ouzilou, I., E. Chiot, I. Pelletier, M.C. Prevost, E. Pringault, and F. Colbere-Garapin. 2002. Poliovirus transcytosis through M-like cells. *J. Gen. Virol.* 83: 2177–2182.

Pascopella, L., B. Raupach, N. Ghori, D. Monack, S. Falkow, and P.L. Small. 1995. Host restriction phenotypes of *Salmonella typhi* and *Salmonella gallinarium. Infect. Immun.* 63: 4329–4335.

Pierce, N.F., J.B. Kaper, J.J. Mekalanos, W.C. Cray Jr. and K. Richardson. 1987. Determinants of the immunogenicity of live virulent and mutant *Vibrio cholerae* 01 in rabbit intestine. *Infect. Immun.* 55: 477–481.

Pospischil, A., R.L. Wood and T.D. Anderson. 1990. Peroxidase-antiperoxidase and immunogold labeling of *Salmonella typhimurium* and *Salmonella cholerae* suis var kunzendorf in tissues of experimentally infected swine. *Am. J. Vet. Res.* 51: 619–624.

Sabin, A.B. 1959. Reoviruses. *Science* 130: 1387–1389.

Uchida, J. 1987. An ultrastructural study on active uptake and transport of bacteria by microfold cells (M cells) to the lymphoid follicles in the rabbit appendix. *J. Clin. Electron Microsc.* 20: 379–405.

Van der Brugge-Gamelkoorn, G., M. van de Ende, and T. Sminia. 1985. Uptake of antigens and inert particles by bronchus-associated lymphoid tissue (BALT) epithelium in the rat. *Cell Biol. Int. Rep.* 9: 524.

Walker, R.I., E.A. Schauder-Chock, and J.L. Parker. 1988. Selective association and transport of *Campylobacter jejuni* through M cells of rabbit Peyer's patches. *Can. J. Microbiol.* 34: 1142–1147.

Wassef, J.S., D.F. Keren, and J.L. Mailloux. 1989. Role of M cells in initial antigen uptake and in ulcer formation in the rabbit intestinal loop model of shigellosis. *Infect. Immun.* 57: 858–863.

Watson, J.L., S. Ansari, H. Cameron, A. Wang, M. Akhter, and D.M. McKay. 2004. Green tea polyphenol (-)-epigallocatechin gallate blocks epithelial barrier dysfunction provoked by IFN-γ but not IL-4. *Am. J. Physiol. Gastrointest. Liver Physiol.* 287: G954–G961.

Wolf, J.L., D.H. Rubin, R. Finberg, R.S. Kauffman, A.H. Sharpe, J.S. Trier, and B.N. Fields. 1981. Intestinal M cells: a pathway for entry of reovirus into the host. *Science* 212: 471–472.

Wolf, J.L., R.S. Kaufman, R. Finberg, R. Dambrauskas, B.N. Fields, and J.S. Trier. 1983. Determinants of reovirus interaction with the intestinal M cells and absorptive cells of murine intestine. *Gastroenterology* 85: 291–300.

Wolf, J.L., R. Dambrauskas, A.H. Sharpe, and J.S. Trier. 1987. Adherence to and penetration of the intestinal epithelium by reovirus type 1 in neonatal mice. *Gastroenterology* 92: 82–91.

Woode, G.N., J.F. Pholenz, N.E. Gourley, and J.A. Fagerland. 1984. Astrovirus and Breda virus infections of dome cell epithelium of bovine ileum. *J. Clin. Microbiol.* 19: 623–630.

Yamamoto, T. and T. Yokota. 1989. Adherence targets of *Vibrio parahaemolyticus* in human small intestines. *Infect. Immun.* 57: 2410–2419.

9 Alteration of Intestinal Function by Xenobiotic Exposure: Animal Models

Shayne C. Gad

CONTENTS

INTRODUCTION

The gastrointestinal (GI) tract shares with the skin and lungs the distinction of being of a major route of both exposure and systemic absorption for environmental chemicals and serving as a target for their actions. Most pharmaceuticals, foods, and water-borne chemicals enter the body via the GI tract, whereas occupational exposure to chemicals occurs primarily through skin and lungs. When the GI tract is injured by ingested materials, their deleterious effects impact the whole organism. In addition, damage to the gastrointestinal barrier may enhance or suppress absorption of other substances. Because an intact GI tract is necessary for the maintenance of the nutritional status, a chemically injured intestinal mucosa may alter the normal and absorptive functions as reflected by poor nutritional status and altered responsiveness to the chemical insult.

The response of the GI tract to viral agents or microorganisms may cause a self-limited diarrheal disease. The limited course of such disease tends to remove chemicals via diarrheal secretions and increased motility. Intestinal toxins that result from interactions of chemicals, nutrients, and microorganisms add another dimension to the possible alterations of intestinal function by chemical exposure. The possible interactions of chemicals, nutrients, and microorganisms continue to be explored.[60] Animal gene knockout models are used to evaluate the identities, membrane locations, and metabolic activities of epithelial ion transporters including the secretory isoforms of the Na(+)/H(+) exchanger and the colonic H(+)-K(+)-ATPase.[79]

NATURE OF XENOBIOTIC EXPOSURE

The numbers and amounts of potentially toxic chemicals entering the environment have increased steadily since the beginning of the Industrial Revolution. Their effects went unnoticed or were of little concern initially, but gradual awareness of risks posed to human health by chemically contaminated food and water has developed.[8] Although the rate of increase in chemical pollution has slowed, thousands of chemicals are still emitted into the air, dumped into rivers and lakes, and buried in the land. It appears that large-scale degradation of surface waters has been stopped, but water quality data indicate that surface water pollution from conventional and toxic pollutants is still widespread.

Ground water has always been considered a pristine resource, but recent information reveals that ground water is contaminated in many locations. This contamination arises from many sources and includes a variety of materials, e.g., synthetic organic chemicals and inorganic chemicals. The concentrations of these synthetic organic chemicals in the ground water are often orders of magnitude higher than concentrations found in raw or surface water supplies. A third of all public supplies and 95% of all rural domestic supplies depend on ground water resources.[22] Based on total use (withdrawal), fresh groundwater is used predominantly for agricultural purposes. The identities of potential pollutants are largely unknown and uncharacterized at present.

Comprehensive surveys reveal a vast array of chemical entities added to foods by humans. These include food additives and residues as well as entities occurring as natural toxicants and contaminants such as the food additives and residues from migration of packaging materials to food. Estimates of the number of compounds included in the food additive and residue category vary, but a 10,000 figure is probably conservative. Since 95% of the food reaching consumers is processed in some way, the intentional food additives consumed have been estimated as 1.5 kg/yr/capita. As a toxicological consideration, the extensiveness of this consumption makes it difficult to draw attention to individual substances or groups of related compounds.

NATURE OF INTESTINAL FUNCTION

The principal function of the GI tract is to modify ingested food so that the nutrients can be absorbed by the intestines, passed into the bloodstream and lymph

TABLE 9.1
Major Gastrointestinal Processes

Process	Description
Secretion	Release of ions, substances, and enzymes
Digestion	Intraluminal breakdown of ingested substances
Absorption	Uptake of molecules across mucosal surface
Metabolism	Intracellular synthesis
Motility	Movement of intraluminal contents along tract

system, and transported throughout the organism. This function involves the processes of secretion, digestion, absorption, metabolism, and motility all working together (Table 9.1). In addition, the intestine serves as a selective barrier to foreign molecules, some of which provoke antigenic responses.

Food- and water-borne chemicals entering the GI tract can injure it and alter these normal functions and modulate their effects. Interactions of these chemicals within the tract reflect the properties of the tract per se, the chemicals and the organisms. Examination of the roles of the GI tract in these interactions requires an understanding of the luminal milieu (bacterial and biochemical components), the dietary factors, the brush border, and the intracellular processes (metabolism of nutrients and chemicals). The ingested chemicals may vary in solubility, size, and reactivity, all of which affect their digestion, absorption, and interactions with the mucosal surface. Specific organism factors such as age, genetic defects, and disease state also influence the interactions of chemicals with the GI tract. The major diseases of the tract are at least, in part, environmentally determined.[68]

Examination of the effects of ingested environmental chemicals on the GI tract as a target organ system may focus on the time course of damage, recovery, repair, and adaptation within this system. To better understand the impacts of these chemicals, model systems are designed to evaluate these effects. The modeling effort develops and exploits animal analogs of the disease processes. A number of approaches have been developed to examine various aspects of GI tract function. The choice of approach reflects the focus of a project and may involve enzymes, isolated cells, intestinal sacs, or whole animals. Recent work examines intraluminal metabolism as well as intracellular metabolism.

APPROACHES TO STUDYING CHEMICAL ALTERATION OF INTESTINAL FUNCTION

The body of knowledge concerning the effects of ingested chemicals on gastrointestinal function is growing rapidly. The approaches utilized in the examination of chemically altered gastrointestinal function include *in vivo* exposure and *in vivo*, *in situ*, or *in vitro* evaluation, or *in vitro* exposure and *in vitro* evaluation.[69] The various methodologies for evaluating gastrointestinal function

TABLE 9.2
Evaluation of Altered Gastrointestinal Function

Method of Exposure/ Method of Monitoring	Function Studied	Environmental Agent	Reference
In vivo/in vivo	Digestion, flora	Methyl mercury	76
	Barrier	Cadmium	77,41
In vivo/in situ	Absorption	Organochlorine compounds	84
	Absorption	Cadmium	85
In vivo/in vitro	Absorption	Dieldrin	47
	Motility	Hexachlorobenzene	64
	Absorption	Lindane; DDT	49,58
In vitro/in vitro	Metabolism	Salicylate	82
	Absorption	Aluminum; DDT; DDE	24
	Motility	Amitraz (pesticide)	33,62

were reviewed previously. Specific examples of these approaches taken from the current literature are given in Table 9.2.

GASTROINTESTINAL FUNCTIONS AFFECTED BY XENOBIOTIC EXPOSURE

Ingested food is processed by the GI tract by mixing with a number of secretions produced primarily by the salivary glands, stomach, pancreas, liver, and intestines. These secretions consist of ions, water, enzymes, and bile. In some instances, the degradation processes are assisted by the intestinal flora. Although the salivary glands and their secretions are not essential to life, the secreted electrolytes, K^+ and HCO_3, and enzymes, a-amylase, lysozyme, and kallikrein, enhance the digestive process. The stomach elaborates electrolytes, intrinsic factor, pepsinogen, and mucus that convert the ingested food into semiliquid form.

More specific enzymes, e.g., trypsin, chymotrypsin, carboxypeptidase, and pancreatic lipase, enter the intestinal lumen from the pancreas. The human liver secretes up to a liter per day of bile containing bile salts, mucin, hemoglobin breakdown products, phospholipids, cholesterol, and electrolytes. Bile salts are essential for the emulsification of the oil and water portions of semidigested food and for the formation of micelles. The intestinal secretions such as mucus play important roles as lubricants.

Examination of the effects of known food and water contaminants and food additives on gastrointestinal secretion and digestion of food is in its infancy. As would be expected, agents identified as liver, pancreatic, stomach, and colon carcinogens would be anticipated to affect these normal functions. Also, agents that are destructive of the mucosa surfaces on contact would be expected to disrupt secretory and digestive functions. Examples of such agents include gastric juices, aspirin,[37] alcohol,[46] and T-2 toxin.[39]

TABLE 9.3

Excretion of Several Chemicals in Feces of Conventional (Control), Germ-Free, and Antibiotic-Treated Animals

Chemical	Conventional	Germ-Free (% of Dose)	Antibiotic-Treated	Reference
Warfarin	24	31	33	63
Inorganic mercury	9.3	—	1.8	77
Diphenylhydantoin	78	—	95	21

The GI tract contains a bacterial system within the lumen, particularly in the colon. These microorganisms contain enzymes that hydrolyze undigested food and chemicals. A well known role of the gastrointestinal flora is the hydrolysis of glucuronide conjugates. Studies have shown that a variety of compounds secreted in the bile as glucuronide conjugates are hydrolyzed by the bacterial α-glucuronidase that allows for reabsorption of the compounds. Facilitation of enterohepatic circulation by rat intestinal bacteria has been reported for phenytoin,[21] phenacetin,[80] diethylstilbesterol,[25] digitoxin,[87] and warfarin.[63] More recently, these microorganisms have been demonstrated to convert methyl mercury to inorganic mercury.[76,77] There are many recent examples of the effects of microorganisms on the concentration of ingested substances in the feces (Table 9.3).

The monitoring of substances in the feces is one approach to measuring the relative absorption of agents such as aliphatic hydrocarbons.[1] The effects of a dioxin on lipid absorption have been examined in detail in rats.[70]

Prior oral exposure to low doses of 2,3,7,8-tetrachlorodibenzo-p-dioxin markedly augmented the appearance of lipid in the serum after a dose of corn oil.[74] Several agents have been used to limit the absorption of lipophilic toxins, e.g., cholestyramine[23] and paraffin.[64] Monitoring radiolabeled carbon dioxide production from radiolabeled nutrients has been utilized to examine malabsorption induced by chemical exposure. In this instance, careful selection of dose and time of monitoring are essential for detecting altered nutrient absorption and subsequent metabolism. Several investigators have used the everted sacs technique for examining alterations in intestinal absorptions of nutrients, e.g., simple sugars and amino acids (Table 9.4).

One aspect of the target organ approach that has changed in emphasis is the recognition that metabolism by an organ is not necessarily synonymous with detoxification. The role of intestinal metabolism of foreign substances by laboratory animals and humans is discussed fully in later chapters.

The intestinal mucosa is an extremely active metabolic tissue. The proliferative nature of the crypt cells and differentiation to well defined absorptive villous tip cells require marked synthesis of macromolecules. For instance, it has been estimated that 50 g of protein is sloughed per day.[55] The active transport and

TABLE 9.4
Altered Absorption of Nutrients by Chemicals

Chemical	Species	Method	Effect	Suggested Mechanism	Reference
DDT	Rats	Everted sacs	Inhibition of active transport of glucose and tyrosine	Inhibition of sodium pump	1,19
Dieldrin	Monkeys	Everted sacs	Augmented glucose and depressed leucine uptake	Increased disaccharidase activity	8,17
Malathion	Rats	Tissue accumulation	Reduced glucose and glycine absorption	Depressed brush border enzyme activities	
TCDD	Rats	Everted sacs	No physiologically significant changes in glucose or leucine active transport	Monosaccharide and amino acid active transport unaffected	16,22

synthetic components of intestinal metabolism entail the production of large amounts of metabolic energy. Intestinal absorptive cells contain increased numbers of apical mitochondria. Isolated mucosal cells have been utilized to monitor the unique energy requirements, e.g., glucose and glutamine, for this tissue.[73,78] Salicylate alters oxidative phosphorylation monitored in isolated gastric mucosal cells.[82] It has been demonstrated that arsenate inhibits mitochondrial oxidative phosphorylation that is pyruvate-mediated.[29] Intestinal pyruvate dehydrogenase has been implicated in that inhibitory process.[71] The full impact of foreign substances on gastrointestinal metabolism is largely unknown.

Control of intestinal motility is complex and involves both cholinergic and adrenergic nervous system components.[54] In general, cholinergic stimulation increases intestinal motility and adrenergic stimulation inhibits motility. Somnolence and constipation are side effects of many antihistamines.[66] A formamidine pesticide, amitraz, is widely used to control ticks but with some toxicity to horses.[66] The effects of amitraz on drug-induced contractions of guinea pig ileum *in vitro* indicate inhibition of the histamine H, agonists which stimulated contractions.[62] This action may be relevant to the intestinal stasis observed in horses.

Recent approaches to monitoring motility rely on marker substances other than polyethylene glycol, chromium sesquioxide, and barium sulfate. Of particular value as marker substances are polystryrene particles that are available in varying sizes (50 to 100 μ and 800 to 1000 μ) and are of low specific gravity.[38] Phenol reds alone and complexed with a high molecular weight anion exchange resin have also been confirmed as appropriate markers for gastrointestinal transit time in mammals[45] and poultry.[30]

A second *in vitro* model, the parallel artificial membrane permeability assay (PAMPA),[6] is more recent. Several caveats are associated with the use of Caco models (e.g., poor predictability for transporter-mediated and paracellularly absorbed compounds, significant nonspecific binding to cells and devices leading to poor recovery, and variability associated with experimental factors) and these must be considered carefully to utilize their full potential.

PAMPA was introduced in 1998[43] and since then numerous reports have been published illustrating the general applicability of this model as a high throughput permeability screening tool.[20,39–41] The model consists of a hydrophobic filter material coated with a mixture of lecithin and phospholipids dissolved in an inert organic solvent such as dodecane to create an artificial lipid membrane barrier that mimics the intestinal epithelium. The rate of permeation across the membrane barrier was shown to correlate well with the extent of drug absorption in humans. The use of 96-well microtiter plates coupled with rapid analysis using a spectro-photometric plate reader makes this system a very attractive model for screening large numbers of compounds and libraries. PAMPA is much less labor intensive than cell culture methods and appears to show similar predictability. One of the main limitations is that PAMPA underestimates the absorption of compounds that are actively absorbed via drug transporters. Despite the limitation, PAMPA may serve as an invaluable primary permeability screen during early drug discovery process because of its high throughput capability.

PAMPA is a non-cell-based permeability model that provides estimates of passive transcellular permeability. The lack of any functional drug transporters and paracellular pores in PAMPA makes it an inappropriate model for compounds that are absorbed via transporter- and pore-mediated processes. However, the lack of transporter- and pore-mediated permeability may be an advantage. Because PAMPA provides uncontaminated transcellular passive permeability data, it could be more useful in constructing structure–permeability relationships at the chemistry bench.

Lipophilicity (most commonly expressed as Log P or Log D values) plays a major role in passive diffusion. Adequate lipophilicity is required for a protein to travel across a phospholipid membrane. However, the PAMPA permeabilities of 22 marketed drugs did not correlate well with lipophilicity alone because other factors (polar surface area, molecular volume and flexibility, hydrogen bonding) are also involved in passive diffusion. Although pharmaceutically important drug transporters (e.g., PEPT 1, OCT, and OAT) are functionally expressed in Caco-2 cells, they are quantitatively unexpressed when compared with *in vivo* situations.

For example, β-lactam antibiotics (e.g., cephalexin, amoxicillin) and ACE inhibitors that are known substrates of dipeptide transporters are poorly permeable across the Caco-2 cell monolayer despite the fact that they are completely absorbed *in vivo*. This model is likely to generate false negatives with drug candidates that are transported by carrier-mediated processes. Caco-2 cells have tight junctions that are significantly tighter compared with human intestine, and thus Caco-2 cells normally under-predict the permeability values of drugs that are absorbed primarily via paracellular pathways. Low molecular weight hydrophilic compounds such as metformin, ranitidine, atenolol, furosemide, and hydrochlo-rothiazide) showed poor permeability (equal to or less than mannitol) in Caco-2 cells despite adequate absorption (more than 50% of dose) in humans. Therefore, models such as PAMPA and Caco-2 cells can serve only as one-way screens such that compounds that show high permeability in these models are typically well absorbed but compounds with low permeability cannot be ruled out as poorly absorbed compounds in humans.

Two *in vitro* models of intestinal absorption in drug development are widely used predictively in various forms. These are the Caco and PAMPA models. The Caco system is a cell culture-based assay of the intestinal mucosa using the human colon carcinoma cell line (Caco-2).[35] It is now widely used by scientists in academia and industry.[5,7,13,15,31,36] The popularity of the Caco-2 cell culture model in studies of intestinal drug transport is due mainly to the ease with which new information is generated. Transport studies using this cell culture model can be performed in large numbers and under controlled conditions, resulting in the generation of a wealth of information. Much of the recent knowledge about transporters in the intestinal mucosa has been derived from *in vitro* cell culture models like the Caco-2 system. The good correlation between passive compound permeation across Caco-2 cell monolayers and that found *in vivo*[5] has made it possible to use this cell culture system (in some situations) to establish structure–transport relationships for drug candidates and predict intestinal mucosal permeation in humans.[5,50] In fact, the U.S. Food and Drug Administration (FDA) is currently evaluating the application of cell culture assays like the Caco-2 in its biopharmaceutical classification systems for drugs (see Internet resources).

To facilitate the use of Caco-2 cell experiments to estimate intestinal perme-ation of lead compounds, many pharmaceutical companies now perform these experiments in an HTS format. Conversion to HTS formats was made possible by technological advances including (1) miniaturization of cell culture apparatus (24-well instead of 6-well inserts); (2) automation of cell culture and transport experiments; (3) coupling of cell culture experiments to sophisticated and sensi-tive analytical methodologies such as liquid chromatography/tandem mass spectrometry; (4) development of standardized methods for quantitation of trans-port data; and (5) development of sophisticated data systems for the analysis, storage, and retrieval of transport data.

In addition to using this cell culture assay to estimate the intestinal mucosal permeation of compounds, the Caco-2 cell culture system has also been used in many mechanistic studies of compound transport and delivery (see Table 9.5 for a summary of applications). The development of cell culture assays represents one of the most exciting advances in the pharmaceutical sciences. These systems, if properly used, can lead to improved understanding of the biochemical basis of the barrier properties of the intestinal mucosa and potentially expedite the pro-cesses of drug discovery and development, thus improving the efficiency of these processes in the pharmaceutical industry. However, in order to maximize the benefits from these technologies, meaningful refinements such as inducing the expression of underexpressed transporters and enzymes to *in vivo* levels by cell

TABLE 9.5
Application of Caco-2 Cell Culture System to Mechanistic Studies of Drug Transport

Applications	Reference
Elucidate pathways of drug transport (paracellular versus transcellular; passive versus carrier-mediated) across intestinal mucosa	44
Determine optimal physiochemical characteristics (hydrogen bonding potential, conformation) of a drug for passive diffusion via paracellular or transcellular pathways across intestinal mucosa	14
Determine structure–transport relationships for carrier-mediated pathways (peptide transporter of drug	34
Determine structure–transport relationships for apically polarized efflux systems (P-glycoprotein) in intestinal mucosa	15
Determine how formulation components (adjuvants) may influence intestinal mucosal transport of drug candidates	61
Assess potential toxic effects of drug candidates or formulation components on intestinal mucosa	83
Elucidate potential pathways of drug metabolism in intestinal mucosa	75
Determine potential drug–drug interactions during intestinal mucosal transport	88

biology methods, shortening culturing times, miniaturizing the cell culture apparatus, and automating the transport and metabolism experiments must be made.[4,11]

Caco-2 cells, when grown to polycarbonate filters, form confluent monolayers that can be used as *in vitro* models of the intestinal mucosa. By measuring the permeability of a compound across these cell monolayers, one can estimate the extent of its permeation through the intestinal mucosa.

INTESTINAL TRANSIT

Drugs that modify intestinal transit include atropine, morphine, clonidine, papaverine, and isoproterenol. In addition to *in vivo* testing, a number of *in vitro* techniques have been developed to evaluate the effects of test compounds on visceral smooth muscle function. Among them, a method for studying peristalsis[86] is particularly valuable in producing results predictive of activity on intestinal transit. However, this test does not meet the requirements of safety pharmacological drug testing intended to assess possible direct and indirect effects of drugs. For these studies, *in vivo* assays are preferable. The intestinal transit assay presented in this unit is very simple, reliable, reproducible, and relatively low in cost; it requires no expensive equipment. The assay is widely used for primary screening and as a test for safety pharmacology.

The effects of drugs on the extent of intestinal transit during a fixed period following oral administration of a test compound can be evaluated in rats. The

TABLE 9.6
Treatment Groups for Measurement of
Intestinal Transit

Group	Treatment
1	Vehicle control
2	Test compound, dose 1
3	Test compound, dose 2
4	Test compound, dose 3
5	Reference compound (positive control)[a]

[a] For measurement of intestinal transit, the reference compounds are atropine sulfate (0.8 mg/ml) and morphine (4.8 mg/ml).

TABLE 9.7
Effects of Test Compounds on Intestinal Transit in Rats

Treatment[a]	Dose	Distance Covered by Charcoal (cm ± SEM)	Percent Transit (± SEM)[b]
Control	0.5% CMC[c]	80 ± 5	70 ± 6
Atropine sulfate	2 mg/kg	54 ± 6	50 ± 2[b]
Morphine hydrochloride	12 mg/kg	51 ± 3	50 ± 3[b]
Test compound	10 mg/kg	68 ± 4	62 ± 3
Test compound	30 mg/kg	66 ± 6	60 ± 4
Test compound	100 mg/kg	72 ± 3	70 ± 3

[a] Single oral dose of vehicle, reference compound (atropine sulfate and morphine hydrochloride), or test compound (glucose) was administered 1 hr prior to administration of charcoal suspension. Values are mean ± standard error of mean (SEM); eight animals per group.

[b] $P \leq 0.001$ for intergroup versus control comparisons.

[c] Control is 0.5% carboxymethylcellulose.

measured endpoint is the extent of passage of a charcoal suspension through the small intestine.[52,27] Atrophine sulfate and morphine hydrochloride (reference compounds) are used as positive controls. For each test compound, five groups of eight animals each are used (Table 9.6). This protocol can also be used with the modifications noted to measure intestinal transit in mice. Typical results are shown in Table 9.7.

ULCEROGENIC ACTIVITY

Mucus acts as a lubricant barrier to protect the surface of the GI tract against acid, pepsin, and the mechanical forces of digestion.[2,28] Nonsteroidal anti-inflammatory

TABLE 9.8
Treatment Groups for Measurement of Ulcerogenic Activity

Group	Treatment	Evaluated on Day
1	Vehicle control	1
2	Vehicle control	4
3	Test compound, dose 1	1
4	Test compound, dose 1	4
5	Test compound, dose 2	1
6	Test compound, dose 2	4
7	Test compound, dose 3	1
8	Test compound, dose 3	4
9	Reference compound (positive control)[a]	1
10	Reference compound (positive control)[a]	4

[a] For measurement of ulcerogenic activity, the reference compound is indomethacin (6.4 mg/ml).

drugs (NSAIDs) decrease the thickness of the mucus gel layer,[57] provoking mucosal erosion and ultimately ulcers. Similarly, a serious side effect of adrenocorticotropic hormone (ACTH) and corticoid therapy in humans is development or reactivation of gastroduodenal ulcers.[65] A variety of other agents including ethanol[56] also cause damage to the GI tract. The ulcerogenic assay is described below; it is simple, reliable, and reproducible and widely used for safety pharmacology studies.

Estimation of luminal mucus in gastric washings has been used as an index of secretion.[10,42] Among the techniques developed for measuring the dimensions of the gastric mucus layer are the slit lamp and pachymeter[9] and direct microscopic methods.[56] Basic Protocol 2 is a rapid assay that allows easy detection and quantification of the ulcerogenic potential of test substances, but it provides no information on the effects of test substances on the gastric mucus layer. The ulcerogenic effects of drugs can readily be evaluated in rats. Test compounds are administered orally to rats once daily for 1 to 4 days, then the stomach and the duodenum are removed and scored for irritation and ulcers. Indomethacin (reference compound) is used as a positive control. For each test compound, ten groups of eight animals each are used: five groups for examination on day 1 and five additional groups for examination on day 4 (Table 9.8).

CONCLUSIONS

Appreciation of the gastrointestinal tract as a target organ system for ingested substances is growing. This appreciation is reflected in the increasing interest in the GI tract as metabolic organ contributing to the homeostasis of an entire organism. The several areas of gastrointestinal research at the forefront include the role of the bacterial ecosystem in the metabolism of nutrients and foreign substances[27,67] and the role of enterohepatic circulation in affecting the absorption of substances from the lumen,[17,20] the role of fiber in digestion, absorption, and protection of the intestines,[81,89] and response of the local gastrointestinal immune system to toxic substances.[18,40] Adaptation normally occurs in the GI tract in response to increasing age, enteral feeding of nutrients, and after surgical removal of a section of intestine.[70] The ability of the GI tract to adapt after toxic insults is being explored. Because of the high metabolic and cell turnover rates of the intestinal mucosa, it is likely that this tissue is particularly susceptible to injury.

REFERENCES

1. Albro, P.W. and Fishbein, L., Absorption of aliphatic hydrocarbons by rats, *Biochim. Biophys. Acta*, 219, 437, 1970.
2. Allen, A. Structure and function of gastrointestinal mucus, in *Physiology of the Gastrointestinal Tract*, Vol. 1, Johnson, R.L., Ed., Raven Press, New York, 1981, p. 617.
3. Artursson, P. and Borchardt, R.T., Intestinal drug absorption and metabolism in cell cultures: Caco-2 and beyond, *Pharm. Res.*, 14, 1655, 1997.
4. Artursson, P. and Karlsson, J., Correlation between oral drug absorption in humans and apparent drug permeability coefficients in human intestinal epithelial (Caco-2) cells, *Biochem. Biophys. Res. Commun.*, 175, 880, 1991.
5. Artursson, P., Palm, K., and Lathman, K., Caco-2 monolayers in experimental and theoretical predictions of drug transport, *Adv. Drug Delivery Rev.*, 22, 85, 1996.
6. Avdeef, A. and Tsinman, Q., PAMPA-A drug absorption *in vitro* model 13: chemical selectivity due to membrane hydrogen bonding: in combo comparisons of HDM-, DOPC-, and DS-PAMPA models, *Eur. J. Pharm Sci.* 28, 43, 2006. Epub Feb. 2006.
7. Bailey, C.A., Bryla, P., and Malik, A.W., The use of the intestinal epithelial cell culture model, Caco-2, in pharmaceutical development, *Adv. Drug Delivery Rev.*, 22, 67, 1996.
8. Ballantyne, B. Assessment of absorptive function of the gastrointestinal tract, *Gen. Appl. Toxicol.* 2003.
9. Bickel, M. and Kauffman, G.L., Gastric mucus gel thickness: effect of distension, 16,16-dimethyl prostaglandin E2 and carbenoxolone, *Gastroenterology*, 80, 770, 1981.
10. Bolton, J.P., Palmer, D., and Cohen, M.M., Stimulation of mucus and non-parietal cell secretion by e2 prostaglandins, *Am. J. Dig. Dis.*, 23, 359, 1978.
11. Borchardt, R.T., The application of cell culture systems in drug discovery and development, *J. Drug Targeting*, 3, 179, 1995.
12. Borchardt, R.T., Wilson, G., and Smith, P., Eds., *Model Systems Used for Biopharmaceutical Assessment of Drug Absorption and Metabolism*. Plenum, New York, 1996.
13. Brayden, D., Human intestinal epithelial cell monolayers as prescreen for oral drug delivery, *Pharm. News*, 4, 11, 1997.

14. Burton, P.S. et al., How structural features influence the permeability of peptides, *J. Pharm. Sci.*, 85, 1336, 1996.

15. Burton, P.S. et al., *In vitro* permeability of peptidomimetics: the role of polarized efflux pathways as additional barriers to absorption, *Adv. Drug Delivery Rev.*, 23, 143, 1997.

16. Carson, R., *Silent Spring*, Houghton Mifflin, Boston, 1962.

17. Chowdhury, J.S. et al., Effect of a single oral dose of malathion on D-glucose and glycine uptake and on brush border enzymes in rat intestine, *Toxicol. Lett.*, 6, 411, 1980.

18. Colburn, W.A., Pharmacokinetic and biopharmaceutic parameters during entero-hepatic circulation of drugs, *J. Pharm. Sci.*, 71, 131, 1982.

19. Dobbins, W.D., Gut immunophysiology: a gastroenterolgists' view with emphasis on pathophysiology, *Am. J. Physiol.*, 242, G1, 1982.

20. Douglas, W.W., Histamine and 5-hydroxytryptamine (serotonin) and their antag-onists, in *The Pharmacological Basis of Therapeutics,* Gillman, L.F. et al., Eds., Macmillan, New York, 1980, p. 609.

21. Duggan, D.E. et al., Enterohepatic circulation of indomethacin and its role in intestinal irritation, *Biochem. Pharmacol.*, 25, 1749, 1975.

22. El-Hawaii, A.M. and Plaa, G.L., Role of the enterohepatic circulation in the elimination of phenytoin in the rat, *Drug Metab. Dispos.*, 6, 59, 1978.

23. Environmental Protection Agency, National Safety Drinking Water Strategy: One Step at a Time (draft report), U.S. Environmental Protection Agency, Washington, D.C., 1975.

24. Ershoff, B.A., Proctective effects of cholestyramine in rats fed low fiber dicts containing toxic doses of sodium cyclamate and amaranth, *Proc. Soc. Exp. Biol. Med.*, 152, 253, 1976.

25. Feinroth, M., Feinroth, M.V., and Berlyne, G.M., Aluminum absorption in the rat everted gut sac, *Miner. Electrolyte Metab.*, 8, 29, 1982.

26. Fichelle, J., Mesure du transit intestinal chez le rat, *J. Pharmacol.* (Paris), 2, 85, 1971.

27. Fischer, L.J., Kent, T.H., and Weissinger, J.L., Absorption of diethylstilbesterol and its glucuronide conjugate from the intestines of five- and twenty-five-day-old rats, *J. Pharmacol. Exp. Ther.*, 185, 163, 1973.

28. Flemström, G. and Garner, A., Gastroduodenal HCO_3 transport: characteristics and proposed role in acidity regulation and mucosal protection, *Am. J. Physiol.*, 242, G183, 1982.

29. Flock, M.H. and Hentges, D.J., Intestinal microecology, *Am. J. Clin. Nutr.*, 27, 1261, 1974.

30. Fowler, B.A., Woods, J.S., and Schiller, C.M., Studies of hepatic mitochondrial structure and function. 1. Morphometric and biochemical evaluation of *in vivo* perturbation by arsenate, *Lab. Invest.*, 41, 313, 1979.

31. Gan, L.S.L. and Thakker, D.R., Application of the Caco-2 model in the design and development of orally active drugs: elucidation of biochemical and physical barriers posed by the intestinal epithelium, *Adv. Drug Delivery Res.*, 23, 77, 1997.

32. Gao, J. et al., Estimating intestinal mucosal permeation of compounds using Caco-2 cell monolayers, in *Current Protocols in Pharmacology*, John Wiley & Sons, New York, 2000, p. 7.2.1.

33. Gonalons, E., Rial, R., and Tur, J. A., Phenol red as indicator of digestive tract motility in chickens, *Poult. Sci.*, 61, 581, 1982.

34. Hidalgo, I.J. and Li, J., Carrier-mediated transport and efflux mechanisms in Caco-2 cells, *Adv. Drug Delivery Res.*, 22, 53, 1996.

35. Hidalgo, I.J., Borchardt, R.T., and Raub, T., Biochemical, histological and physiochemical characterization of human adenocarcinoma cells (Caco-2) as a model system for studying mucosal transport and metabolim of drugs, *Gastroenterology,* 96, 736, 1989.

36. Hillgren, K.M., Kato, A., and Borchardt, R.T., *In vitro* systems for studying intestinal drug absorption, *Med. Res. Rev.*, 15, 83, 1995.

37. Iiboshi, Y. et al., Asia Pacific, *J. Clin. Nutr.,* 6, 111, 1997.

38. Iturri, S.J. and Wolff, D., Inhibition of the active transport of D-glucose and L-tyrosine by DDT and DE in the rat small intestine, *Comp. Biochem. Biophys.,* 71, 131, 1982.

39. Jacobson, E. D., The gastrointestinal system, in *Essentials in Human Physiology,* Ross, G., Ed., Year Book Medical Publishers, Chicago, 1978, p. 370.

40. Jilge, B., Rate of movement of marker substances in the digestive tract of the rabbit, *Lab. Anim.*, 16, 7, 1982.

41. Joffe, A.Z., Alimentary toxic aleukia, in *Microbial Toxins*, Vol. 7, Kadis, S. et al., Eds., Academic Press, New York, 1971, p. 139.

42. Johansson, C. and Kollberg, B., Stimulation by intragastrically administered E$_2$ prostaglandins of human gastric mucus output, *Eur. J. Clin. Invest.*, 9, 229, 1979.

43. Kansy, M., Senner, F., and Bubernator, K., Physiochemical high throughput screening: parallel artificial membrane permeation assay in the description of passive absorption processes, *J. Med. Chem.*, 41, 1007, 1998.

44. Knipp, G.T. et al., Paracellular diffusion in Caco-2 monolayers: effect of perturbants on the transport of hydrophilic compounds that vary in charge and size, *J. Pharm. Sci.*, 86, 1105, 1997.

45. Katz, A. J. et al., Gluten-sensitive enteropathy: inhibition by cortisol of the effect of gluten protein *in vitro*, *New Engl. J. Med.*, 295, 131, 1976.

46. Keino, H. and Aoki, E., Scanning electrgn microscopic and enzyme histochemical observations on the cadmium-affected gastrointestinal villi of mice, *J. Toxicol. Sci.*, 6, 191, 1981.

47. Kunihara, M. and Meshi, T., Measurement of gastrointestinal transit of solid food using a colestipol-phenol red complex as a marker, *J. Pharmacobiodyn.*, 4, 916, 1981.

48. LaCroix, D. and Guillaume, P., Gastrointestinal models: intestinal transit and ulcerogenic activity in the rat, in *Current Protocols in Pharmacology*, John Wiley & Sons, New York, 1998.

49. Langman, M.J. and Bell, G.D., Alcohol and the gastrointestinal tract, *Br. Med. Bull.*, 38, 71, 1982.

50. Lennernas, H. et al., Correlation between paracellular and transcellular drug permeability in the human jejunum and Caco-2 monolayers, *Int. J. Pharm.*, 127, 103, 1996.

51. Lwoff, J.M., Activité ulcérigéne chez le rat, *J. Pharmacol.* (Paris), 2, 81, 1971.

52. Macht, D.I. and Barba-Gose, J., Two methods for pharmacological comparison of insoluble purgatives, *J. Am. Pharmacol. Assoc.*, 20, 558, 1931.

53. Mahmood, A. et al., Acute dieldrin toxicity: effect on the uptake of glucose and leucine and on brush border enzymes in monkey intestine, *Chem. Biol. Interact.*, 37, 165, 1981.

54. Mahmood, A. et al., Effects of DDT (chlorophenotane) administration on glucose uptake and brush border enzymes in monkey intestine, *Acta Pharmacol. Toxicol.*, 43, 99, 1978.

55. Mayer, S.E., Neuroburnoral transmission and the autonomic nervous system, in *The Pharmacological Basis of Therapeutics*, Gilman, A.F. et al., Eds., Macmillan, New York, 1980, p. 56.

56. McQueen, S. et al., Gastric and duodenal surface mucus gel thickness in rats: effects of prostaglandins and damaging agents, *Am. J. Physiol.*, 245, G388, 1983.

57. Menguy, R. and Masters, Y.F., The effects of aspirin on gastric mucus secretion, *Surg. Gynecol. Obstet.*, 92, 1, 1965.

58. Munro, H.N., Protein secretion into the gastrointestinal tract, in *Postgraduate Gastroenterology*, Thompson, T.J., Eds., Balliere, Tindall, and Cassell, London, 1966, p. 58.

59. Nedkova-Bratanova, N. et al., Effect of the pesticides phosalone and lindane on the activity of some dipeptidases and disaccharidases in rat intestinal mucosa, *Enzymes*, 24, 281, 1979.

60. Nelson, N., Human Health and the Environment: Some Research Needs, U.S. Government Printing Office, Washington, D.C., 1976.

61. Nerurkar, M.A., Burton, P.S., and Borchardt, R.T., The use of surfactants to enhance the permeability of peptides through Caco-2 cells by inhibition of an apically polarized efflux system, *Pharm. Res.*, 13, 528, 1996.

62. Pass, M. A. and Seawright, A.A., Effect of amitraz on contractions of the guinea pig ileum *in vitro.*, *Comp. Biochem. Physiol.*, 73C, 419, 1982.

63. Remmel, R.P., Pohl, L.R., and Elmer, G.W., Influence of the intestinal microflora on the elimination of warfarin in the rat, *Drug Metab. Dispos.*, 9, 410, 1981.

64. Richter, E. and Schafer, S.G., Intestinal excretion of hexachlorobenzene, *Arch. Toxicol.*, 47, 233, 1981.

65. Robert, A. and Nezamis, J.E., Ulcerogenic property of steroids, *Proc. Soc. Exp. Biol. Med.*, 99, 443, 1958.

66. Roberts, M.C. and Seawright, A.A., Armitraz induced large intestinal impaction in the mouse, *Aust. Vet. J.*, 55, 553, 1979.

67. Savage, D.C., The microbial flora in the gastrointestinal tract, *Prog. Clin. Biol. Res.*, 77, 893, 1981.

68. Schedl, H.R., Environmental factors and the development of disease and injury to the alimentary tract, *Environ. Health Perspect.*, 20, 39, 1977.

69. Schiller, C.M., Chemical exposure and intestinal function, *Environ. Health Perspect.*, 33, 91, 1979.

70. Schiller, C.M, Effects of toxins on gastrointestinal function: developing systems, *Banbury Rep.*, 11, 43, 1982.

71. Schiller, C.M., Fowler, B. A., and Woods, J. S., Pyruvate metabolism after *in vivo* exposure to oral arsenic, *Chem. Biol. Interact.*, 22, 25, 1978.

72. Schiller, C.M. et al., Alterations; in lipid assimilation induced by 2,3,7,8-tetrachlorodibenzo-p-dioxin (TCDD) in male Fischer rats, *Fed. Proc.*, 42, 355, 1983.

73. Schiller, C.M., Southern, L S., and Walden, R., Glutamine and glutamate utilization by the hamster small intestine, *J. Appl. Biochem.*, 3, 147, 1981.

74. Schiller, C.M., Walden, R., and Shoaf, C. R., Studies on the mechanism of 2,3,7,8-tetrachlorodibenzo-p-dioxin toxicity: nutrient assimilation, *Fed. Proc.*, 41, 1426, 1982.

75. Schmiedlin-Ren, P. et al., Expression of enzymatically active CYP3A4 by Caco-2 cells grown on extracellular matrix-coated permeable supports in the presence of 1,25-dihydroxyvitamin D3, *Mol. Pharmacol.*, 51, 741, 1997.

76. Seko, Y., Miura, T., and Takahashi, M., Reduced decomposition and fecal excretion of methyl mercury in cecum-resected mice, *Acta Pharmacol. Toxicol.*, 50, 117, 1982.

77. Seko, Y., Miura, T., Takahashi, M., and Kayama, T., Methyl mercury decomposition in mice treated with antibiotics, *Acta Pharmacol. Toxicol.*, 49, 259, 1981.

78. Shirkey, R.J. and Schiller, C.M., Preparation and properties of epithelial cell suspensions from rat small intestine, *J. Appl. Biochem.*, 2, 196, 1980.

79. Shull, G.E., Miller, M.L. and Schulterheirs, P.J., Lessons learned from genetically engineered animal models VIII. Absorption and secretion of ions in the gastrointestinal tract, *Am. J. Physiol. Gastrointest. Liver Physiol.* 278, G185, 2000.

80. Smith, G.E. and Griffiths, L.A., Metabolism of a biliary metabolite of phenacetin and the acetanilides by the intestinal microflora, *Experientia*, 32, 1556, 1976.

81. Story, J.A., The role of dietary fiber in lipid metabolism, *Adv. Lip. Res.*, 18, 229, 1981.

82. Tanaka, K. and Fromm, A., Effects of bile acid and salicylate on isolated surface and glandular cells of rabbit stomach, *Surgery*, 93, 660, 1983.

83. Tang, A.S. et al., Utilization of a human intestinal epithelial cell culture system (Caco-2) for evaluating cytoprotective agents, *Pharm. Res.*, 10, 1620, 1993.

84. Turner, J.C. and Shanks, V., Absorption of some organochlorine compounds by the rat small intestine *in vivo*, *Bull. Environ. Contain. Toxicol.*, 24, 652, 1980.

85. Valberg, L.S. et al., Cadmium-induced enteropathy: comparative toxicity of cadmium chloride and cadmium thionein, *J. Toxicol. Environ. Health*, 2, 963, 1977.

86. Van Nueten, J.M. et al., An improved method for studying peristalsis in the isolated guinea pig ileum, *Arch. Int. Pharmacodyn. Ther.*, 203, 411, 1973.

87. Volp, R.E. and Lage, G.L., The fate of a major biliary metabolite of digitoxin in the rat intestine, *Drug Metab. Dispos.*, 6, 418, 1978.

88. Wacher, V.J., Salphati, L., and Benet, L.Z., Active secretion and enterocytic drug metabolism barriers to drug absorption, *Adv. Drug Delivery Rev.*, 20, 99, 1996.

89. Walsh, C.T., Methods in gastrointestinal toxicology, in *Principles and Methods of Toxicology*, 4th ed.., Taylor & Francis, Philadelphia, 2001, p. 1215.

10 Intestinal Absorption and Metabolism of Xenobiotics in Laboratory Animals

William J. Brock

CONTENTS

INTRODUCTION

In toxicologic evaluation of xenobiotics in laboratory animals, treatment by the oral route of administration is a typical means of exposure. Oral administration of drugs or chemicals is an easily accessible route and, with training, ensures complete delivery of a test article. Considerations of dosing formulations and solubility of the test article, although important, can usually be overcome by encapsulation, divided dosing or other means that are less easily accomplished when drugs, for example, are administered intravenously, by inhalation, or via some other route.

Exposure of humans to environmental or therapeutic agents is most often by the oral route of administration. Hence, in assessing the potential for adverse health effects in humans, an understanding of the similarities in absorption and the physiology of systemic distribution and metabolism of these agents in animals is of prime importance. Changes in regional blood flow to the gastrointestinal (GI) tract, the presence of food and nutrients, and disease states will all have some influence on the degree of absorption and the biological fate of an agent. Therefore, a great deal of time and energy has been devoted to furthering our knowledge relative to *in vitro* and *in vivo* models used in toxicological assessment of environmental and therapeutic agents.

Since this topic was covered about 20 years ago (Chhabra and Eastin, 1984), there has been considerable advancement in our knowledge of intestinal absorption and metabolism of xenobiotics. This chapter will review the state of this knowledge since the original 1984 review by Chhabra and Eastin although an in-depth review is beyond the scope of this chapter. The reader is referred, however, to reviews cited by Chhabra and Eastin in addition to Kaminsky and Zhang (2003), Carriere et al. (2001), Klaassen and Slitt (2005), Ioannides and Lewis (2004), and Schuetz (2001).

MECHANISMS OF INTESTINAL ABSORPTION OF XENOBIOTICS

The GI system should be viewed as a long tube that is open to the outside environment. Absorption occurs along the entire length of the GI tract. The cellular makeup of this system is described elsewhere in this book. Because of this cellular environment, the surface areas available for absorption of xenobiotics are very large. Absorption across gastrointestinal tissue can occur via several processes — the same processes used for absorption of nutrients. Furthermore, absorption of xenobiotics is dependent on the molecular size of a compound, the microenvironment of the gastrointestinal lumen, and the lipophilicity of the agent, i.e., the greater the lipid solubility of the agent the greater potential for absorption.

Absorption of xenobiotics and nutrients from the GI tract occurs primarily by passive diffusion or active transport. Other means of absorption, however, include filtration, facilitated transport, pinocytosis, etc.

Passive Diffusion

Permeation of xenobiotics across biological membranes occurs primarily by diffusion, with absorption into systemic circulation dependent on the concentration gradients across the gastrointestinal epithelium. Small molecules of molecular weights below 600 are readily absorbed across the epithelia through aqueous pores within the membrane whereas larger molecules are absorbed across the gastrointestinal epithelium based primarily on the physiochemical properties of the agent, e.g., hydrophobicity. The degree of gastrointestinal absorption tends to increase with an increase in hydrophobicity.

TABLE 10.1
Octanol: Water Partition
Coefficients of Selected
Agents

Compound	Log P
Glucose	−3.24
Glutathione	−3.05
Citric acid	−1.72
p-Aminohippuric acid	−0.25
2-Butanone	0.3
Aniline	0.9
Methylene chloride	1.25
Benzoic acid	1.9
Trichloroethylene	2.61
1,4-Dichlorobenzene	3.4
Phenanthrene	4.5
Vitamin A	5.68
DDT	6.2

Estimation of absorption has historically been associated with an assessment of the octanol:water partition coefficient, Log P, and is the equilibrium ratio of the solute concentrations in the two solvents:

$$K_{ow} = [\text{solute}]_{oct}/[\text{solute}]_{w}$$

Very lipid soluble compounds that can readily traverse biological membranes have high positive values of Log P (Table 10.1).

Absorption across biological membranes is based also on the ionization of molecules because many compounds are organic acids or bases. The ionized form of a molecule will be more water soluble and less likely to be absorbed although some absorption will occur through aqueous pores. In contrast, the un-ionized form of the molecule will have greater absorption with the limit of that absorption based on molecular size and lipid solubility as noted above. The degree of ionization is dependent on the pKa and pH of the solution according to the Henderson–Hasselbalch equation. This basic principle of ionization that we all learned in introductory chemistry was that the pKa is the ratio of the concentration of the un-ionized form of the molecule to the concentration of the ionized form of the molecule.

$$\text{For acids: pKa} - \text{pH} = \log \frac{[\text{un-ionized}]}{[\text{ionized}]}$$

$$\text{For bases: pKa} - \text{pH} = \log \frac{[\text{ionized}]}{[\text{un-ionized}]}$$

At acidic pH as encountered in the stomach, organic acids would be largely un-ionized and readily available for absorption. For example, benzoic acid (pKa 4) is about 50% ionized at stomach pH. As the compound is moved into the small intestines, the local pH increases to about 7 and greater so that the proportion of the molecule becomes largely ionized. For organic bases, the opposite occurs. At low pH, the organic base would be highly ionized with very little of the compound available for absorption whereas within the intestines, the degree of ionization declines and absorption potential increases.

ACTIVE TRANSPORT

Although most xenobiotics will be absorbed across the gastrointestinal epithelium by simple diffusion, a number of compounds including many nutrients are absorbed via active transport mechanisms. Overall, these mechanisms require an expenditure of energy, and transport into and out of cells is against a concentration gradient.

Active transport is the movement of a molecule across a membrane that is driven by energy in the form of expenditure of ATP and against a concentration gradient. In addition, specific transport proteins that facilitate transport are often present so that even large molecules can be moved across the membrane. Active transport results in greater concentrations of compounds within cells. Indeed, active transport of compounds into cells becomes particularly important when structurally related toxicants, e.g., 5-fluorouracil, compete with a nutrient, for example, for the transporter protein. This competition can be used for therapeutic benefits.

In the last decade, a great deal of research has been reported on protein transporters. Several gastrointestinal protein transporters have been identified. The multi-drug resistant protein (mdr) was one of the first families of protein transporters identified. This transporter was found to transport chemotherapeutic agents out of gastrointestinal cells and cells of other organs. Other gastrointestinal transporters that have been identified include nucleotide (nt), divalent-metal ion (dmt), and peptide (pept) transporters.

FILTRATION

Passage of small solutes can occur with movement of water through pores and tight epithelial junctions within the GI tract. Transport of molecules with molecular weights below 200 is carried through by the hydrostatic forces of water. This phenomenon is known as solvent drag (Blanchard, 1975). Although filtration is more common in the kidney, it can occur to a limited extent in the GI tract, e.g., calcium absorption.

FACILITATED DIFFUSION

Facilitated diffusion is a carrier-mediated process of absorption similar to active transport. However, absorption does not occur against a concentration gradient,

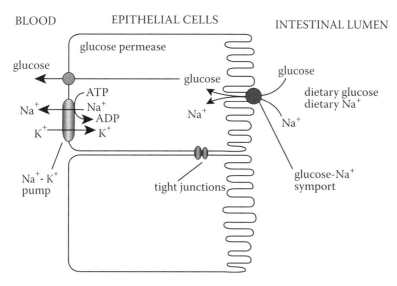

FIGURE 10.1 Facilitated glucose transport across gastrointestinal epithelium.

thereby distinguishing this process from active transport. Furthermore, facilitated diffusion does not require the expenditure of cellular energy and is not subject to inhibition by cell poisons.

The transport of glucose into the cell occurs with the Na^+–K^+ pump that generates a Na^+ gradient across the cell membrane. The glucose–Na^+ symport protein uses that Na^+ gradient to transport glucose into the cell (Figure 10.1).

In the GI tract, cells take in glucose and Na^+ from the intestine and transport them through the cell into the bloodstream by the Na^+ glucose transporter, glucose permease (a glucose-facilitated diffusion protein), and Na^+–K^+ pumps. A similar mechanism for glucose transport occurs in the central nervous system.

PINOCYTOSIS

Cells have the ability to transport macromolecules (proteins, polysaccharides, polynucleotides) to their interiors through endocytosis — a broad term that includes phagocytosis and pinocytosis. Phagocytosis is the process of enveloping a particle by modifying its membrane to form a phagosome around the particle. Phagosomes are then pulled by cytoskeleton motion of the cytosol into one or more lysosomes for digestion of the particles.

In contrast, pinocytosis transports liquid substances into cells. A pocket in a given area of a cell membrane captures the liquid and forms vesicles that are then pulled by cytoskeleton motion into the cytoplasm. Pinocytosis may be selective or non-selective. Selective pinocytosis occurs in two stages. The liquid substance adheres initially to membrane receptors and is then transferred to vesicles that leave the membrane surface and transport their content to the cytoplasm. In non-selective pinocytosis, the vesicles envelop all the solutes eventually present in the extracellular fluid.

Absorption of nutrient biomolecules occurs via this route, and the disposition of particles, e.g., cadmium, is absorbed via this mechanism. Uptake of proteins via pinocytosis has been observed in neonatal rats, guinea pigs, and rabbits (Leece and Broughton, 1973). Interestingly, immune complexes responsible for food allergies may be absorbed into systemic circulation by pinocytosis (Walker and Bloch, 1983; Sasser and Jarboe, 1980; LeFevre and Joel, 1984).

FACTORS AFFECTING INTESTINAL ABSORPTION

Normal physiological functioning of the GI tract (food intake and bodily responses to food intake) can affect the systemic absorption of xenobiotics as well as nutrients. In addition, absorption into the systemic circulation from the GI tract is affected by the metabolism of the agent by intestinal microflora or metabolic enzymes present in the gastrointestinal epithelium.

FOOD AND DRUG INTERACTIONS

Food has long been recognized as a factor that influences absorption drugs, chemicals, and other nutrients. Indeed, in routine acute oral toxicity testing of substances, fasting of animals is often utilized as suggested by regulatory guidance (OECD 1987). The influence of foods on absorption has been recognized for many years. Dahan and Altman (2004) and Palumbo et al. (2005) reported that grapefruit juice co-administered with drugs will alter the pharmacokinetics of some drugs due to inhibition of cytochrome P4503A4 in the small intestine. These authors have also suggested that grapefruit juice may inhibit P-glycoprotein (P-gp), a transporter that carries drugs from the enterocytes back into the lumen, resulting in greater absorption. Flavanols appear to affect various gastric transporters for drugs and other substances with the multi-drug-transporter P-gp being the more characterized transporter (Wagner et al., 2001). Edwards et al. (1996) also identified 6′,7′-dihydroxybergamottin, a furancoumarin in grapefruit juice, as a potent inhibitor of cytochrome P4503A4 that may be responsible for the altered pharmacokinetics of certain drugs.

Foods can modify the absorption of substances including other foods, by changing dissolution and solubility, enhancing binding to food-containing materials, changing gastric residence time, altering blood flow, etc. In an extensive review of the subject, Singh (1999) classified drugs into decreased, delayed, accelerated, increased, and unaffected categories in terms of the effects of foods on gastrointestinal absorption (Table 10.2).

The classification is based on an alteration of the maximum blood concentration (Cmax) and the area under the blood concentration and time curve (AUC) of the pharmaceutical. For decreased and delayed absorption, the author indicates that the extent of absorption is not affected, but the time course of absorption is changed. Whether such a change is due to a direct interaction of the food with

TABLE 10.2
Classification of Therapeutic Substances Based on Effects of Food

Therapeutic Class	Decreased Effects	Delayed Effects	Accelerated Effects	Increased Effects	Unaffected
Cardiovascular	Desmopressin, furosemide, hydralazine	Isosorbide mononitrite, verapamil, isradipine	Diltiazem	Diprafenone, lovastatin, quinidine glucuonate	Atorvastatin, digoxin, pravastatin
Anti-Infective	Ciprofloxacin, ethambutol, rifampicin	Fluconazole, ketoconazole, levofloxacin	Temafloxacin	Albendazole, atovaquone, clofazimine	Adefovir, artemisinin, azithromycin
CNS	Levodopa, carbidopa, avitripan	Pyridoxal, rizatriptan, dolasetron	Oxybutynin	Morphine, ziprasidone, dixyrazine	Oxycodone, valproic acid, bromocriptine
Respiratory	Theophylline	Domitroban, salbutamol, procaterol	Theophylline*	Montelukast	Loratadine, phenylpropanolamine, pseudoephedrine
Antineoplastic	Estramustine, mercaptopurine, methotrexate	Letrozole*		Cyclosporin	Bicalutamide, finasteride

* Modified release formulation.

Source: From Singh, N.M. (1999). *Clin. Pharmacokinet.* 37: 213–255.

the pharmaceutical or whether there is a delay in gastric emptying time from the stomach to the intestine remains possible and appears to largely depend on the pharmaceutical.

In contrast, drugs that show accelerated or increased absorption appear to be those with poor solubility. Furthermore, the altered absorption results from a greater gastric residence time, allowing for increased dissolution in the presence of, for example, bile acids. Overall, however, a majority of the drugs that Singh (1999) examined were unaffected by the co-administration of foods, with only a few drugs showing accelerated absorption in the presence of foods.

Weber and Ehrlein (1998) also showed that gastric emptying time affects intestinal absorption. In their studies, carbohydrates were absorbed at a higher rate compared to fats and proteins although there continued to be a large absorptive reserve within the intestine. Numerous authors have examined the effects of foods and beverages on the absorption of drugs and nutrients, with the outcome of the research showing a great deal of disparity among drugs and food substances (Lee et al., 1997; Fraser, 1997; Kinoshita, et al., 1996; Watkins, et al., 1992).

In addition to the literature on the influence of foods on gastrointestinal absorption, a large number of publications concern the interactions between drugs and other substances on absorption. Choi et al. (2004) demonstrated that co-administration of flavone enhanced the pharmacokinetics of paclitaxel, prolonging the half-life and increasing the AUC. The authors suggested that the alteration in the pharmacokinetics of paclitaxel was related to the inhibition of cytochrome P450 and the P-gp efflux pump. Similarly, Zhang et al. (2003) had previously suggested that Tween 80, a common solvent for drug delivery, inhibits P-gp, resulting in increased absorption of digoxin administered to rats.

Alteration of gastrointestinal absorption by inhibition of transporters or altering the metabolism of substances is clearly recognized as one means of enhancing or inhibiting absorption. However, other factors will be of importance and include binding of gastrointestinal contents, as described above for foods, and chelation. In *in vitro* studies, Tanaka et al (1993) demonstrated that levofloxacin and other quinolones will bind to different aluminum salts, resulting in a lower bioavailability. Mechanistically, the authors suggested that the absorption of quinolones by aluminum hydroxide re-precipitation may be responsible for the reduced bioavailability. Similarly, absorption of inorganic ions such as iron is disrupted by the presence of other cations such as copper. Iturri and Nunez (1998) found that cadmium and copper, manganese, or lead, but not mercury, inhibited the uptake of iron in perfused mouse duodenal preparations. Furthermore, the inhibition by copper and cadmium was dependent on the iron redox state, since neither cation inhibited Fe^{3+} uptake. The authors proposed that Fe^{2+} and Fe^{3+} are transported from the GI tract by different mechanisms, or that Fe^{3+} is reduced to Fe^{2+} in enterocytes and the subsequent absorption is not inhibited by either cadmium or copper.

REGIONAL DIFFERENCES IN ABSORPTION

As stated previously, the GI tract is a tube open to the environment with absorption occurring along its entire length. The extent of absorption is dependent on a variety of factors but the epithelial lining, regional blood flow along the tube, and local environment within the lumen exert a certain amount of influence on absorption.

Absorption from the buccal cavity has long been recognized as a way to achieve high therapeutic levels quickly, and has been an advantageous route for administration of nitrites for treatment of cardiovascular disorders such as angina. More recently, a number of investigators have examined buccal absorption of insulin as a means of treatment for diabetes (Oh and Ritschel, 1990; Hoffman and Ziv, 1997; Chetty and Chien, 1998). However, this route has not yet proven completely efficacious and continues to be the subject of research for a variety of drugs and over-the-counter (OTC) preparations such as steroids, anti-inflammatory agents, etc.

Although absorption across the esophageal tissue has not been examined thoroughly, absorption does occur following the principles of absorption outlined above. However, absorption from the stomach occurs to a very great extent and is a primary site for the absorption of nutrients and many substances (see Chapter 5).

Intestinal absorption of xenobiotics has received the greatest attention. A number of investigators have examined jejunal and ileal absorption of compounds as these segments of the gastrointestinal tract represent those areas where the greatest absorption of pharmaceutical agents occurs. Studies with Caco-2 cells, intestinal perfusion, everted intestinal sacs, and other membrane systems have been used to examine the active transport of xenobiotics (Berggren et al., 2004). In these studies the *in vitro* models were predictive of jejunal and ileal absorption of compounds such as digoxin, verapamil, bile acids, etc. (Amelsberg, et al., 1996; Johnson et al., 2003; Berggren et al., 2004). In a review by Bohlen (1998), he showed that the role of intestinal blood flow and other physiological factors and cellular mechanisms influence intestinal absorption. Such a conclusion was similarly reached by Winne (1980) more than 25 years ago.

Absorption from the colon has a clear benefit in certain disease cases, and has long been recognized as means to avoid first-pass liver metabolism. The degree of absorption depends on the many factors described above, and this route has proven useful for many therapeutic agents. Calcagno et al. (2006) compared the gene expression of Caco-2 cell line to normal colon to determine whether the cell line was predictive of colonic absorption. They found that the gene expression pattern of the cell line closely patterned the transporter profile of normal colon, but was distinctly different from tumor samples. Hence, colonic drug absorption will parallel normal colon but caution must be utilized in predicting absorption in colon cancer.

INTESTINAL METABOLISM

Historically, the metabolism of xenobiotics has been classified as either a Phase 1 or Phase 2 reaction. Although such terminology is outdated, these classes remain convenient for the purposes of description of the mechanisms of metabolism. Phase 1 reactions result primarily in the oxidation of parent compounds but also involve reduction reactions. These cytochrome P450 reactions often result in an increased polarity of the parent molecule and generally precede conjugation reactions (Phase 2 metabolism). These enzyme systems are responsible for the metabolism of xenobiotics, but also are responsible for the metabolism of nutrients and endogenous compounds.

Over the last 10 to 20 years, different isoforms of cytochrome P450 have been characterized for their metabolic specificity. For example, cytochrome P4503A4 is the major isoform that metabolizes most drugs whereas halogenated hydrocarbons are generally substrates for cytochrome P4502E1. Parkinson (2001) described the different isoforms of cytochrome P450 with regard to substrate specificity and inhibitors and inducers of these enzyme systems. The liver contains the highest concentration of the metabolic enzymes, and the enzymes are located within the endoplasmic reticulum.

Distribution studies by Chhabra and Fouts (1976) revealed that enzyme activity declines from the proximal end of the intestine to the distal-colonic end of the intestine. These authors examined aniline hydroxylase, aminopyrine N-demethylase, and aryl hydrocarbon hydroxylase in intestinal microsomes and found these enzymes along the entire length of small intestine. Maximal activity was present in the proximal 60 cm of the intestine. Mizuma et al. (1997) examined the intestinal transport and metabolism of kyotorphin (KTP) in everted small intestines in rats. They found that KTP on the mucosal side was metabolized within 60 min. No metabolism was detected on the serosal side of the intestine. In intestinal homogenates, KTP was metabolized and metabolism was decreased by peptidase inhibitors, bestatin, o-phenanthrolin, and tryptophan hydroxamate.

In perfusion studies of the rat small intestine, regional differences in intestinal metabolism and elimination of cimetidine were observed (Piyapolrungroj et al., 2000). The metabolite cimetidine S-oxide was formed to a greater extent in the jejunum compared with the ileum, and the occurrence of the metabolite was a function of the pH-dependent intracellular uptake. Perfusion studies with inhibitors of cimetidine mucosal transport and inhibitors of microsomal S-oxidation provided an inhibition profile suggesting that jejunal cimetidine permeability decreases with increasing intracellular cimetidine concentration.

Inhibitors and inducers of cytochrome P450 enzymes have been extensively examined. In the original article by Chhabra and Eastin (1984), the authors presented data from their laboratory demonstrating induction of intestinal metabolism in various species. They found (Table 10.3) that intestinal cytochrome P450 activity was refractory to induction by phenobarbital or 3-methylcholantrene although it is well known that hepatic cytochrome P450 isozymes are well induced by either substance (Parkinson, 2001).

TABLE 10.3
Intestinal Cytochrome P450 Activity in Animals Treated with Phenobarbital (PB) or 3-Methylcholanthrene (3-MC)*

Species	Control	PB	Control	3-MC
Guinea pig	0.22 ± 0.02	0.231 ± 0.03	0.26 ± 0.014	0.26 ± 0.004
Rabbit	0.41 ± 0.06	0.40 ± 0.04	0.54 ± 0.12	0.34 ± 0.03

* Values = mean (± SE) expressed as nmol/mg protein

Source: From Chhabra, R.S. and Eastin, W.C. (1984). In *Intestinal Toxicology*, Schiller, C.M., Ed., Raven Press, New York.

As discussed above, dietary components have an influence on the absorption of xenobiotics. Similarly, diet will influence the metabolism of xenobiotics, and the literature is full of examples (Domeneghini et al., 2006; Ramesh et al., 2004). Furthermore, we have long recognized that gut microflora play a major role in the metabolism of xenobiotics in the GI tract (Goel et al., 2005; Smith et al., 2005). Local interactions at the cellular level between bacteria and food constituents, therefore, may have dramatic influence on the metabolism of xenobiotics, thereby influencing the absorption and hence toxicity.

REFERENCES

Amelsberg, A., Schteingart, C.D., Ton-Nu, H.T. and Hofman, A.F. (1996). Carrier-mediated jejunal absorption of conjugated bile acids in the guinea pig. *Gastroenterology* 110: 1098–1106.

Berggren, S., Hoogstraate, J., Eagerholm, U. and Lennernas, H. (2004). Characterization of jejunal absorption and apical efflux of ropivacaine, lidocaine and bupivacaine in the rat using *in situ* and *0* absorption models. *Eur. J. Pharm. Sci.* 21: 553–560.

Blanchard, J. (1975). Gastrointestinal absorption I. Mechanisms. *Am. J. Pharm. Sci.* 147: 135–146.

Bohlen, H.G. (1998). Integration of intestinal structure, function, and microvascular regulation. *Microcirculation* 5: 27–37.

Calcagno, A.M., Ludwig, J.A., Fostel, J.M., Gottesman, M.M. and Ambudkar, S.V. (2006). Comparison of drug transporter levels in normal colon, colon cancer and Cacco-2 cells: impact on drug disposition and discovery. *Mol. Pharm.* 3: 87–93.

Carriere, V., Chambaz, J. and Rousset, M. (2001). Intestinal responses to xenobiotics. *Toxicol. In Vitro* 15: 373–378.

Chetty, D.J. and Chien, Y.W. (1998). Novel methods of insulin delivery: an update. *Crit. Rev. Therap. Drug Carrier Syst.* 15: 629–670.

Chhabra, R.S. and Fouts, J.R. (1976). Biochemical properties of some microsomal xenobiotics-metabolizing enzymes in rabbit small intestine. *Drug Metabol. Dispos.* 4: 208–214.

Chhabra, R.S. and Eastin, W.C. (1984). Intestinal absorption and metabolism of xenobiotics in laboratory animals, in *Intestinal Toxicology*, Schiller, C.M., Ed., Raven Press, New York.

Choi, J.S., Choi, H.K. and Shin, S.C. (2004). Enhanced bioavailability of paclitaxel after oral co-administration with flavone in rats. *Int. J. Pharmacol.* 275: 165–170.

Dahan, A. and Altman, H. (2004). Food-drug interaction: grapefruit juice augments drug bioavailability: mechanisms, extent and relevance. *Eur. J. Clin. Nutr.* 58: 1–9.

Domenenghini, C., DiGiancamillo, A., Arrighi, S. and Bosi, G. (2006). Gut-trophic feed additives and their effects upon the gut structure and intestinal metabolism: state of the art in the pig and perspective toward humans. *Histol. Histopathol.* 21: 273–283.

Fraser, A.G. (1997). Pharmacokinetic interactions between alcohol and other drugs. *Clin. Pharmacokinet.* 33: 79–90.

Goel, G., Puniya, A.K., Agular, C.N. and Singh, K. (2005). Interaction of gut microflora with tannins in feeds. *Naturwissenschaften* 92: 497–503.

Hoffman, A. and Ziv, E. (1997). Pharmacokinetic considerations of new insulin formulation and routes of administration. *Clin. Pharmacokinet.* 33: 285–301.

Ioannides, C. and Lewis, D.F. (2004). Cytochromes P450 in the bioactivation of chemicals. *Curr. Topics Med. Chem.* 4: 1767–1788.

Iturri, S. and Nunz, M.T. (1998). Effect of copper, cadmium, mercury, manganese and lead on Fe^{2+} and Fe^{3+} absorption in perfused mouse intestine. *Digestion* 59: 671–675.

Johnson, B.M., Chen, W., Borchardt, R.T., Charman, W.N. and Porter, C.J. (2003). A kinetic evlauatin of the absorption, efflux, and metabolism of verapamil in the autoperfused rat jejunum. *J. Pharmacol. Exp. Therap.* 305: 151–158.

Kaminsky, L.S. and Zhang, Q.Y. (2003). The small intestine as a xenobiotic-metabolizing organ. *Drug Metabol. Dispos.* 31: 1520–1525.

Kinoshita, H., Ijiri, I., Ameno, S., Fuke, C., Fujisawa, Y. and Ameno, K. (1996). Inhibitory mechanism of intestinal ethanol absorption induced by high acetaldehyde concentrations: effect of intestinal blood flow and substance specificity. *Alcohol Clin. Exp. Res.* 20: 510–513.

Klaassen, C.J. and Slitt, A.J. (2005). Regulation of hepatic transporters by xenobiotic receptors. *Curr. Drug Metabol.* 6: 309–328.

Lee, K.H., Xu, G.X., Schoenhard, G.L. and Cook, G.S. (1997) Mechanisms of food effects of structurally related antiarrhythmic drugs, disopyramide and bidisomide in the rat. *Pharm. Res.* 14: 1030–1038.

Leece, J.W. and Broughton, C.W. (1973). Cessation of uptake of macromolecules by neonatal guinea pig, hamster and rabbit intestinal epithelium (closure) and transport into blood. *J. Nutr.* 103: 744–750.

LeFevre, M.E. and Joel, D.D. (1977). Intestinal absorption of particulate matter. *Life Sci.* 21: 1403–1408.

Mizuma, T., Koyanagi, A. and Awazu, S. (1997). Intestinal transport and metabolism of analgesic dipeptide, kyotorphin: rate-limiting factor in intestinal absorption of peptide as drug. *Biochim. Biophys. Acta* 1335: 111–119.

Organization for Economic Cooperation and Development (OECD). (1987). Acute oral toxicity. *OECD Guideline* 401.

Oh, C.K. and Ritschel, W.A. (1990). Biopharmaceutic aspects buccal absorption of insulin. *Method Find. Exp. Clin. Pharmacol.* 12: 205–212.

Palumbo, G., Bacchi, S., Palumbo, P., Primavera, L.G. and Sponta, A.M. (2005). Grapefruit juice: potential drug interaction. *Clin. Ter.* 156: 97–103.

Parkinson, A. (2001). Biotransformation of xenobiotics, in *Casarett and Doull's Toxicology: The Basic Science of Poisons.* C.D. Klaassen, Ed., McGraw-Hill, New York.

Piyapolrungroj, N., Zhou, Y.S., Li, C., Liu, G., Zimmermann, E. and Fleisher, D. (2000) Cimetidine absorption and elimination in rat small intestine. *Drug Metabol. Dispos.* 28: 65–72.

Ramesh, A., Walker, S.A., Hood, D.B., Guillen, M.D., Schneider, K. and Weyand, E.H. (2004). Bioavilability and risk assessment of orally ingested polycyclic aromatic hydrocarbons. *Int. J. Toxicol.* 23: 301–333.

Sasser, J.E. and Jarboe, G.E. (1980). Intestinal absorption and retention of cadmium in neonatal pigs compared to rats and guinea pigs. *J. Nutr.* 110: 1641–1647.

Schuetz, E.G. (2001) Induction of cytochromes P450. *Curr Drug Metab.* 2: 139–147.

Singh, B.N. (1999). Effects of food on clinical pharmacokinetics. *Clin. Pharmacokinet.* 37: 213–255.

Smith, A.H., Zoetendal, E. and Mackie, R.I. (2005). Bacterial mechanisms to overcome inhibitory effects of dietary tannins. *Microbiol. Ecol.* 50: 197–205.

Tanaka, M., Kurata, T. Fujisawa, C., Ohshima, Y., Aoki, H., Okazaki, O. and Hakusui, H. (1993). Mechanistic study of inhibition of levofloxacin absorption by aluminum hydroxide. *Antimicrob. Agents Chemother.* 37: 2173–2178.

Wagner, D., Spahn-Langguth, H., Hanafy, A., Koggel, A. and Langguth, P. (2001). Intestinal drug efflux: formulation and food effects. *Adv. Drug Dev. Rev.* 50: S13–S31.

Walker, W.A. and Bloch, K.J. (1983). Intestinal uptake of macromolecules: *in vitro* and *in vivo* studies. *Ann NY Acad Sci.* 409: 593–602.

Watkins, D.W., Jahangeer, S., Floor, M.K. and Alabaster, O. (1992). Magnesium and calcium absorption in Fischer-344 rats influenced by changes in dietary fibre (wheat bran), fat and calcium. *Magnes. Res.* 5: 15–21.

Weber, E. and Ehrlein, H.J. (1998). Relationships between gastric emptying and intestinal absorption of nutrients and energy in mini pigs. *Dig. Dis. Sci.* 43: 1141–1153.

Winne, D. (1980). Influence of blood flow on intestinal absorption of xenobiotics. *Pharmacology* 21: 1–15.

Zhang, H., Yao, M., Morrison, R.A. and Chong, S. (2003). Commonly used surfactant, Tween 80, improves absorption of P-glycoprotein substrate, digoxin, in rats. *Arch. Pharm. Res.* 26: 768–782.

11 Normal and Abnormal Intestinal Absorption by Humans

David W. Hobson and Valerie L. Hobson

CONTENTS

In humans as in most animal species, the primary function of the gastrointestinal (GI) tract is to process food materials and absorb nutrients from these materials required for cellular metabolism and maintaining normal systemic functions. The process of digestion and absorption in the GI tract is thus essential both in terms of maintaining the nutritional status and homeostasis of the entire body. The GI tract is the primary organ system responsive initially to the composition of the diet and mediates as well as modulates variations in dietary consumption and composition. Since the processing and absorption of nutrients within the GI tract is highly dependent on normal intestinal function, it is important to understand the processes involved as well as how intestinal absorption affects the human GI response under both normal and abnormal conditions. It is critical for studies to show how toxicants and toxins may affect GI function and the overall metabolic response by the whole organism.

The digestive and absorptive functions of the GI system depend on a variety of mechanisms that soften the food, propel it through the GI tract, and mix it with hepatic bile stored in the gallbladder and digestive enzymes secreted by the salivary glands and pancreas. Some of these mechanisms depend on intrinsic properties of the intestinal smooth muscle; others involve the operation of reflexes involving the neurons intrinsic to the gut, reflexes involving the central nervous system (CNS), paracrine effects of chemical messengers, and GI hormones. The hormones are humoral agents secreted by cells in the mucosa and transported in the circulation to influence the functions of the stomach, intestines, pancreas, and gallbladder, and can act in a paracrine fashion. Some of the principal functions within the GI tract critical to its role in nutrition and human health are shown by principal regions in Table 11.1.

The diets of early humans were extremely varied due to a wide range of plant species and plant organs consumed [1]. Foods of animal origin included combinations of those taken opportunistically, such as invertebrates, amphibians,

TABLE 11.1
Regional Functions of Human GI Tract in Absorption of Nutrients and Maintenance of Fluid and Electrolyte Balance

Gastrointestinal Location	Normal Absorption Function(s) and pH
Oral cavity	Mastication, maceration of food, fluid intake, saliva production; pH 6 to 7
Esophagus	Food and fluid transport to stomach; pH 4 to 6
Stomach	Digestive processing (acidic and enzymatic) to absorbable units; pH 1 to 2.5
Pylorus	Muscular control of absorbable unit entry from stomach into small intestine
Small intestine (duodenum)	Mixing with bile and pancreatic secretions; iron and calcium absorption; bicarbonate secretion; pH 4 to 8
Small intestine (jejunum)	Intestinal digestion; pH 6.5 to 8
Small intestine (ileum)	Absorption of fat soluble vitamins (B_{12} especially), other nutrients, fatty acids and bile salts; pH 7 to 8
Cecum	Separates intestinal contents from microbial-laden colon contents; pH 5.7 to 7
Colon (ascending)	Fluid absorption; some protein absorption; liquid to solid conversion; pH 6 to 7
Colon (transverse)	Fluid absorption; liquid to solid stool formation; pH 6 to 7
Colon (descending)	Stool formation; fluid absorption; pH 6 to 7
Colon (sigmoid)	Stool formation and storage; some fluid absorption; pH 6 to 7
Rectum	Stool formation and storage; stool retention and expulsion control; pH 6 to 7
Anus	Stool release; stool retention and expulsion control

reptiles, small mammals, birds and their eggs, and the scavenging and hunting of larger mammals. All these types of foods have characteristic nutritional compositions. Studies of the compositional features of the diets of early humans reveal that an adequate diet could be obtained in a variety of ways. Obtaining adequate water and energy are likely to have been the main physiological drives and the selection of fat-containing foods probably had substantial advantages in reducing the amount of plant foods that had to be gathered due to their ability to provide essential nutrients and a higher degree of satiety.

Then, just as now, many plant foods contained, in addition to nutrients, natural toxicants that needed to be recognized and either avoided or eliminated by processing in some fashion or by cooking. Although it is certain that primitive humans must have possessed a vast knowledge of the consequences of consuming acutely toxic plants, it has also been surmised that a preference for sweet tastes may have played a role in protecting early humans from consuming sometimes bitter toxic plants [1].

TABLE 11.2
Estimated Daily Nutrient
Intakes for Adults[a]

Nutrient	Amount
Protein, g	91
Carbohydrate, g	271
Total fat, g	65
Saturated fat, g	17
Monounsaturated fat, g	24
Polyunsaturated fat, g	20
Linoleic acid, g	18
Alphalinolenic acid, g	1.7
Cholesterol, mg	230
Total dietary fiber, g	31
Potassium, mg	4,044
Sodium, mg	1,779
Calcium, mg	1,316
Magnesium, mg	380
Copper, mg	1.5
Iron, mg	18
Phosphorus, mg	1,740
Zinc, mg	14
Thiamin, mg	2.0
Riboflavin, mg	2.8
Niacin equivalents, mg	22
Vitamin B_6, mg	2.4
Vitamin B_{12}, µg	8.3
Vitamin C, mg	155
Vitamin E, mg	9.5
Vitamin A, µg	1,052

[a] *U.S. Department of Agriculture Food Guide* nutrient values based on population-weighted averages of typical food choices within each food group or subgroup at 2000-calorie level.

Although some primitive populations continue to consume traditional foodstuffs regularly in the modern world, it is still the case and is well known that the sources and estimated daily amounts of essential nutrients ingested by adults vary worldwide. This is primarily due to differences in dietary preferences and the types and natures of available foodstuffs. Current values estimated by the U.S. Department of Agriculture are shown in Table 11.2 [2]. The recommended daily water consumption is 2 to 3 liters. The data shown in Table 11.2 pertain to dietary solids only and do not include the absorption of water and fluids from endogenous secretions that are processed and absorbed daily. It has been estimated that endogenous secretions account for about 6 to 7 liters of water overall, an additional 35 to 100 g of protein, and 20 to 30 g of fat [2].

The GI tract has a very high nutrient demand, in large part due to the high turnover of epithelial cells along the villi and the daily synthesis and secretion of protein as a digestive enzyme. Protein turnover in the GI tract is estimated to account for about 20% of total body protein turnover, although the GI tract typically constitutes less than 5% of total tissue mass in the body. The intestinal organs are able to derive part of their nutrient needs from the nutrients present in the lumen during digestion. In fact, the hormones released during the gastric and intestinal phases of digestion to stimulate secretion and motility also have trophic effects that ensure cell and enzyme renewal during the postprandial phase [3].

The luminal presence of nutrients is requisite to maintaining normal GI tract function. Research comparing enteral and parenteral feeding demonstrates that atrophy of intestinal tissue occurs when luminal nutrients are not present to support growth [4]. Because of high nutrient requirements, GI function may be severely compromised during malnutrition. The potential consequences of malnutrition on GI function include:

- Decreased digestion of food materials by pancreatic enzymes
- Mucosal surface atrophication
- Impairment of immune functions of the GI tract
- Increased microbial activity in the colon due to decreased intestinal motility and a greater presence of undigested substrates

In a malnourished state, the GI tract can fail to function effectively to provide nutrients to other tissues. Restoration of normal GI function is critical because the loss of digestive and absorptive capacity in the malnourished state can result in serious consequences [5].

RESPONSE TO DIET

The GI response to diet is mediated by neural and hormonal stimuli. An important part of the neural stimulation of GI function occurs during the cephalic phase of digestion, when food is seen and smelled. This response essentially prepares the GI tract for the presence of food. Neural stimulation, primarily mediated by the vagus nerve, elicits acid and pepsin secretion in the stomach, gallbladder contraction, and secretion of enzyme-rich fluid from the pancreas. Neural reflexes are also known to be involved in mediating motility of the small and large intestines.

GI smooth muscle responses to stimulation of nonadrenergic noncholinergic inhibitory nerves are thought to be mediated by polypeptides, ATP, or another unidentified neurotransmitter [6]. Nitric oxide (NO), an inorganic, gaseous molecule, appears to act as an inhibitory neurotransmitter on GI smooth muscle. The "nitrergic" nerves appear to play major roles in the control of smooth muscle tone, motility, and fluid secretion in the GI tract. This knowledge is currently revising our understanding of GI tract neural response. NO-induced GI smooth muscle relaxation is mediated not only by cyclic GMP directly or indirectly via hyperpolarization, but also by cyclic GMP-independent mechanisms. Understanding nitrergic innervation and responses in the GI tract may to lead to a new understanding of its regulation, physiology, and pathophysiology and may also demonstrate how this sort of smooth muscle control affects GI motility and intestinal absorption overall.

In addition to the innervation of the gut, the GI tract contains various hormones and regulatory peptides that can be released by the presence of food and elicit responses from organs in the gut, which is one of the richest endocrine organs in the body. Insulin and glucagon are examples of hormones that are released from the GI tract whose peripheral effects on organs other than those of the GI tract have been well studied. The potential effects of other gut hormones on non-GI tissues have not been well characterized. The distribution of hormones and regulatory peptides along the gut is regional as shown in Table 11.3.

The release of hormones is mediated by the presence of protein or amino acids, fats, and carbohydrates in the GI tract. Protein is a potent stimulant of gastrin, cholecystokinin (CCK), and gastric inhibitory peptide (GIP) release; fat is a stimulant of CCK, secretin, and GIP release as well as enteroglucagon, neurotensin, and peptide YY release. Carbohydrate presence is involved in the release of GIP as well as the endocrine hormones, insulin, and glucagon and the magnitude of carbohydrate exposed surface area is also important [7–9].

The pancreas contains a range of hydrolytic enzymes that digest the macromolecules that are ingested in the diet. These enzymes include proteases (e.g., trypsinogen, chymotrypsinogen, proelastase, procarboxypeptidases), [α]-amylase, lipase, colipase, phospholipase, and cholesterol esterase. The proteases and possibly the lipid digestive enzymes are secreted from the pancreas in an inactive form and are activated in the small intestine by the action of enterokinase or trypsin. The secretion of an enzyme-rich fluid from the pancreas can be stimulated by the gastrin hormone released from the stomach and CCK released from the duodenum [10,11]. Thus, during the cephalic and gastric phases of digestion, pancreatic secretion is initiated, and while nutrients are in the small intestine, CCK has an important role in sustaining sufficient enzyme secretion for digestion to occur.

Dietary constituents can also stimulate enzyme secretion from the pancreas by feedback mechanisms. For example, dietary composition and content can stimulate pancreatic enzyme secretion via a vagal cholinergic pathway. This response is mediated by differences in the release of GI hormones [12,13].

The effect of diet on the secretion of digestive enzymes other than the proteases differs. The pancreas can adapt to a high fat, low carbohydrate diet by increasing the activity of lipase and decreasing the activity of amylase [14]. The mechanism for this adaptation is not known but may be mediated by the

TABLE 11.3
Regional Distribution of Gastrointestinal Hormones

Origin	Hormone(s)	Function
Stomach	Gastrin	Acid release/pH regulation
Duodenum and proximal jejunum (upper small intestine)	Cholecystokinin (CCK-A)	Stimulates pancreatic enzyme delivery
		Stimulates bile delivery from gallbladder
	Secretin	Bicarbonate release/pH regulation
	Gastric inhibitory peptide (GIP)	Inhibits gastric motility and acid secretion
		Enhances insulin release
	Motilin	Controls upper GI pattern of contraction
	Enkephalins	Opiate-like actions
	Bombesin-like immunoreactivity	Stimulates CCK and gastrin release
Distal intestine (ileum and colon)	Neurotensin	Modulates motility
		Relaxes the lower esophageal sphincter
		Blocks stimulation of acid and pepsin secretion
	Glucagon-like-peptide 1	Enhances the release of insulin in response to glucose
	Glucagon-like-peptide 2	Stimulation of intestinal cell proliferation
	Oxyntomodulin	Inhibition of gastric secretion and motility
		Inhibition of pancreatic secretion
	Peptide YY	Regulates appetite control/obesity regulation
Pancreas	Insulin	Regulates carbohydrate metabolism
	Glucagon	Blood glucose regulation
	Pancreatic polypeptide	Increases gastric emptying and secretion
		Relaxes pyloric and ileocecocolic sphincters
		Relaxes the gall bladder and colon
	Somatostatin	Inhibits release of GIP, motilin, secretin, gastrin, CCK-A
		Lowers gastric emptying rate
		Inhibits release of insulin and glucagon
	Vasoactive intestinal peptide	Smooth muscle relaxation
		Stimulates pancreatic secretion
Entire GI tract	Substance P	Pain (nociception)
		Vomit reflex
		Induces vasodilation
		Stimulates salivary secretion

absorption of lipid and carbohydrate digestion products rather than release of a specific hormone.

It has long been known that dietary proteins and fats are potent stimulants of GI function, but until recently the carbohydrate portion of the diet, whether the digestible carbohydrates (starch and sugars) or the nondigestible polysaccharides associated with dietary fiber, have been viewed as somewhat neutral. However, it is now known that glucose is a potent releaser of GIP, which augments insulin release [8].

Some sources of dietary fiber such as pectins and gums have been associated with slower digestion and absorption of carbohydrates and fats due to their ability to interfere with digestive enzyme activity, to increase the viscosity and volume of the intestinal contents, and to bind micellar components [15,16]. Dietary fiber and undegraded starch have been shown to be primary sources of fermentable substrate for the microflora of the large intestine [17]. The products of dietary fiber fermentation such as short-chain fatty acids can be absorbed and utilized by the body. Increases in plasma triglycerides after a meal originate from both intestinal and hepatic sources [18,19]. In contrast, plasma cholesterol concentrations do not change significantly during the alimentary period after a meal [18–20].

NORMAL INTESTINAL ABSORPTION

During the process of digestion, large, naturally occurring carbohydrates, proteins, and fats are hydrolyzed by catalytic enzymes to simple sugars, amino acids, and fatty acids, respectively. These smaller compounds are more efficiently absorbed in the small intestine and provide the necessary building blocks and energy content to be used by the cells of the body. Besides the absorption of dietary nutrients, the intestinal mucosa functions in the absorption of water, electrolytes, vitamins, and minerals. Electrolytes, water, and metabolic substrates are absorbed into the blood and distributed to cells throughout the body for their use. Figure 11.1 shows how different dietary components are processed and absorbed by the intestines.

As shown in Figure 11.1, intestinal absorption essentially involves the transport of nutrients from digested food and water from the gut lumen, across the intestinal epithelium, into the lymph or venous blood. Basic mechanisms of absorption into an intestinal cell are by three different mechanisms: simple diffusion, facilitated diffusion, and active transport. Diffusion does not use metabolic energy, and the solute is not transported against a gradient. It does not need a transport protein and velocity-versus-substrate concentration is linear. Facilitated diffusion involves a transport protein, demonstrates substrate specificity, and the reaction is saturable. The solute is not transported against a gradient and does not need metabolic energy. Active transport involves transport proteins and demonstrates substrate specificity. Transport is against a concentration gradient and metabolic energy is necessary.

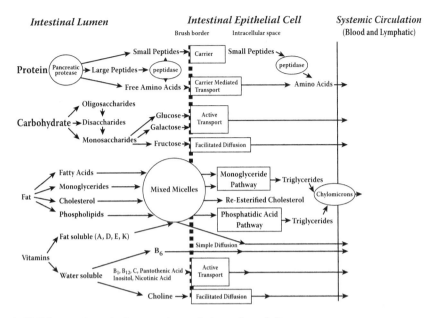

FIGURE 11.1 Intestinal processing and absorption of dietary components.

Most absorption takes place in the small intestine. The surface area of the intestine is well suited to its function: the structural adaptations of mucosal folds, villi, and microvilli give a total absorptive area for the small intestine of 200 to 500 m², or a 600-fold increase over the projected surface area of a smooth-surfaced tube of equivalent length. On average, for adults, total daily intestinal absorption amounts to 200 to 300 g of carbohydrates, about 100 g of amino acids, about 100 g of fat, about 100 g of electrolytes, and 7 or 8 liters of water. Under normal conditions and with few exceptions, much of what is ingested is absorbed. It has been estimated that the intestinal tract has enough reserve capacity to allow five to ten times more food substances and two to three times more water to be absorbed per day over recommended average consumption [21].

The human small intestine villar absorptive surface and mucosal structure greatly increase the total surface area for highly efficient absorption. The lining of the stomach, in contrast, has a poor absorptive area because it lacks a villar absorptive surface and has tight junctions between its epithelial cells. Only alcohol and some drugs such as aspirin are absorbed in the stomach and the amount of absorption is low.

The mucosa of the human small intestine has structures called folds of Kerckring that increase the surface area of the mucosa about three-fold. The millions of villi covering the surface of the mucosa enhance this absorptive surface area by perhaps another ten-fold. Furthermore, each intestinal mucosal cell in the villus is characterized by a brush border that consists of approximately 600 microvilli per cell that substantially increase the total absorptive surface area of the small intestine perhaps another twenty-fold [22].

In addition to diffusion and active transport of digested materials across the cells of the intestinal epithelium, small amounts of substances are also taken into the cells via pinocytosis [21].

Actin filaments contract intermittently and cause continual movement in the microvilli, keeping mucosal cells exposed to new quantities of intestinal fluid, enhancing opportunities for absorption. Absorbed materials can be sent directly into the portal circulation or lymphatic system. Each intestinal villus contains a vascular system with an artery, a vein, blood capillaries, and a central lacteal for absorption into the lymph.

FLUIDS AND ELECTROLYTES

The small intestine is the primary site of fluid and solute absorption in the GI tract and absorbs approximately 85% of the fluid, with the colon absorbing the remaining 15%. It is estimated that an adult human ingests about 2 liters of fluid daily, not including the volume of fluid from internal secretions. The secreted volumes are approximately three to four times the amount of fluid ingested or between 6 and 8 liters of which approximate proportional amounts of the different components of secreted fluid are saliva, 15%; gastric juice, 25%; pancreatic juice 10%; bile 20%; and intestinal secretions 30%. During GI absorption, the small intestine absorbs the majority of this fluid and the colon a lesser amount. It is estimated that of the total fluid entering the GI tract only 1% or less is excreted via fecal matter [21,23].

Water is transported through the intestinal membrane by osmosis. Partially digested solubilized food (chyme) delivered from the stomach into the intestinal tract is hypertonic and is adjusted to isotonicity in the duodenum. The opposite occurs when chyme is hyperosmotic. Water then is transferred to the chyme, making it iso-osmotic with blood plasma. When dissolved substances are absorbed, the osmotic pressure of the chyme is decreased. Water diffuses rapidly through the membranes of the intestine and is absorbed immediately into the blood with any associated ions. Water absorption by the jejunum is greater than the ileum; however, the colon is most efficient and absorbs more water than any other part of the GI tract.

Due to the handling of electrolytes, the small intestinal mucosal cell may be considered a polarized epithelial cell. The plasma membrane consists of the brush border facing the lumen and the basolateral membrane facing the blood. The Na^+–K^+–ATPase is located exclusively on the basolateral membrane. Its function is to transport K^+ into the cell and Na^+ out of the cell. Both of these transport processes occur against a concentration gradient requiring metabolic energy. The Na^+–K^+–ATPase is a transport protein as well as an ATPase. The energy released after ATP hydrolysis is used to energize the transport. The stoichiometry between the transported ions is 3 Na^+:2 K^+. This results in Na^+ and K^+ gradients across the basolateral membrane. It also produces a chemical gradient across the membrane (inside-negative). Under normal conditions, luminal fluid contains high concentrations of Na^+ (from diet, intestinal, and pancreatic secretions), so an electrochemical gradient is created across the brush border membrane.

CARBOHYDRATE ABSORPTION

Luminal and membrane digestion of dietary carbohydrates produces glucose, galactose, and fructose. Fructose is absorbed by facilitated diffusion, so there is no need for metabolic energy, but a specific carrier is required. Once inside the cell, fructose is phosphorylated and converted to glucose prior to entering the portal blood.

Galactose and glucose are actively transported into mucosal cells by a common transport protein [24]. The energy for this active transport is provided by the electrochemical Na^+ gradient. The glucose carrier has binding sites for Na^+ and glucose. When both sites are occupied, it translocates across the membrane. The Na^+ and glucose are released into the cytoplasm of cells and the unloaded, empty carrier returns to the original position to start the transport cycle again. Stoichiometry between Na^+ and glucose is 2:1 or 1:1. The transport of glucose and Na^+ via the carrier results in the transfer of a positive charge across the membrane. Both the electrical and chemical components of the electrochemical Na^+ gradient provide energy for glucose transport. This process is known as Na^+–glucose co-transport. Galactose shares the glucose binding site and can be absorbed in a manner similar to that outlined for glucose [24].

The electrochemical Na^+ gradient is the direct energy source for glucose transport, but ATP ultimately is necessary for the transport. The hydrolysis of ATP via the Na^+–K^+–ATPase system generates the electrochemical Na^+ gradient. In the intact cell, glucose transport is inhibited by metabolic poisons such as dinitrophenol (causes a reduction of ATP synthesis), hypoxia (synthesis of ATP is reduced), ouabain (Na^+–K^+–ATPase is inhibited), and phlorizen (blocks glucose from binding to its site on the carrier) [25,26]. Absorbed glucose leaves the cell across the basolateral membrane to enter mucosal capillaries. This process occurs via a facilitated glucose transport system, GLUT 2 [27]. The transporter is Na^+-independent and is inhibited by phlorizen. In a healthy human fed a meal containing 20 to 60 g of starch, as much as 10% of the starch metabolic product escapes absorption in the small intestine. This starch passes on to the colon, where it provides a carbon source for bacteria of the colon.

AMINO ACIDS AND PEPTIDES

Intact proteins and large peptides are not appreciably absorbed in the human intestinal tract. Several different types of peptide and amino acid transport proteins have been characterized in the luminal membranes of intestinal epithelial cells [28–31,48]. Dipeptides and tripeptides are transported across the brush border membrane. A single-membrane transport system with broad specificity is responsible for such small peptides. It has a high affinity for dipeptides and tripeptides with physiologic L-amino acids. This membrane transport system has greater affinity for peptides with amino acids containing bulky side chains [31].

The brush border mucosal cells of the small intestine have an active peptide transport system and there may be multiple systems. The transport system is energized by an electrochemical H^+ gradient and not by a Na^+ gradient. It accepts dipeptides and tripeptides as substrates. The H^+ gradient across the brush border membrane is generated by the action of the Na^+–H^+ exchanger. The total amount of each amino acid that enters intestinal epithelial cells in the form of dipeptides and tripeptides is considerably greater than the amount that enters as a single amino acid.

Amino acids are transported across the brush border plasma membrane into the intestinal mucosal cells by way of certain specific amino acid transport systems. There are three main sodium-dependent active transport systems for amino acids in brush border membranes. The neutral brush border (NBB) system transports most of the neutral amino acids, both hydrophobic and hydrophilic. The amino acid transport system handles proline and hydroxyproline. The PHE system transports phenylalanine and methionine. The dicarboxylic amino acid transporter transports aspartate and glutamate [32,33,47].

Two facilitated transport systems are independent of Na^+. The Y^+ system transports basic amino acids such as arginine and lysine, while the L system transports neutral amino acids, preferably those with hydrophobic side chains [35]. At the basolateral membrane are two different types of sodium-dependent transport systems. One system prefers small, hydrophobic amino acids and the other system prefers small neutral amino acids. The sodium-independent L system transports neutral hydrophobic amino acids [36]. This basolateral membrane is more permeable to amino acids than is the brush border membrane. Therefore, diffusion is an important pathway for transport across the basolateral plasma membrane. This is especially true for amino acids with hydrophobic side chains.

FAT ABSORPTION

Fat digestion products, i.e., monoglycerides, fatty acids, cholesterol, and phospholipids, are present in the intestinal lumen in the form of micelles (aggregates). Micelle formation is aided by the presence of bile acids. These products are absorbed into the intestinal mucosal cell from these micelles. On the surface of the brush border, pH is acidic due to secretion of H^+ from cells by the Na^+–H^+ exchanger. This acidic pH causes the dissociation of micelles and these products can now pass freely through the brush border membrane by diffusion, largely dependent on lipid solubility. Free fatty acids, 2-monoglycerides, and other products of lipid digestion can diffuse across the brush border membrane very rapidly. Cholesterol is absorbed more slowly than the other lipid products associated with micelles. As the micelles travel down the small intestine, they become more concentrated with cholesterol. Although the duodenum and jejunum are active in absorbing fatty components, most of the ingested fat is absorbed at the mid-jejunum.

The absorbed monoglycerides and free fatty acids are converted back into triglycerides within the intestinal cell. A recently discovered cytoplasmic fatty acid-binding protein plays a role in transporting fatty acid to the smooth endoplasmic reticulum. This protein has a higher affinity for unsaturated fatty acids than for saturated fatty acids, and it binds long-chain fatty acids more tightly than medium- or short-chain fatty acids. In the smooth endoplasmic reticulum, the 2-monoglycerides are re-esterified with fatty acids at the 1 and 11 carbons to reform triglycerides. Cholesterol is largely re-esterified, although some free cholesterol remains. Lysophospholipids are reconverted to phospholipids, such as lecithin. Some *de novo* synthesis of lipids can take place in intestinal epithelial cells [37]. Triglyceride synthesis occurs via two pathways: the monoglyceride pathway and the phosphatidic acid pathway.

The monoglyceride pathway accounts for about 70% of intestinal triglyceride synthesis. The reprocessed lipids and lipids that have been synthesized *de novo* accumulate in the vesicles of the smooth endoplasmic reticulum. Phospholipid covers the external surfaces of these droplets (vesicles). Their polar head groups face toward the aqueous exterior and hydrophobic acyl chains face the fatty interior. The lipid droplets thus formed, some as large as 1 mm in diameter, are known as chylomicrons. About 10% of the surface is covered by -lipoprotein, which is synthesized by intestinal epithelial cells.

The resynthesized triglycerides leave the cell in the chylomicron form. They form a milky fluid, the chyle, which diffuses into lymphatic lacteals, passes via lymphatic vessels to the thoracic duct, and into systemic circulation. Chylomicrons may now be as large as 750 nm in diameter. They are macromolecular particles containing 80 to 90% triglycerides, about 10% phospholipids, 3% cholesterol, and 2% protein. This protein needed for chylomicron synthesis is called apoprotein. If protein synthesis is inhibited in the intestinal cell, fewer chylomicron forms and triglycerides accumulate in the cytoplasm of the cell.

The majority of absorbed fatty acids larger than 10-carbon atoms are absorbed as esterified fatty acids in the lymph. Fatty acids smaller than 10-carbon atoms are transported into the portal venous blood. Glycerol and medium-chain fatty acids are water-soluble and can be transported into blood without going through the chylomicron pathway [37].

Bile Acids

The ileum is the principal site of bile acid absorption. Bile acids cross the brush border plasma membrane by simple diffusion or active transport. The active process is a secondary active transport powered by a Na^+ gradient across the brush border plasma membrane. Na^+ is co-transported with bile acids. Conjugated bile acids (bile salts) are substrates for active absorption. Deconjugated bile acids are less polar and can be absorbed by simple diffusion. Absorbed bile acids leave the intestinal cell via the basolateral membrane and enter the portal circulation. Hepatocytes take up the bile acids and reconjugate most deconjugated bile acids and rehydroxlate some secondary bile acids. These reprocessed bile acids, along with newly synthesized bile acids, are secreted into the bile [37].

VITAMINS

Fat-Soluble Vitamins

The fat-soluble vitamins (A, D, E, and K) partition into mixed micelles formed by bile acids and lipid digestion products. Fat-soluble vitamins diffuse across the brush border plasma membranes of intestinal epithelial cells. Bile acids and lipid digestion products enhance the absorption of fat-soluble vitamins. Fat-soluble vitamins diffuse into intestinal mucosal cells and enter the chylomicrons that leave the intestine in the lymph. If bile acids are not present, a good proportion of fat-soluble vitamins leave the intestine in the portal blood.

Vitamin A (retinol) is absorbed better than -carotene (provitamin A) and retinal; -carotene and retinal are converted to retinol in the intestine. In the thoracic duct, vitamin A is present as fatty acid esters of retinol. Vitamin A is absorbed independently of bile acid and leaves the intestine in the portal blood. Vitamin D is absorbed as the free vitamin in the jejunum. Many esters of vitamin D are hydrolyzed in the intestinal lumen before absorption, and 55 to 99% of ingested vitamin D is absorbed. The absorption of vitamin E requires the presence of bile-acid mixed micelles [37]. Although small quantities of ingested vitamin E are absorbed, significant amounts are not absorbed if ingested in larger quantities, and will appear in feces. This vitamin also leaves the intestine in the lymph.

Vitamins K_1 and K_2 contain hydrophobic side chains partitioned into bile-acid mixed micelles and leave the intestine through lacteals into lymphatic vessels. Vitamin K_3 lacks a side chain and is absorbed independently of the mixed micelles. It leaves the intestine via portal blood.

Water-Soluble Vitamins

Most water-soluble vitamins, if consumed in high doses, are absorbed by simple diffusion. However, specific transport mechanisms also play an important role in absorption of these vitamins under other conditions. Vitamin C (ascorbic acid) is absorbed in the proximal ileum by active transport. Na^+ and ascorbate are co-transported into cells [37]. The energy for this transport comes from the Na^+ electrochemical potential gradient. Biotin is transported by facilitated diffusion in the upper small intestine by a mechanism involving Na^+ presence in the lumen. Folic acid as 5-methyltetrahydrofolate is absorbed by simple diffusion [45]. Folic acid also is absorbed by carrier-mediated active transport via an H^+ gradient supplying energy in the jejunum.

Thiamine (vitamin B_1) is absorbed in free form by a Na^+-dependent active transport in the jejunum. Some thiamine is phosphorylated in mucosal cells of the jejunum. Riboflavin (vitamin B_2) is absorbed in the proximal small intestine by facilitated transport; absorption is increased if bile acids are present. Pyridoxine (vitamin B_6) is most likely absorbed by simple diffusion. Nicotinic acid also is absorbed by the jejunum by a Na^+-dependent mechanism. Pantothenic acid and inositol are actively transported by the small intestine via a Na^+ gradient providing the energy. Choline absorption is by facilitated diffusion.

Vitamin B_{12} absorption involves an active transport process. Four physiologically important forms of vitamin B_{12} are cyanocobalamin, hydroxycobalamin, methylcobalamin, and deoxyadenosylcobalamin. Up to 5 mg of vitamin B_{12} is stored in the liver. About 70% of the vitamin B_{12} present in the bile is reabsorbed. This liver storage is thought to be sufficient for 3 to 6 years [37]. Most cobalamins are bound to proteins and absorbed in the intestine. The low pH of the stomach and pepsin release cobalamins that are bound to R proteins, i.e., haptocorrin (HC) secreted from salivary glands and gastric juice. Intrinsic factor (IF) is a cobalamin-binding protein secreted by the gastric parietal cells [38]. Its secretory rate usually parallels that of HCl. Dietary cobalamin bound to food proteins is released in the stomach by pepsin and acid pH and more free cobalamin binds to HC than IF.

The cobalamin–HC complex moves to the intestinal lumen, is digested by pancreatic proteases, and the liberated cobalamin complexes with IF. The cobalamin–IF complex moves through the small intestine and binds to a transmembrane receptor (IFCR) in the ileum. After endocytosis of the complex, cobalamin is released intracellularly and transferred to transcobalamin II (TC II). This cobalamin–TC II complex leaves the ileal mucosal cell and enters the circulation.

SODIUM AND CHLORIDE

The Na^+–H^+ exchange system in the brush border of small intestinal and colonic cells is the principal means of Na^+ absorption from the intestinal lumen. This process is responsible for the acid pH microclimate at the surface of the brush border membrane and transports Na+ from the lumen into the cell and H^+ from the cell into the lumen. The electroneutral NaCl transport across the brush border membrane of the small intestine is due to two exchangers: the Na^+–H^+ exchanger and the Cl–HCO_3^- exchanger. The transport is inhibited by acetazolamide, an inhibitor of carbonic anhydrase that reduces HCO_3^- within cells. Na^+ is often co-transported with glucose, bile salts, amino acids, and water-soluble vitamins in the small intestine. In addition, a small amount of Na^+ may enter small intestine cells by passive diffusion [37].

The sodium pump, Na^+–K^+–ATpase, is responsible for active transport of Na^+ from the intestinal cell to the capillary. This pump is found in the basolateral membrane of the small intestinal cell. It is inhibited by ouabain, a cardiac glycoside.

Finally, in aldosterone-stimulated Na^+ transport, the transport occurs at the apical (luminal) membrane of the distal colon. This is due to a Na^+ channel that allows Na^+ to move passively down the electrochemical Na^+ gradient. Aldosterone stimulates the Na^+ channel. Chloride ions in the duodenum and jejunum are absorbed by passive diffusion.

CHLORIDE AND BICARBONATE

HCO_3 secreted into the proximal duodenum moves to the jejunum where both Cl^- and HCO_3^- are absorbed in large amounts. Most HCO_3^- is absorbed in the distal jejunum. Cl^- is absorbed and HCO_3^- is secreted in the ileum. Cl^- is absorbed and HCO_3^- secreted in the colon [37].

POTASSIUM

In the jejunum and in the ileum, the net flux of K^+ is from the lumen to the blood. As the intestinal contents are reduced through the absorption of water, the K^+ concentration increases and K^+ moves across the intestinal mucosa into the blood. Active transport of K^+ is absent in the small intestine, but in the colon K^+ may be secreted or absorbed. Usually K^+ is secreted in the colon [37]. Most K^+ absorption is due to its enhanced concentration in the lumen, caused by the absorption of water. K^+ loss may occur in diarrhea. If diarrhea is prolonged, the K^+ level falls in the body's extracellular fluid. Normal K^+ levels are needed for the heart to function properly, or cardiac dysrhythmias may occur

CALCIUM

Abnormal or inadequate intestinal calcium absorption is a contributing factor in certain disease states, e.g., osteoporosis. The quantity of calcium absorbed in the intestine is controlled by the amount of calcium in the diet during recent periods. Calcium is absorbed by two distinct mechanisms, and their relative magnitude of importance is set by dietary calcium "history." Active transcellular absorption occurs only in the duodenum when calcium intake has been low. This process involves import of calcium into enterocytes, transport across the cells, and export into extracellular fluid and blood. Calcium enters the intestinal epithelial cells through voltage-insensitive channels and is pumped out of the cell via calcium–ATPase. The rate limiting step in transcellular calcium absorption is transport across epithelial cells, which is greatly enhanced by the carrier protein calbindin, the synthesis of which is totally dependent on vitamin D [39,40,46].

Passive paracellular absorption occurs in the jejunum and ileum, and to a much lesser extent, in the colon when dietary calcium levels have been moderate or high. In this case, ionized calcium diffuses through tight junctions into the basolateral spaces around enterocytes, and hence into blood. Such transport depends on having higher concentrations of free calcium in the intestinal lumen than in blood.

Calcium ions are actively absorbed throughout the small intestine, especially in the duodenum and jejunum, where Ca^{++} can be concentrated against a greater than ten-fold concentration gradient. Although the absorption rate of Ca^{++} is greater than that of other divalent ions, it is 50 times slower than Na^+ absorption. Intestinal absorption of Ca^{++} is stimulated by hormonal vitamin D (1,25 dihydroxycholecalciferol) and parathyroid hormone. Ca^{++} moves from the brush border of the mucosal cell of the small intestine down its electrochemical potential gradient into the cytosol. This Ca^{++} is bound to an intestinal membrane calcium-binding protein (IMCal) that most likely is the transporter for Ca^{++}. The cytosol of the intestinal epithelial cells contains a cytosolic calcium-binding protein (CaBP) that binds two calcium ions with high affinity. CaBP is an essential component of Ca^{++} absorption. Its synthesis is stimulated by hormonal vitamin D. Free and bound Ca^{++} are in dynamic exchange with Ca^{++} in the mitochondria and endoplasmic reticulum.

Within cells, Ca^{++} is stored in the mitochondria and endoplasmic reticulum, and it can be mobilized by the action of a secondary messenger inositol triphosphate. The basolateral cell membrane contains two transport proteins that are capable of ejecting Ca^{++} against its electrochemical potential gradient. Ca^{++}–ATPase in the basolateral membrane is the primary transport protein that splits ATP and uses the energy to transport Ca^{++}. The Na^+–Ca^{++} exchanger uses this energy of the Na^+ gradient to exude Ca^{++} by active transport. Ca^{++} stimulates the activity of Ca^{++}–ATPase by binding to calmodulin, a calcium-binding protein. The calcium–calmodulin complex then stimulates a protein kinase that phosphorylates the Ca^{++}–ATPase, thereby activating it and enhancing its enzymatic and transport activities.

Hormonal vitamin D is essential for normal calcium absorption, binds to nuclear receptors, and stimulates messenger RNA that codes for a particular protein. Vitamin D induces the synthesis of Ca^{++}-binding protein, the absorption of Ca^{++} into intestinal mucosal cells, and exocytosis out of mucosal cells into capillaries at the level of the basolateral membrane. A Na^+–Ca^{++} exchanger may also be involved at the basolateral membrane, but this is not regulated by hormonal vitamin D.

IRON

Iron homeostasis is regulated at the level of intestinal absorption, and it is important that adequate but not excessive quantities of iron be absorbed from the diet. Inadequate absorption can lead to iron deficiency disorders such as anemia. On the other hand, excessive iron is toxic because mammals do not have physiologic pathways for its elimination. Iron is absorbed by villus enterocytes in the proximal duodenum. Efficient absorption requires an acidic environment, and antacids or other conditions that interfere with gastric acid secretion can interfere with iron absorption.

Ferric iron (Fe^{+++}) in the duodenal lumen is reduced to its ferrous (Fe^{++}) form through the action of a brush border ferrireductase. Iron is then co-transported with a proton into enterocytes via the divalent metal transporter DMT-1. This transporter is not specific for iron, and also transports other divalent metal ions [41].

Once inside an enterocyte, iron follows one of two major pathways. The path taken depends on a complex programming of the cell based on both dietary and systemic iron loads:

Iron abundance states — Iron within the enterocyte is trapped by incorporation into ferritin and hence not transported into blood. When the enterocyte dies and is shed, this iron is lost.

Iron-limiting states — Iron is exported out of the enterocyte via a transporter (ferroportin) located in the basolateral membrane. It then binds to the iron carrier transferrin for transport throughout the body.

Iron in the form of heme, from ingestion of hemoglobin or myoglobin, is also readily absorbed. In this case, it appears that intact heme is taken up by small intestinal enterocytes via endocytosis. Once inside enterocytes, iron is liberated and essentially follows the same pathway for export as absorbed inorganic iron. Some heme may be transported intact into the circulation [28,37,51,52].

Dietary iron contains both inorganic iron and heme. The duodenum actively absorbs both forms. Iron is released from heme inside mucosal cells and transferred into the body as inorganic iron. Fe^{++} is absorbed faster than Fe^{+++} because ferric iron is insoluble above pH 3, whereas ferrous iron remains soluble at pH 8. Dietary constituents such as phosphates, carbonates, and oxalates reduce iron absorption because they form insoluble complexes with iron. These iron complexes are more soluble at low pH. Therefore, HCl secreted by the stomach enhances iron absorption; ascorbate also promotes iron absorption. The quantity of iron in the body is maintained by controlled absorption from the duodenum. Iron deficiency enhances erythropoiesis, and hypoxia increases intestinal iron absorption. Iron is stored in the mucosal cell as a ferritin complex. When iron absorption is increased, no ferritin complex is formed and the iron is rapidly delivered into the plasma. When iron absorption is depressed, more iron is trapped in the form of a ferritin complex and retained in the mucosal cell. When Fe^{++} leaves the mucosal cell, transferrin in the circulating blood is the carrier that delivers it to other tissues via transferrin receptors in the plasma membrane [37].

OTHER IONS

Copper

Two processes appear responsible for copper absorption: a rapid, low capacity system and a slower, high capacity system. The processes may be similar to the two processes involved with calcium absorption. Many molecular details of copper absorption remain to be elucidated. Inactivating mutations in the gene encoding an intracellular copper ATPase have been shown responsible for the failure of intestinal copper absorption in Menkes' disease.

A number of dietary factors have been shown to influence copper absorption. For example, excessive dietary intake of either zinc or molybdenum can induce secondary copper deficiency states. Copper is absorbed in the jejunum with about 50% efficiency. Some copper is secreted in the bile bound to certain bile acids and then lost in the feces. Magnesium is absorbed from the entire length of the small intestine, with about half of the dietary intake absorbed. Phosphate is absorbed all along the small intestine. Some phosphate may be absorbed by active transport [37,42,43].

Phosphorus

Phosphorus is predominantly absorbed as inorganic phosphate in the upper small intestine. Phosphate is transported into the epithelial cells by co-transport with sodium, and expression of the transporters is enhanced by vitamin D [37].

Zinc

Zinc homeostasis is largely regulated by its uptake and loss through the small intestine. Although a number of zinc transporters and binding proteins have been identified in villus epithelial cells, a detailed picture of the molecules involved in zinc absorption is not yet in hand. Intestinal excretion of zinc occurs via shedding of epithelial cells and in pancreatic and biliary secretions [50]. A number of factors modulate zinc absorption. Some animal proteins in the diet enhance zinc absorption. Phytates from dietary plant materials (including cereal grains, rice, and corn) can chelate zinc and inhibit its absorption. Subsistence on phytate-rich diets is thought responsible for a considerable fraction of human zinc deficiencies [44].

ABNORMAL INTESTINAL ABSORPTION

A wide variety of conditions and agents can adversely affect intestinal absorption. These range from a variety of disease conditions that cause malabsorption of many nutrients to conditions that produce abnormal absorption of only one or a few specific nutrients [53].

A comprehensive treatise on all known causes of abnormal intestinal absorption in humans is beyond the scope of this chapter. Some conditions may have little relevance to toxicology and are beyond the scope of this chapter. However, many of the major causes of abnormal intestinal absorption including malabsorption syndrome are presented below including selected naturally occurring agents and agents of abuse that may be taken into the GI tract. The effects of synthetic drugs, biomolecules, and other xenobiotics on intestinal absorption and function are covered elsewhere in this text.

MALABSORPTION SYNDROME

Malabsorption syndrome is typically characterized by weight loss and steatorrhea that may occur from a number of conditions (see Table 11.4) that may be classified by mechanism or cause. Most of these conditions produce malabsorption of many or most nutrients but some conditions cause malabsorption of specific nutrients and may or may not produce malabsorption syndromes [49,53]. Some of these are listed in Table 11.5. Unless a condition is quite severe, in many cases the large amount of reserve capacity within the GI tract for nutrient absorption often

TABLE 11.4
Conditions That Cause Malabsorption Syndrome

Diseases of small intestinal wall	a-β-lipoproteinemia
	Blind-loop syndrome
	Celiac disease
	Gluten enteropathy
	Infiltrative disease-amyloid, lymphoma
	Intestinal lymphangiectasia
	Jejunal resection
	Small bowel ishmeia-athersclerosis vasculitis
	Myotonic dystrophy
	Celiac sprue
	Tropical sprue
	Whipple's disease
Drugs	Alcohol
	Cathartics
	Cholestyramine
	Clofibrate
	Colchicine
	Neomycin
	Phenindione
	P-aminosalicylate
Insufficient bile acid	Extrahepatic biliary obstruction
	Intestinal stasis syndromes
	Intrahepatic biliary obstruction
	Short bowel syndrome
Insufficient pancreatic enzyme activity	Chronic pancreatitis
	Cystic fibrosis
	Enterokinase deficiency
	Isolated lipase deficiency
	Pancreatic carcinoma
	Pancreatic resection
Conditions requiring further diagnosis or mechanism unknown	Adrenal insufficiency
	Crohn's disease
	Bacterial enteritis
	Food anaphylaxis
	Carcinoid
	Diabetes mellitus
	Irritable bowel syndrome
	Hyperthyroidism
	Immune deficiencies
	Mast cell disease
	Parasitic infections (i.e., giardiasis, cryptosporidiosis)

TABLE 11.4 (CONTINUED)
Conditions That Cause Malabsorption Syndrome

Multiple defects	Gastrin-secreting tumor
	Ileal dysfunction
	Radiation enteritis
	Scleroderma
	Steatorrhea following gastric surgery

TABLE 11.5
Conditions That Cause Malabsorption of Nutrients

Amino acid malabsorption	Cystinuria
	Hartnup's disease
	Methionine malabsorption
	Proline malabsorption
Folic acid malabsorption	Alcohol
	Dilantin
	Oral contraceptives
Monosaccharide malabsorption	Fructose malabsorption
	Glucose malabsorption
Primary disaccharidase deficiency	Acquired lactase deficiency
	Congenital lactase deficiency
	Congenital sucrase–isomaltase deficiency
Vitamin B_{12} malabsorption	Alcohol
	Congenital B_{12} malabsorption
	Pernicious anemia

may compensate to a substantial degree and normal health continues. This can make the selection and interpretation of various tests for the diagnosis of malabsorption difficult.

In general, the digestion and absorption of food materials can be divided into three major phases.

1. During the luminal phase, dietary fats, proteins, and carbohydrates are hydrolyzed and solubilized by secreted digestive enzymes and bile.
2. The mucosal phase relies on the integrity of the brush border membranes of intestinal epithelial cells to transport digested products from the lumen into the cells.
3. In the postabsorptive phase, reassembled lipids and other key nutrients are transported via lymphatics and portal circulation from epithelial cells to other parts of the body.

Perturbation by disease processes in any of these phases frequently results in malabsorption. Most patients with malabsorption experience diarrhea and weight loss with perhaps other symptoms such as weakness, amenorrhea, bone pain, tetany, a tendency for bruising or bleeding, sore mouth or tongue, or peripheral neuritis. Since conditions that could produce these symptoms and signs are numerous and may or may not involve malabsorption, macroscopic and microscopic stool examination is generally a part of any investigation of malabsorption.

The stool is examined for the presence of undigested material, particularly meat fibers, and the presence of fecal fat by counting lipid droplets in the stool and by using quantitative analysis procedures from a 72-hour stool collection when the patient has been ingesting 50 to 100 g of fat per day for at least 48 hours before initiating collection [54,55]. This test is commonly called the "stool fat test" and is based on the assumption that when secretions from the pancreas and liver are adequate, emulsified dietary fats are almost completely absorbed in the small intestine. When a malabsorption disorder or other cause disrupts this process, excretion of fat in the stool increases.

The test evaluates digestion of fats by determining excessive excretion of lipids in patients exhibiting signs of malabsorption, such as weight loss, abdominal distention, and scaly skin [54]. Reference values may vary from laboratory to laboratory, but are generally found within the range of 5 to 7 g/24 hours for a normal human. Measuring the difference between ingested fat and fecal fat and expressing that difference as a percentage results in a "fat retention coefficient." The coefficient is 95% or more in healthy children and adults. A low value is indicative of steatorrhea [55].

Increased fecal fat levels are found in cystic fibrosis, malabsorption secondary to other conditions like Whipple's disease or Crohn's disease, maldigestion secondary to pancreatic or bile duct obstruction, and "short gut" syndrome secondary to surgical resection, bypass, or congenital anomaly [56].

The management of patients with malabsorption addresses two principal factors: (1) the correction of nutritional deficiencies and (2) the treatment of causative disease if possible. With regard to nutritional deficiencies the following treatments are considered most important [56,57].

- Supplementation with essential vitamins and minerals such as calcium, magnesium, iron, and vitamins that may be deficient
- Caloric and protein replacement
- Administration of medium-chain triglycerides as fat substitutes as they do not require micelle formation for absorption and their transport is portal rather than lymphatic
- Parenteral nutrition in severe cases of intestinal disease

Treatment of causative disease may include the following as necessary:

- Consumption of a gluten-free diet to help correct celiac disease
- Consumption of a lactose-free diet to correct lactose intolerance

- Administration of protease and lipase supplements for pancreatic insufficiency
- Administration of antibiotics are the treatment for bacterial overgrowth
- Administration of corticosteroids and other anti-inflammatory agents to treat regional enteritis

OTHER TESTS FOR MALABSORPTION

Most available methods for measuring intestinal fat absorption have a common limitation in that the results depend on digestion as well as on absorption of the ingested lipid. These techniques have other practical disadvantages when applied to infants and children because they may require adjustment of the amount of fat consumed; because the test requires a few days to complete, loss of stool collection can be a problem. There is also considerable variability in the recommended dosage and in the interpretation of what constitutes abnormal response. Table 11.6 lists additional tests that may be useful in the investigation of malabsorption conditions. References are included to provide further information about how the tests were conducted.

CARBOHYDRATE MALABSORPTION SYNDROMES

Lactose malabsorption syndrome is due to a lack of lactase in the brush borders of the duodenum and jejunum. Individuals who have this condition — at least 50% of human adults — are lactose intolerant. Lactose intolerance is almost universal in oriental countries. To circumvent it, some lactose-intolerant individuals simply avoid using dairy products or take lactase pills along with dairy products and get along quite well. Some infants have rare congenital lactose intolerance. If they are fed a formula rich in sucrose or fructose, they do well [58].

Sucrose–isomaltase deficiency in the small intestine is an autosomal-recessive inherited disorder. Significant portions of the Eskimo population in Greenland have this type of deficiency. If placed on low sucrose diets, they show few problems. A glucose–galactose malabsorption syndrome arises from a defect in active transport for these monosaccharides, although fructose is well tolerated and can be substituted [59].

PROTEIN ENERGY MALNUTRITION

Protein energy malnutrition (PEM) is associated with atrophy of the gastric mucosa and pancreas and morphological changes in the intestine. Intestinal changes are not distinguishable from morphological and functional abnormalities termed "sprue" or tropical enteropathy. The highest prevalence of PEM is in tropical locations lacking adequate sanitation [60,61]. Clinically the intestinal changes may present as hypo- or achlorhydria, bacterial proliferation in the stomach and upper intestine, and malabsorption. Acute and chronic diarrhea and tropical enteropathy, often with colonization by enteric pathogens and subclinical malabsorption, are often superimposed on PEM.

TABLE 11.6

Other Tests Used to Investigate Malabsorption Conditions in Humans

Test	Basis	References
D-xylose test	Proximal intestine primarily absorbs D-xylose; documents integrity of intestinal mucosa	40
Small bowel biopsy	Direct histopathological evaluation	111
Fructose breath test	Detects fructose malabsorption as unabsorbed fructose that results in elevated hydrogen content in expired air from microbial degradation in colon	112, 113
Schilling test	Evaluates vitamin B_{12} absorption using radiolabelled B_{12}	114, 115
Double-contrast small bowel enteroclysis radiographic	Detects short gut, giant diverticula, fistulae, etc. via radiographic imaging	119, 120
Video capsule endoscopy	Detects small bowel Crohn's disease using capsule imaging technology; capable of detecting limited mucosal lesions	117, 118, 126
Magnetic resonance imaging (MRI)	Detects small bowel Crohn's disease using capsule imaging technology	117
CT scan of abdomen	Detects evidence of chronic pancreatitis; enlarged lymph nodes are seen in Whipple's disease and lymphoma; intussusception	120, 121
^{14}C-triolein breath test	Amount of label expired as $^{14}CO_2$	116
Endoscopic retrograde cholangiopancreatogram (ERCP):	Detects malabsorption due to pancreas or biliary-related disorders	122
Lactose/hydrogen breath test	Detects lactose malabsorption as unabsorbed lactose results in elevated hydrogen content in expired air	123, 124
^{14}C-Bile salt breath test	Determines integrity of bile salt metabolism	125
Upper GI endoscopy	Direct visual with biopsy for mucosal histopathological examination	126, 127, 128
Multidetector-row helical CT enteroclysis	Workup of patients with symptoms of intermittent small bowel obstruction, history of prior abdominal surgery for malignant tumor or radiation treatment	120

Malabsorption associated with acute, infectious diarrheas can result in the loss of 7% of yearly food energy; subclinical malabsorption nutrient losses in adults might equal 4 to 6% of yearly food energy. The consequences vary with the adequacy of nutrient intake and presence or absence of concurrent infection. Protein–energy interactions include: (1) at any given energy intake, increasing protein will improve nitrogen retention until physiologic needs for nitrogen balance are approached, (2) at any given protein intake, increasing energy will improve nitrogen retention, (3) the efficiency of nitrogen retention will parallel the degree of malnutrition, and (4) in the hypermetabolic phases of infection, there will be less nitrogen retention for any given energy and protein intake because of increased catabolism. Special attention should be given to situations in which caloric intake is normal while protein intake is inadequate. This has been associated with more marked intestinal morphological changes than when both protein and caloric intakes are decreased. Outcomes in investigations designed to assess nutritional needs in clinical or subclinical malabsorption should be evaluated under usual living conditions and dietary intake to avoid erroneous conclusions regarding prevalence or nutritional consequences.

WHIPPLE'S DISEASE

Whipple's disease is a rare infectious disease caused by a bacterium, *Tropheryma whippelii*. It can affect any system but occurs most often in the small intestine and interferes with the body's ability to absorb certain nutrients. Whipple's disease causes weight loss, incomplete break-down of carbohydrates or fats, and malfunctions of the immune system. Diagnosis is based on symptoms and the results of a biopsy of tissue from the small intestine or other organs that are affected. When recognized and treated with antibiotics, Whipple's disease can usually be cured. It may be fatal if untreated. Full recovery of the small intestine may take years and relapses are not uncommon [62].

CROHN'S DISEASE

Crohn's disease is an inflammatory bowel disease (IBD) that causes chronic inflammation of the intestinal tract. It is estimated that 500,000 Americans have this condition. It is similar to another common IBD, ulcerative colitis [63,64]. Crohn's disease and ulcerative colitis are often mistaken for one another. Both cause many of the same symptoms: diarrhea, abdominal pain and cramping, bloody stools, ulcers, reduced appetite, and weight loss. Crohn's disease begins with inflammation, most often in the lower part of the small intestine (ileum) or in the colon, but sometimes in the rectum, stomach, esophagus, or mouth. Unlike ulcerative colitis, in which inflammation occurs uniformly throughout an affected area, Crohn's disease can develop in several places simultaneously, with healthy tissue in between. In time, large ulcers that extend deep into the intestinal wall may develop in the inflamed areas.

A virus or bacterium may cause Crohn's disease and inflammation occurs when the immune system responds to the infection. The microorganism may also be more directly causal to the inflammatory response. *Mycobacterium avium* subspecies paratuberculosis (MAP), a bacterium that causes intestinal disease in cattle, has been suggested as a possible candidate because MAP is often isolated from the blood and intestinal tissue of patients with Crohn's disease, but only rarely in people with ulcerative colitis. It is also thought genetic susceptibility may trigger an abnormal response to the bacteria in some people, whereas it is also possible that the disease is caused by an abnormal immune response to bacteria present in the normal intestinal microflora. Approximately 20% of those with Crohn's disease have a parent, sibling, or child who also has the disease. Mutations in a gene, NOD2/CARD15, occur with significant frequency in people with Crohn's disease and appear to be associated with the early onset of symptoms and a high risk of relapse following surgery for the disease. Demographically, Crohn's disease occurs more often among people living in urban areas and in industrialized nations; therefore factors associated with such environments such as a diet high in fat or refined foods may also have some involvement [65].

AGING

As people age, gastric motility volume and acid content of gastric juice diminish. This causes hypochlorhydria (insufficient hydrochloric acid) and delayed gastric emptying. Intestinal absorption, motility, and blood flow decrease, impairing drug absorption, along with a proportionate decline in lean mass and blood volume. This results in higher serum drug levels in the elderly if not dosed appropriately [66–68].

Geriatric patients appear to be at increased risk for developing GI problems associated with the use of non-steroidal anti-inflammatory drugs (NSAIDs). It has been estimated that 3 to 4% of patients aged 60 or older using NSAIDs develop gastrointestinal bleeding, as compared with 1% of the general population [66,70,71].

EFFECTS OF TOXIC SUBSTANCES

Toxins

Various naturally occurring toxins can affect intestinal absorption. These toxins can be of microbial origin or from fungal, plant or animal sources. Diarrheal diseases caused by microorganisms and their toxins are major causes of mortality and morbidity throughout the world [75]. Acute diarrhea characterized by increased intestinal secretion is commonly a result of infection with enterotoxin producing organisms (enterotoxigenic *Escherichia coli*, *Vibrio cholera*, etc.) or due to decreased intestinal absorption from infection with organisms that damage the intestinal epithelium (enteropathogenic *E. coli* sp., *Shigella* sp., *Salmonella* sp.).

Most bacterial toxins exert their effects through involvement of ADP ribosylation proteins essential for several cellular functions, while other toxins involve guanylate cyclase systems or calcium and protein kinases for their ultimate actions. Many of these toxins are of microbial origin and play significant roles in enteral infectious disease outbreaks. For example, cholera toxin affects the human jejunum by reducing the absorption of water and electrolytes progressively and induces secretion in a dose-dependent fashion [71,75].

Shiga toxin (Stx)-producing *Escherichia coli* (STEC) colonizes the large intestine, causing a spectrum of disorders including watery diarrhea, bloody diarrhea (hemorrhagic colitis), and hemolytic–uremic syndrome [72]. Stx is a multimeric toxin composed of one A subunit and five B subunits. The Stx2 B subunit induces fluid accumulation independently of A subunit activity by altering the usual balance of intestinal absorption and secretion toward net secretion.

Clostridium perfringens type A produces a 35-kDa enterotoxin (CPE) that is an important cause of food poisoning, human non-foodborne GI disease, and some veterinary GI diseases. CPE action involves formation of complexes in mammalian plasma membranes. One such complex of approximately 155 kDa is responsible for plasma membrane permeability alterations that result in enterotoxin-treated mammalian cell death.

Such membrane permeability changes also damage the epithelium, allowing the enterotoxin to interact with the tight junction (TJ) protein occludin. CPE and occludin interact to form an approximately 200 kDa CPE complex and the internalization of occludin into the cytoplasm. Removal of occludin (and possibly other proteins) damages TJs and disrupts the normal paracellular permeability barrier of the intestinal epithelium and may contribute to CPE-induced diarrhea. Low CPE doses kill mammalian cells by inducing a classic apoptotic pathway involving mitochondrial membrane depolarization, cytochrome C release, and caspase 3/7 activation. High enterotoxin doses, however, induce oncosis, that is a proinflammatory event. CPE is a unique, multifunctional toxin with cytotoxic, TJ-damaging, and potentially significant proinflammatory action [73].

Botulism occurs from consumption or inhalation of preformed botulinum toxin or growth of *Clostridium botulinum* bacteria in the GI tract or within a wound. Growth of *C. botulinum* in the GI tract releases botulinum toxin that reaches the circulation. All forms of botulism cause progressive weakness, bulbar signs (blurred vision, diplopia, mydriasis, dysphagia, and dysarthria), and respiratory failure with normal sensation and mentation. Patients can recover normal muscle strength within weeks to months, but usually complain of fatigue for years [74].

Fungal toxins, such as amatoxins and orellanine, can cause severe organ damage in the human body. Amatoxins are bicyclic octapeptides occurring in some *Amanita*, *Galerina*, and *Lepiota* species. They induce deficient protein synthesis resulting in cell death and also may exert toxicity by inducing apoptosis. Target organs are the intestinal mucosa, liver, and kidneys.

Poisoning generally results in dehydration and electrolyte imbalance, liver necrosis, and possibly kidney damage. Amatoxins from *Amanita phalloides* and related species of mushrooms are associated with severe morbidity and high mortality. Circulating amatoxins can be detected in the sera of poisoned patients as long as 30 hours after ingestion. Toxic effects are particularly high in susceptible cells such as hepatocytes. The administration of cathartics, adsorbent agents, and gastroduodenal lavage are of value in preventing further absorption of toxins from the GI tract [76,77].

Recently, the number of blooms of algae that produce toxins has increased in frequency, intensity, and geographical distribution. Illnesses resulting from toxins from marine algae, fish, and shellfish contaminated with toxins may also be increasing. Scombrotoxic poisoning from toxins in the tissues of certain fish is currently the most common cause of food poisoning associated with the consumption of fish and shellfish. Poisoning results from the consumption of spoiled fish of the families Scomberesocidae or Scombridae — in particular tuna, mackerel, skipjack, and bonito — that naturally contain high levels of histidine. Incorrect storage of fish allows bacterial histidine decarboxylase to convert histidine to histamine. The ensuing symptoms are thought to result from the ingestion and GI absorption of large amounts of histamine [78,79].

Pharmaceuticals and Toxicants

Many pharmaceutical agents and toxic chemicals can affect intestinal absorption; to attempt to list or discuss them all is beyond the scope of this chapter and will be covered elsewhere in this text. Some are encountered unintentionally or by accident and the result is intoxication while others are employed pharmacologically to affect some form of localized intestinal effect or absorbed by any of the avenues of absorption discussed previously to systemically distribute and act therapeutically. Examples of agents that affect intestinal absorption significantly are listed below.

Acetazolamide — Inhibitor of carbonic anhydrase in intestinal epithelial cells involved with HCO_3^- production.

Belladonna (atropine) — Competitive antagonist of acetylcholine at muscarinic receptors; antisecretory agent; decreases GI motility.

Clonidine — -Adrenergic stimulating agent with antisecretory and antidiarrheal properties.

Domperidone — Blocks inhibitory effects of dopamine and increases GI motility.

Ezetimibe — Cholesterol absorption inhibitor that blocks the translocation of dietary and biliary cholesterol from the gastrointestinal lumen into the intracellular spaces of jejunal enterocytes [80].

Histamine-2 receptor antagonists (cimetidine, ranitidine, famotidine) — Reduce gastric acid output that may affect subsequent intestinal absorption processes.

Loperamide — Opioid receptor agonist; antisecretory agent that slows colonic motility.

Opiates — Antisecretory effects from relaxation of intestinal smooth muscle.

Ouabain — Inhibits the $Na^+–K^+–ATPase$ pumps of intestinal epithelial cells.

Prokinetic drugs (cisapride, metoclopramide, erythromycin, bethanechol) — Increase GI motility in selected portions of the GI tract or less selectively over the entire tract, depending on pharmacologic action and mechanism of the agent.

Proton pump inhibitors (lansoprazole, rabeprazole, esomeprazole, omeprazole) — Inhibit gastric acid secretion that may affect subsequent intestinal absorption and motility events.

Somatostatin — Regulatory peptide that inhibits the release of insulin and glucagon from the pancreas and exerts a general inhibitory effect on many other GI hormones including gastrin, gastric inhibitory peptide, cholecystokinin, secretin, vasoactive intestinal polypeptide, and motilin; hormonal action reduces exocrine secretions and slows digestion, decreases GI motility, and decreases absorption of nutrients.

EFFECTS OF NATURALLY OCCURRING STIMULANTS, DEPRESSANTS, AND SUBSTANCES OF ABUSE

Alcohol

Many alcohols can reach the intestinal tract either intentionally or unintentionally. Common alcohols include ethanol, isopropanol, and methanol. Ethanol (ethyl alcohol) can be used as a solvent, antiseptic, or beverage. Alcoholic beverages such as beer, wine, and distilled spirits all contain ethanol. It is the single most widely used drug in the world and therefore its effects on the digestive system have been studied extensively. It may cause decreased absorption of D-xylose, folic acid, and thiamin. In alcoholics, it may cause decreased absorption of essential nutrients such as vitamin B_{12} and methionine.

Ethyl alcohol is one of the most commonly abused drugs. Consumption averages 10 liters per person per year in the United States. Alcohol is distributed throughout the tissues of the body by means of water; therefore, major organs of the body such as the heart and the brain receive the same blood alcohol concentration. Alcohol is not digested; instead it is absorbed into the mucus linings of the digestive system. Rate of absorption differs, depending on different factors such as body size, sex, and concentration of alcohol. Alcohol dehydrogenase, the principal enzyme involved in the metabolism and detoxification of alcohol, is typically less abundant in women. Therefore some women may have less resistance to the effects of alcohol than most men.

Carbonated drinks contain carbon dioxide that appears to affect the gastrointestinal epithelium in a manner that results in a higher rate of alcohol absorption. Mucosal absorption begins within 10 minutes after the first sip of the beverage, and absorption is completed in the small intestine. The majority of absorption (80%) occurs in the small intestine because of its large surface area and concentration of villi and microvilli. More specifically, the duodenum and jejunum contain the largest surface areas and the ileum contains the least amount of surface area. Consumption of large quantities of alcohol may lead to impaired intestinal absorption of nutrients, vitamins, sodium, and water that may lead to diarrhea.

Additionally, alcoholics may be inhibited from absorbing other nutrients such as vitamin B_{12}, folic acid, thiamin, amino acids, calcium, and magnesium. The consumption of alcohol may also inhibit the absorption of some drugs such as cephalosporins, chlorpropamides, and sulfonamides. Metabolism of antihistamines, barbiturates, and narcotics may be slowed with alcohol intoxication.

Damage to the mucus of the digestive system due to alcohol consumption may lead to duodenal erosions and bleeding. It can also lead to greater permeability that may allow bacterial toxins to enter the blood from the digestive tract that can cause additional damage to digestive and other organs. Another consequence of excessive consumption of alcohol is the relaxation of the esophageal sphincter that deters gastric contents from damaging the esophageal mucus. Alcohol reduces the pressure of the esophageal sphincter leading to increased heartburn.

Alcoholics have more relaxed esophageal muscles and thus have greater increases in acid reflux and are more prone to esophageal tears due to vomiting. Membranes in the mouth may become irritated due to consumption of alcohol and eventually cause throat or mouth cancer. Consumption of alcohol has also been linked to increased risks of tumors in the pharynx, colon, mouth, stomach, and esophagus. Tumors may also develop in the GI tract due to free radicals such as preservatives and additives found in alcoholic beverages. The risk of developing these cancers may increase linearly with the addition of tobacco usage.

Low alcohol-containing beverages such as wine and beer, when consumed in small amounts, may contain substances that induce gastric motility. Higher quantities may delay gastric emptying and thus cause a feeling of fullness or nausea [81]. Appetite is increased with consumption of small quantities of alcohol because it stimulates the production of stomach juices; over time, appetite may become dulled, which can lead to malnutrition. An influx of gastric juices due to alcohol consumption may also lead to ulcers on the stomach lining.

The toxicity of isopropanol is almost twice that of ethanol. Symptoms of poisoning may include catatonia and ketonuria with the loss of metabolic acidosis. Methanol is generally considered nontoxic and can be found in items such as antifreeze, fuel, solvent, and paint remover.

Betel

It is common for people in countries of South and Southeast Asia to chew a combination of betel, areca nut, and tobacco packaged into "quids." Nuts of the Areca palm are wrapped in leaves and spread with lime paste to form small packets that can be inserted into the mouth. In some populations, tobacco may also be inserted. Betel chewing is the fourth most common habit in South Asia, behind smoking, alcohol, and caffeine usage. Some diseases that are linked to the use of betel chewing are oral submucous fibrosis, oral leukoplakias, and oral cavity, head, and neck cancers [82]. Betel chewing may lead to the development of esophageal cancer and may increase the carcinogenetic effects of smoking and alcohol.

Although the effects of betel on the development of cancer are well known, the effects of betel quids on vitamin D metabolism and calcium homeostasis in the GI tract are only now being studied. It is likely that this practice has other effects on intestinal motility and absorption that are worthy of study given the commonality of use in some parts of the world.

Caffeine

Caffeinated coffee stimulates colonic motor activity with a magnitude similar to that of a meal. It is 60% stronger than water and 23% stronger than decaffeinated coffee [83]. Coffee contains a multitude of substances, many of which are potentially biologically active, although the main physiologic effects resulting from consumption are usually ascribed to the presence of caffeine. Coffee is also an extremely rich source of chlorogenic acids (CGAs), an important group of biologically active dietary phenols, the best known of which is 5-caffeoylquinic acid (5-CQA).

The daily intake of CGA by coffee drinkers ranges from 0.5 to 1.0 g (3,6). Olthof et. al. [84] showed that 33% of a 2.8-mmol load of CGA was absorbed by ileostomy patients. Plasma glucose concentrations were significantly higher after consumption of caffeinated coffee than after consumption of a control beverage or decaffeinated coffee. Caffeine is an adenosine receptor antagonist [107] and inhibits muscular glucose uptake, even in the presence of insulin [108]. Moreover, Sharp and Debnam [106] showed that acute luminal exposure of GI cells to cAMP has stimulatory effects on sugar transport. The secretion of the GIP and GLP-1 hormones is significantly altered in response to the consumption of caffeinated beverages.

Cannabinoids

The human nervous system contains cannabinoid CB1 receptors that decrease the functions of the GI tract. CB1 receptors depress gastrointestinal motility by inhibiting ongoing contractile transmitter release. This results in a relaxation of the sphincters of the lower esophagus that in turn retards gastric emptying and inhibition of the transit of materials through the small intestine. The inhibitory effects of cannabinoid receptor agonists on gastric emptying and intestinal transit are mediated to some extent by CB1 receptors in the brain and by enteric CB1 receptors.

Acid production in the stomach is also inhibited by the activation of CB1 receptors. In clinical trials, marijuana was found to aid in colon functioning, intestinal dysfunction, and diarrhea. In the future, cannibinoids may be used to help treat gastrointestinal dysfunction, diarrhea, vomiting, nausea, colon cancer and inflammation of the bowels [85].

Evidence also indicates that cannabinoid receptor agonists can suppress increases in gastrointestinal activity precipitated by naloxone in morphine-dependent animals. Ä9-THC (but not cannabidiol) produces a dose-related blockade of naloxone-induced signs of heightened gastrointestinal activity (diarrhea and increased defecation) and other abstinence signs in morphine-dependent rats. These findings indicate that cannabinoids may have potential for the management of opioid withdrawal in human clinical settings [86].

Catechins

Recently, the benefit to metabolism from drinking green and black tea has been widely publicized. Green and black tea both originate from the leaves of *Camellia sinensis*. The leaves of tea plants contain large amounts of monomeric flavonoids called catechins. Green tea is made by inactivating the enzymes in the freshly picked leaves while black tea is produced from fresh green teas through a fermentation process. Tea catechins have been shown to reduce plasma cholesterol and suppress hypertriacylglycerolemia by reducing triglyceride absorption. However, the mechanism is not yet clear.

One of the possible mechanisms is that tea polyphenols may modify dietary fat emulsification in the GI tract. The digestive enzyme (lipase) acts on specific emulsion interface properties (droplet size and surface area). Therefore, changes in these properties may modify emulsification and lead to changes in dietary fat digestion and absorption. The effects of both green and black tea on changes of emulsification were examined *in vitro* by measuring droplet size and the surface area [87]. Using a model emulsion system containing olive oil, phosphatidylcholine (PC), and bile salt developed to simulate small intestinal conditions, initial changes in droplet size (from 1.4 to 52.8 μ and from 1.4 to 25.9 μ) of the emulsion were observed in the presence of 1.04 mg/mL and 0.10 mg/mL of total catechins prepared from green and black tea, respectively. Both teas caused similar changes of emulsion properties; however, black tea was more effective than green tea.

Flavonoids that are not absorbed in the small intestine are metabolized by the bacterial flora in the colon [97–99]. Colonic microorganisms mediate fission of the central C3 rings of catechins. This type of fission is decisive for the basic structure of the resulting metabolites, i.e., hydroxyphenyl-valerolactones and phenolic acids [98]. These metabolites are absorbed from the colon, and their urinary concentrations exceed that of the intact flavonoid [84,100–102]. In addition, dietary flavonoids may have significant effects on colonic flora [103] and thus confer a type of prebiotic effect.

It has been noted that drinking tea and also wine [102], cider [104], and coffee [84] can result in increases in urinary hippuric acid excretion, which indicates that polyphenols from different dietary sources may have similar effects on colonic flora. Green tea consumption and black tea consumption result in absorption of similar amounts of microbial degradation products by the body. These microbial metabolites, and not the native tea flavonoids, may be responsible for at least some of the health effects attributed to tea consumption. [105].

Cocaine

Historically, cocaine was utilized by Native Americans and other indigenous people because of its ability to suppress hunger and was taken orally by chewing on the leaves of the plant. Current data suggests a rise in the number of deaths attributed to cocaine by means of oral ingestion. A popular means of drug smuggling involves the swallowing of several balloons, condoms, or small vials containing cocaine. This practice is commonly termed "body packing" and is also used to smuggle other drugs of addiction such as cannabis and heroin. However, most research on the effects of body packing has been conducted on individuals who smuggle cocaine.

In the past, it was assumed that cocaine was harmless when ingested orally [88], but current studies have shown the opposite [89]. On occasion, a swallowed vessel may rupture in the stomach of a body packer and may cause severe complications of digestion and normal gastric functioning. Thirty minutes after ingestion, cocaine begins to be absorbed into the GI tract and becomes ionized due to the acid in the stomach. The cocaine may pass through the stomach, but it does not become appreciably absorbed until it reaches the more alkaline small intestine. After a ruptured package is discovered through x-ray or sonogram, an emergency surgical exploration may ensue or, in the absence of complications, the individual may be administered laxatives. Complications due to ingestion of cocaine may include status epilepticus, wide and narrow complex bradyarrhythmias, ventricular arrhythmias, and delayed hyperthermia [89].

Although the most common application of cocaine is through the nasal passage, a study conduced by van Dyke and colleagues [90] concluded that oral administration produced the quickest high (15 to 60 minutes) versus intranasal application (45 to 90 minutes). The highs experienced by users who chose intranasal application may be attributed to the passage of cocaine through the nasopharynx into the GI tract.

Nicotine

Smoking has been found to have both negative and positive consequences on the gastrointestinal system. Cigarette smoking presents a high risk factor for developing gastroduodenal ulcers and gastric carcinoma. Smoking may also tighten the gastric mucosa in smokers and is associated with a smaller increase of gastric permeability induced by alcohol [91].

Smokeless tobacco users consume a significantly larger amount of nicotine into the GI tract because they may swallow small amounts of tobacco juice. Most of the absorbed nicotine is converted to cotinine during first pass hepatic metabolism [92]. Smoking can have detrimental and beneficial effects on gastrointestinal disease — it has a polarizing effect in patients with Crohn's disease and ulcerative colitis. Studies of tobacco smokers have not clearly identified which agents are responsible for these effects, but research on the action of nicotine alone may help explain some of the positive and negative links between smoking and gastrointestinal disease [93].

Unlike cigarette smokers, spit tobacco (ST) users absorb significant amounts of nicotine through the GI tract while swallowing tobacco juice. This process potentially compromises the utility of cotinine as a biomarker for systemic nicotine exposure in ST users. To investigate this question, Ebert [92] correlated nicotine and cotinine concentrations with clinical measures of ST use in 68 daily ST users enrolled in a non-nicotine pharmacologic intervention trial. It was found that a higher frequency of swallowing tobacco juice (P = 0.007) was an independent predictor of higher serum cotinine concentrations. Serum nicotine concentrations, on the other hand, were not correlated with a higher frequency of swallowing. In the absence of a reliable way to measure frequency of swallowing, it was concluded that cotinine should not be used for guiding clinical decisions that depend upon a precise quantification of systemic nicotine exposure such as tailored nicotine replacement therapy.

Glycyrrhizic acid is widely applied as a sweetener in food products and chewing tobacco. In addition, it is of clinical interest for possible treatment of chronic hepatitis C. In some highly exposed subjects, side effects such as hypertension and symptoms associated with electrolyte disturbances have been reported. Glycyrrhizic acid is mainly absorbed after presystemic hydrolysis as glycyrrhetic acid.

Because glycyrrhetic acid is a 200 to 1000 times more potent inhibitor of 11-beta-hydroxysteroid dehydrogenase compared to glycyrrhizic acid, the kinetics of glycyrrhetic acid are relevant in a toxicological perspective. Once absorbed, glycyrrhetic acid is transported and taken into the liver by capacity-limited carriers, where it is metabolized into glucuronide and sulfate conjugates. These conjugates are transported efficiently into the bile. After outflow of the bile into the duodenum, the conjugates are hydrolyzed to glycyrrhetic acid by commensal bacteria; glycyrrhetic acid is subsequently reabsorbed, causing a pronounced delay in terminal plasma clearance.

Pharmacokinetic modeling shows that in humans the transit rate of gastrointestinal contents through the small and large intestines predominantly determines to what extent glycyrrhetic acid conjugates will be reabsorbed. Parameters that can be estimated noninvasively may serve as useful risk estimators for glycyrrhizic-acid-induced adverse effects because glycyrrhetic acid may accumulate after repeated intake in subjects with prolonged gastrointestinal transit times [94].

Clinical evaluation, upper gastrointestinal endoscopy, and electron microscopy of mucosal biopsies from the antrum, body, and fundus of stomach from control subjects and habitual tobacco chewers show marked differences. Electron microscopic abnormalities such as discontinuous fragmented basement membranes with reduction in hemidesmosomes and widened intercellular spaces filled with clusters of desmosomes were found in the gastric mucosa of habitual tobacco chewers; these were similar to those reported in experimental carcinogenesis and leukoplakia. It is concluded that habitual chewing of tobacco produces electron microscopic alterations in the human gastric mucosa that may be important precursors for gastric malignancy. [95].

Smoking cessation aids include nicotine patches, chewing gums, and lozenges. Nicotine lozenges have been available over the counter for over 15 years. Studies have found that they contain substantial amounts of nicotine and may provoke irritation in the GI tract that may result in vomiting [96].

Opium and Opioids

Opioid receptors in the GI tract mediate the effects of endogenous opioid peptides and exogenously administered opioid analgesics on a variety of physiological functions associated with motility, secretion, and visceral pain.

INTESTINAL ABSORPTION MODELING

Human intestinal absorption is an important roadblock in the formulation of new drug substances. In many cases obtaining direct information for evaluating the intestinal absorption of new candidate drug compounds is (1) time consuming due to the need for clinical study design and conduct, (2) expensive due to the cost of conducting clinical studies with several candidate compounds, or (3) potentially dangerous if a compound has not been well characterized toxicologically. For these reasons computational models are constantly developed and utilized for the rapid estimation and prediction of the human intestinal absorption of various substances and compounds.

Generally, the initial parameter estimates are determined via *in vivo* animal experiments or *in vitro* permeability studies. Currently, permeability through human Caco-2 cells is a method in common use. Several different methods are available for the development of predictive models and statistical quality is of importance in their selection and use [109]. As pharmaceutical and biotechnology companies strive to reduce the enormous costs and time required to bring new drugs to market, computational modeling methods have become important and necessary parts of drug discovery and development. These computational models range from simple spreadsheet routines to sophisticated supercomputer molecular dynamics models. Modeling procedures to predict human intestinal absorption generally have one or more of the following objectives.

- Rapid analysis and understanding of the behaviors of drug candidates in animals and humans
- Rapid ability to test hypotheses regarding formulation, changing physicochemical parameters, fasted and fed state effects, ionization effects on solubility and absorption
- Ability to quickly estimate the best dosing for toxicity studies in animals
- Ability to fit absorption and pharmacokinetic models to Phase I data in humans and use those models to determine optimum dosing for later phases

The ability of these models to predict human intestinal absorption depends on the quality of the input information but generally have the ability to predict absorption with 70 to 90% percent success on a qualitative basis using datasets from compounds that have known or subsequently determined human intestinal absorption data.

More than 100 computational packages are commercially available for the development of absorption models. Some are used more widely than others and some claim to be "validated." In quality control terms, this typically indicates that each keystroke has been checked and each module has been tested with a standard dataset and returned a computed value within acceptable numerical limits. One popular software package, GastroPlus™ (Simulations Plus, Inc., Lancaster, CA) is widely used as are packages designed to make building of physiologically based pharmacokinetic (PBPK) models for humans relatively simple by building in collections of human parameter data from the literature so that each model is built on a relatively similar set of initial physiological parameter estimates. Commercial software packages for PBPK model development include commercial turn-key packages such as PBPK Modeling™ (The Lifeline Group, Annandale, VA) and acslExtreme® (Aegis Technologies Inc., Huntsville, AL). Other computational methods employ various molecular structure-based approaches such as the topological substructural approach (TOPS-MODE) used by Pérez et al. [110].

These *in silico* methods of estimating human intestinal absorption of a variety of substances are rapidly gaining international popularity and the quality, quantity, and variety of information in databases available to develop these models is increasing such that modeling methods are becoming accepted and regular fixtures in many current pharmaceutical development projects.

SUMMARY

Intestinal absorption encompasses many highly significant and important processes in health and disease. As our understanding of normal intestinal function improves so will our ability to recognize and potentially treat or correct abnormal intestinal function. Advances in genomics, proteomics, computational modeling, and nanotechnology are certain to have major impacts toward advancing both our knowledge of human intestinal function and the quality of life of those with conditions involving abnormal intestinal function. The sciences of gastroenterology and toxicology will be important contributors to these advancements.

REFERENCES

1. Southgate DA. Nature and variability of human food consumption. *Philos Trans R Soc Lond B Biol Sci* 334: 281. 1991.
2. U.S. Department of Health and Human Services and U.S. Department of Agriculture, *Dietary Guidelines for Americans*. 2005.
3. Johnson LR. Regulation of gastrointestinal mucosal growth. *Physiol Rev* 68: 456. 1982.
4. Lo CW and Walker WA. Changes in the gastrointestinal tract during enteral and parenteral feeding. *Nutr Rev* 47: 193. 1989.
5. U.S. Department of Health and Human Services. *Surgeon General's Report on Nutrition and Health*. Publication 88-50210, Washington, D.C., 1988.

6. Toda N and Herman AG. Gastrointestinal function regulation by nitrergic efferent nerves. *Pharmacol Rev* 57: 315. 2005.

7. Go VLW. Role of gastrointestinal hormones in adaptation, in Halsted CH and Rucker RB, Eds., *Nutrition and Origins of Disease: Bristol-Myers Nutrition Symposia*. Academic Press, New York, 1989, p. 321.

8. Little TJ et al. The release of GLP-1 and ghrelin, but not GIP and CCK, by glucose is dependent upon the length of small intestine exposed. *Am J Physiol Endocrinol Metab.* May 9, 2006.

9. Holst JJ. Glucagon-like peptide-1: from extract to agent. *Diabetologia.* 49: 253. 2006.

10. Rehfeld JF. Clinical endocrinology and metabolism: cholecystokinin. *Best Pract Res Clin Endocrinol Metab* 18: 569. 2004.

11. Rozengurt E, Guha S, and Sinnett-Smith J. Gastrointestinal peptide signalling in health and disease. *Eur J Surg Suppl* 587: 23. 2002.

12. Owyang C. Physiological mechanisms of cholecystokinin action on pancreatic secretion. *Am J Physiol.* 271 (Pt 1), GL1. 1996.

13. Liddle RA, Goldfine ID, and Williams JA. Bioassay of plasma cholecystokinin in rats: effects of food, trypsin inhibitor, and alcohol. *Gastroenterology* 87: 542. 1984.

14. Sabb JE, Godfrey PM, and Brannon PM. Adaptive response of rat pancreatic lipase to dietary fat: effects of amount and type of fat. *J Nutr* 116: 892. 1986.

15. Leeds AR. Dietary fibre: mechanisms of action. *Int J Obes* 11 (Suppl 1): 3. 1987.

16. Schneeman BO. Macronutrient absorption, in Kritchevsky D et al., Eds., *Dietary Fiber.* Plenum Press, New York, 1990. p. 157.

17. Cummings JH. Effect of dietary fiber on fecal weight and composition, in Spiller GA, Ed., *Handbook of Dietary Fiber in Human Nutrition.* CRC Press, Boca Raton, FL. 1986. p. 211.

18. Cohn JS. Postprandial lipid metabolism. *Curr Opin Lipidol* 5: 185. 1994.

19. Cohn JS, Lam CWK, Sullivan DR, and Hensley WJ. Plasma lipoprotein distribution of apolipoprotein (a) in fed and fasted states. *Atherosclerosis* 90: 59. 1991.

20. Cohn JS et al. Role of triglyceride-rich lipoproteins from the liver and intestine in the etiology of postprandial peaks in plasma triglyceride concentration. *Metabolism* 38: 484. 1989.

21. Madara JL. Functional morphology of epithelium of small intestine, in Field M et al., Eds., *Handbook of Physiology.* American Physiological Society, Bethesda, MD, 1991, chap. 3.

22. Corazza GR, Caletti G, Brocchi E, and Gasbarrini G. Duodenal folds in celiac disease. *Gastroenterology* 95: 1518. 1988.

23. Hendrix TR and Bayless TM. Digestion: intestinal secretion. *Annu Rev Physiol* 32: 139. 1970.

24. Reuss L. One hundred years of inquiry: the mechanism of glucose absorption in the intestine. *Annu Rev Physiol* 62: 939. 2000.

25. Bray GA and Greenway FL. Pharmacological approaches to treating the obese patient. *Clin Endocrinol Metab* 5: 455. 1976.

26. Henry C et al. Cellular uptake and efflux of trans-piceid and its aglycone trans-resveratrol on the apical membrane of human intestinal Caco-2 cells. *J Agric Food Chem* 9: 798. 2005.

27. Leturque A et al. The role of GLUT2 in dietary sugar handling. *J Physiol Biochem* 61: 529. 2005.

28. Shayeghi M et al. Identification of an intestinal heme transporter. *Cell* 122: 789. 2005.

29. Li T, Ghishan FK, and Bai L. Molecular physiology of vesicular glutamate transporters in the digestive system. *World J Gastroenterol* 11: 1731. 2005.

30. Buddington RK and Diamond JM. Ontogenetic development of intestinal nutrient transporters. *Annu Rev Physiol* 51: 601. 1989.

31. Dawson DC. Gastrointestinal physiology: molecular basis of GI transport. *Annu Rev Physiol* 55: 571. 1993.

32. Malo C. Multiple pathways for amino acid transport in brush border membrane vesicles isolated from the human fetal small intestine. *Gastroenterology* 100: 1644. 1991.

33. Ruhl A et al. Functional expression of the peptide transporter PEPT2 in the mammalian enteric nervous system. *J Comp Neurol* 12: 490. 2005.

34. Anderson CM et al. H$^+$/amino acid transporter 1 (PAT1) is the amino acid carrier: an intestinal nutrient/drug transporter in human and rat. *Gastroenterology* 127: 1410. 2004.

35. Meng Q et al. Regulation of amino acid arginine transport by lipopolysaccharide and nitric oxide in intestinal epithelial IEC-6 cells. *J Gastrointest Surg* 9: 1276. 2005.

36. Fraga S, Serrao MP, and Soares-da Silva P. L-type amino acid transporters in two intestinal epithelial cell lines function as exchangers with neutral amino acids. *J Nutr* 132: 733. 2002.

37. Ganong WF, Ed. *Review of Medical Physiology*, 7th ed., Lange Medical Publishers, Los Altos, CA.1975.

38. Wuerges J et al. Structural basis for mammalian vitamin B$_{12}$ transport by transcobalamin. *Proc Natl Acad Sci USA* 103: 4386. 2006.

39. Lambers TT, Bindels RJ, and Hoenderop JG. Coordinated control of renal Ca^{2+} handling. *Kidney Int* 69: 650. 2006.

40. Bronner F. Mechanisms of intestinal calcium absorption. *J Cell Biochem* 88: 387. 2003.

41. Simovich M et al. Localization of the iron transport proteins mobilferrin and DMT-1 in the duodenum: the surprising role of mucin. *Am J Hematol* 74: 32. 2003.

42. Sharp P. The molecular basis of copper and iron interactions. *Proc Nutr Soc* 63: 563. 2004.

43. Schweigel M and Martens H. Magnesium transport in the gastrointestinal tract. *Front Biosci* 5: D666. 2000.

44. Mazariegos M et al. Zinc absorption in Guatemalan schoolchildren fed normal or low-phytate maize. *Am J Clin Nutr* 83: 59. 2006.

45. Said HM and Mohammed ZM. Intestinal absorption of water-soluble vitamins: an update. *Curr Opin Gastroenterol* 22: 140. 2006.

46. Bronner F. Calcium absorption: paraadigm for mineral absorption. *J Nutr* 128: 917. 1998.

47. Christenson HN. Regulation of amino acid and sugar absorption by diet. *Nutr Rev* 42: 237. 1984.

48. Gray GM. Dietary protein processing: intraluminal and enterocyte surface events, in Field M and Frizzell BA, Eds., *Handbook of Physiology*, American Physiological Society, Bethesda, MD, 1991.

49. VanDyke RW. Mechanisms of digestion and absorption of food, in Sleisenger MH and Fordtran H, Eds., *Gastrointestinal Disease*, 4th ed., W.B. Saunders, Philadelphia, 1991.

50. Krebs NF. Overview of zinc absorption and excretion in the human gastrointestinal tract. *J Nutr* 130: 1374S. 2000.

51. Miret S, Simpson RJ, and McKie AT. Physiology and molecular biology of iron absorption. *Annu Rev Nutr* 23: 283. 2003.

52. Wessling-Resnick M. Iron transport. *Annu Rev Nutr* 20: 129. 2000.

53. Weser E. Intestinal adaptation to parenteral nutrition, in Halsted C. and Rucker RB, Eds., *Nutrition and Origins of Disease: Bristol-Myers Nutrition Symposia.* Academic Press, New York. 1989, p. 343.

54. Cahill M. *Handbook of Diagnostic Tests.* Springhouse Corporation, Springhouse, PA. 1995.

55. Pagana KD. *Mosby's Manual of Diagnostic and Laboratory Tests.* Mosby, St. Louis. 1998.

56. Parekh N, Seidner D, and Steiger E. Managing short bowel syndrome: making the most of what the patient still has. *Cleveland Clin J Med* 72: 833. 2005.

57. Thomas PD et al. Guidelines for the investigation of chronic diarrhoea. *Gut* 52 (Suppl 5): 1. 2003.

58. Montalto M et al. Management and treatment of lactose malabsorption. *World J Gastroenterol* 12: 187. 2006.

59. McNair A, Gudmand-Hoyer E, Jarnum S, and Orrild L. Sucrose malabsorption in Greenland. *Br Med J* 2: 19. 1972.

60. Nath SK. Tropical sprue. *Curr Gastroenterol Rep* 7: 343. 2005.

61. Westergaard H. Tropical sprue. *Curr Treat Opt Gastroenterol* 7: 7. 2004.

62. Monkemuller K, Fry LC, Rickes S, and Malfertheiner P. Whipple's disease. *Curr Infect Dis Rep* 8: 96. 2006.

63. Ahmed FE. Role of genes, the environment and their interactions in the etiology of inflammatory bowel diseases. *Expert Rev Mol Diagn* 6: 345. 2006.

64. Domenech E. Inflammatory bowel disease: current therapeutic options. *Digestion* 73 (Suppl 1): 67. 2006.

65. Ekbom A, Helmick C, Zack M, and Adami HO. The epidemiology of inflammatory bowel disease: a large, population-based study in Sweden. *Gastroenterology* 100: 350. 1991.

66. Turnheim K. When drug therapy gets old: pharmacokinetics and pharmacodynamics in the elderly. *Exp Gerontol* 8: 843. 2003.

67. Holt PR. Diarrhea and malabsorption in the elderly. *Gastroenterol Clin North Am* 30: 427. 2001.

68. Holt PR. Gastrointestinal diseases in the elderly. *Curr Opin Clin Nutr Metab Care* 6: 41. 2003.

69. Pilotto A. Aging and upper gastrointestinal disorders. *Best Pract Res Clin Gastroenterol* 18: 73. 2004.

70. Greenwald DA. Aging, the gastrointestinal tract, and risk of acid-related disease. *Am J Med.* 117: 8S. 2004.

71. Petritsch W et al. Effect of cholera toxin on the human jejunum. *Gut* 33: 1174. 1992.

72. Creydt VP et al. The Shiga toxin 2 B subunit inhibits net fluid absorption in human colon and elicits fluid accumulation in rat colon loops. *Braz J Med Biol Res* 37: 799. 2004.

73. McClane BA and Chakrabarti G. New insights into the cytotoxic mechanisms of *Clostridium perfringens* enterotoxin. *Anaerobe* 10: 107. 2004.

74. Davis LE. Botulism. *Curr Treat Opt Neurol* 5: 23. 2003.

75. Kaur T and Ganguly NK. Modulation of gut physiology through enteric toxins. *Mol Cell Biochem* 253: 15. 2003.

76. Vesconi S et al. Therapy of cytotoxic mushroom intoxication. *Crit Care Med* 13: 402. 1985.

77. Karlson-Stiber C and Persson H. Cytotoxic fungi: overview. *Toxicon* 42: 339. 2003.

78. Brett MM. Food poisoning associated with biotoxins in fish and shellfish. *Curr Opin Infect Dis* 16: 461. 2003.

79. McLauchlin J, Little CL, Grant KA, and Mithani V. Scombrotoxic fish poisoning. *J Pub Health (Oxf)* 28: 61. 2006.

80. Toth PP and Davidson MH. Cholesterol absorption blockade with ezetimibe. *Curr Drug Targets Cardiovasc Haematol Disord* 5: 455. 2005.

81. Pfeiffer A, Holgl B, and Kaess H. Effect of ethanol and commonly ingested alcoholic beverages on gastric emptying and gastrointestinal transit. *Clin Invest* 70: 487. 1992.

82. Mazahir, S et al. Socio-demographic correlates of betel, areca and smokeless tobacco use as a high risk behavior for head and neck cancers in a squatter settlement of Karachi, Pakistan. *Subs. Abuse Treat Prev Policy* 1: 10. 2006.

83. Rao SS et al. Is coffee a colonic stimulant? *Eur J Gastroenterol Hepatol* 10: 113. 1998.

84. Olthof MR et al. Chlorogenic acid, quercetin-3-rutinoside and black tea phenols are extensively metabolized in humans. *J Nutr* 133: 1806. 2003.

85. Izzo AA and Coutts AA. Cannabinoids and the digestive tract. *Hanb Exp Pharmacol* 168: 573. 2005.

86. Pertwee RG. Cannabinoids and the gastrointestinal tract. *Gut* 48: 859. 2005.

87. Mulder TP, Rietveld AG, and van Amelsvoort JM. Consumption of both black tea and green tea results in an increase in the excretion of hippuric acid into urine. *Am J Clin Nutr* 81: 256S. 2005.

88. Ashley R. *Cocaine: Its History, Uses and Effects.* St. Martin's Press, New York, 1975, p. 150.

89. Tanen DA, Graeme KA, and Curry SC. Crack cocaine ingestion with prolonged toxicity requiring electrical pacing. *J Toxicol Clin Toxicol* 38: 653. 2000.

90. van Dyke et al. Oral cocaine: plasma concentrations and central effects. *Science* 200: 211. 1978.

91. Gotteland M et al. Effect of acute cigarette smoking, alone or with alcohol, on gastric barrier function in healthy volunteers. *Dig Liver Dis* 34: 702. 2002.

92. Ebbert JO. Cotinine as a biomarker of systemic nicotine exposure in spit tobacco users. *Addictive Behav* 29: 349. 2004.

93. Thomas GA, Rhodes J, and Ingram JR. Mechanisms of disease: nicotine: a review of its actions in the context of gastrointestinal disease. *Nat Clin Pract Gasteoenterol Hepatol* 2: 536. 2005.

94. Ploeger B et al. A population physiologically based pharmacokinetic/pharmacodynamic model for the inhibition of 11-beta-hydroxysteroid dehydrogenase activity by glycyrrhetic acid. *Toxicol Appl Pharmacol* 170: 46. 2001.

95. Shankaran K et al. Electron microscopic observations in gastric mucosa of habitual tobacco chewers. *Indian J Med Res* 99: 267. 1994.

96. Foulds J et al. Nicotine absorption and dependence in unlicensed lozenges available over the counter. *Addiction* 93: 1427. 1998.

97. Meselhy MR, Nakamura N, and Hattori M. Biotransformation of epicatechin 3-*O*-gallate by human intestinal bacteria. *Chem. Pharm. Bull (Tokyo)* 45: 888. 1997.

98. Hollman PC and Katan MB. Absorption, metabolism and bioavailability of flavonoids, in *Flavonoids in Health and Disease,* Rice-Evans C et al., Eds. Marcel Dekker, New York, 1997.

99. Meng X, Sang S, and Zhu N. Identification and characterization of methylated and ring-fission metabolites of tea catechins formed in humans, mice, and rats. *Chem Res Toxicol* 15: 1042. 2002.

100. Li C et al. Structural identification of two metabolites of catechins and their kinetics in human urine and blood after tea ingestion. *Chem Res Toxicol* 13: 177. 2000.

101. Rechner AR et al. The metabolism of dietary polyphenols and the relevance to circulating levels of conjugated metabolites. *Free Radic Res* 36: 1229. 2002.

102. Gonthier MP et al. Microbial aromatic acid metabolites formed in the gut account for a major fraction of the polyphenols excreted in urine of rats fed red wine polyphenols. *J Nutr* 133: 461. 2003.

103. Hara H et. al. Effect of tea polyphenols on fecal flora and fecal metabolic products of pigs. *J Vet Med Sci* 57: 45. 1995.

104. DuPont MS et al. Polyphenols from alcoholic apple cider are absorbed, metabolized and excreted by humans. *J Nutr* 132: 172. 2002.

105. Mulder TP et al. Analysis of tea flavins in biological fluids using liquid chromatography–electrospray mass spectrometry. *J Chromatogr B Biomed Sci Appl* 760: 271. 2002.

106. Sharp PA and Debnam ES. The effect of rapid changes in plasma sugar concentration on the brush border potential difference in rat jejunum. *Exp Physiol* 79: 415. 1994.

107. Leblanc J and Soucy J. Hormonal dose-response to an adenosine receptor agonist. *Can J Physiol Pharmacol* 72: 113. 1993.

108. Vergauwen L et al. Adenosine receptors mediate synergistic stimulation of glucose uptake and transport by insulin and by contractions in rat skeletal muscle. *J Clin Invest* 93: 974. 1994.

109. Subramanian G and Kitchen DB. Computational approaches for modeling human intestinal absorption and permeability. *J Mol Model* (online). April 1, 2006.

110. Pérez MA ct al. A topological sub-structural approach for predicting human intestinal absorption of drugs *Eur J Med Chem* 39: 905. 2004.

111. Sempoux C. Role of the pathologist in the differential diagnosis of malabsorption. *Acta Gastroenterol Belg* 69: 49. 2006.

112. Nucera G et al. Abnormal breath tests to lactose, fructose and sorbitol in irritable bowel syndrome may be explained by small intestinal bacterial overgrowth. *Aliment Pharmacol Ther* 21: 1391. 2005.

113. Romagnuolo J, Schiller D, and Bailey RJ. Using breath tests wisely in a gastroenterology practice: an evidence-based review of indications and pitfalls in interpretation. *Am J Gastroenterol* 97: 1113. 2002.

114. Adams JF and Seaton DA. Reproducibility and reliability of the Schilling test. *J Lab Clin Med* 58: 67. 1961.

115. Ward PC. Modern approaches to the investigation of vitamin B^{12} deficiency. *Clin Lab Med* 22: 435. 2002.

116. Mylvaganam K, Hudson PR, Herring A, and Williams CP. 14C triolein breath test: an assessment in the elderly. *Gut* 30: 1082. 1989.

117. Albert JG et al. Diagnosis of small bowel Crohn's disease: a prospective comparison of capsule endoscopy with magnetic resonance imaging and fluoroscopic enteroclysis. *Gut* 54: 1721. 2005.

118. Eisen GM. The economics of PillCam. *Gastrointest Endosc Clin N Am* 16: 337. 2006.

119. La Seta F et al. Radiology and adult celiac disease: current indications of small bowel barium examinations. *Radiol Med* (Torino) 108: 515. 2004.

120. Maglinte DD et al. Multidetector row helical CT enteroclysis. *Radiol Clin North Am* 41: 249. 2003.

121. Gayer G et al. Intussusception in adults: CT diagnosis. *Clin Radiol* 53: 53. 1998.

122. Epstein RJ et al. Role of ERCP in the diagnosis of pancreatic malignancy presenting as steatorrhea. *Gastrointest Endosc* 26: 98. 1980.

123. Pimentel M, Kong Y, and Park S. Breath testing to evaluate lactose intolerance in irritable bowel syndrome correlates with lactulose testing and may not reflect true lactose malabsorption. *Am J Gastroenterol* 98: 2700. 2003.

124. Casellas F and Malagelada JR. Applicability of short hydrogen breath test for screening of lactose malabsorption. *Dig Dis Sci* 48: 1333. 2003.

125. Hellemans J et al. Positive 14CO2 bile acid breath test in elderly people. *Age Ageing* 13: 138. 1984.

126. Kesari A, Bobba RK, and Arsura EL. Video capsule endoscopy and celiac disease. *Gastrointest Endosc* 62: 796. 2005.

127. Sundar N, Mukhtar A, and Finnie IA. Ileocolonoscopic diagnosis of coeliac disease. *Endoscopy* 35: 374. 2003.

128. Olds G et al. Celiac disease for the endoscopist. *Gastrointest Endosc* 56: 407. 2002.

12 Intestinal Absorption and Metabolism of Xenobiotics in Humans

William J. Brock and David W. Hobson

CONTENTS

INTRODUCTION

In previous chapters to this text, gastrointestinal (GI) absorption and metabolism of xenobiotics in animals were reviewed, as were normal and abnormal intestinal functions in humans. Those chapters described the various physiological and biochemical mechanisms of absorption, including factors that influence xenobiotic absorption. In the original work to this series, Hoensch and Schwenk (1984) extensively reviewed the biochemical and cellular processes of absorption and metabolism of agents and described in detail the factors that influenced gastrointestinal absorption and metabolism of xenobiotics. It is quite clear that the processes are essentially the same for animals and humans although quantitative and qualitative differences of absorption are expected.

Because the earlier work of this series addressed the fundamental concepts of absorption, and this topic is very well described in textbooks of toxicology (Klaassen, 2001; Hayes, 2001), these concepts will not be discussed in too much detail. Furthermore, readers are urged to review the prior chapters on gastrointestinal anatomy and physiology and the processes involved in absorption and the text book of Yamada (2004). In the current chapter, we will briefly review the absorption of agents, primarily pharmaceutics, and the biochemical and physiological factors that modulate gastrointestinal absorption and metabolism in humans.

HUMAN INTESTINAL TRACT

The intestine can absorb vast quantities of fluid from the intestinal lumen to maintain normal homeostasis. More than 98% is absorbed to preserve health, with a majority of the fluid secreted rather than ingested. The balance between absorptive and secretory functions is a highly regulated process that is disrupted by disease states or conditions that can result in excessive fluid secretion. Under certain conditions, the secretory function can exceed the absorptive function, leading to diarrhea and loss of fluid. An extreme example has been noted in cholera patients, where fluid loss can be up to 20 L per day (Montrose, et al., 2003).

Over decades of study, the scientific understanding of the intestinal tract has seen dramatic advances. We have gained new appreciation of the molecular transport and the regulatory and structural proteins involved in normal absorption and malabsorption of nutrients and xenobiotics. Through advances in biochemistry, we have identified various protein transporters and how these transporters interact with secondary messenger pathways and with the cytoskeleton to allow the intestinal epithelium to respond to changes in the extracellular environment.

In the stomach, gastric juice contains a variety of substances, e.g., ions, enzymes, etc. and about 2500 mL are secreted daily. The hydrochloric acid secreted by the gastric tissue kills ingested bacteria, provides the necessary pH for pepsin to start protein digestion, and stimulates bile flow. The mucosal cells of the stomach secrete HCO_3^- to maintain pH gradients of 1 to 2 at the luminal side and 6 to 7 at the surfaces of the epithelial cells.

The previous chapter covered normal and abnormal intestinal absorption in humans and provided a review of human intestinal functions and malabsorption syndromes. The differential pH ranges of the human GI tract cited in the previous chapter should be consulted for an appreciation of the overall ranges involved and the regional nature of the pH gradients along the human GI tract, both of which are important issues for understanding the forms in which pH-sensitive substances are absorbed.

Lui et al. (1986) examined differences in stomach pH levels of humans and dogs because dogs are often used to examine absorption pharmacokinetics. In this investigation, pH was continuously recorded through the use of Heidelberg capsules that transmit data through a radio frequency transmitter. Gastric pH was significantly higher in dogs compared to humans, although gastric emptying time was similar (Table 12.1). The intestinal pH of the dogs was also greater.

The authors suggested that the differences between dogs and humans related to differences in gastric secretion and pancreatic bicarbonate secretion, with gastric secretion lower in dogs and pancreatic secretion higher in humans. Hence, it would be expected that dogs would have higher gastric and intestinal pH levels. The implications of this difference could be that xenobiotic absorption may differ. However, the time–pH profiles for dogs and humans tend to be similar such that absorption of compounds would not significantly differ. Clearly, where the pKa values of poorly soluble drugs fall within the range of pH 5 to 8, there may be discrepancies in absorption between dogs and humans. The purest specimens of parietal cell secretion that have been obtained contain approximately 0.17 N HCl, with pH as low as 0.87 (Montrose et al., 2003). The pH of the cytoplasm of the parietal cells, like that of other cells, is 7.0 to 7.2.

Acid secretion is stimulated by histamine (H_2 receptors) and by acetylcholine (M_3 muscarinic receptors). The H_2 receptors increase intracellular cAMP, and the muscarinic receptors and the gastrin receptors exert their effects by increasing

---

TABLE 12.1
Gastric pH and Emptying Time in Dogs and Humans[a]

Measure	Dog	Human
Gastric pH	1.8 ± 0.07	1.1 ± 0.15
Gastric emptying time (min)	99.8 ± 27.2	59.7 ± 14.8
Intestinal pH	7.3 ± 0.09	6.0 ± 0.05

[a] Values = mean ± standard deviation.

Source: From Lui, C.Y. et al., *J. Pharmaecut. Sci.* 75: 271, 1986.

intracellular free Ca^{2+}. Gastrin also acts by stimulating the secretion of histamine from enterochromaffin-like (ECL) cells, vesicle- and granule-containing cells that are the predominant endocrine cell type in the acid-secreting portion of the stomach.

The presence of food in the mouth reflexively stimulates gastric secretion. Vagal nerve stimulation increases in gastric secretion. In humans, for example, the sight, smell, and thought of food increase gastric secretion, a Pavlovian response. Food in the stomach accelerates the increase in gastric secretion produced by the sight and smell of food and the presence of food in the mouth. Although gastrin-containing cells are present in the small intestine and stomach, instillation of amino acids directly into the duodenum does not increase circulating gastrin levels (Montrose, et al., 2003). Fats, carbohydrates, and acid in the duodenum inhibit gastric acid and pepsin secretion and gastric motility. Gastric acid secretion increases with surgical removal of large parts of the small intestine and tends to be proportionate in degree to the amount of intestine removed.

The rate at which the stomach empties into the duodenum depends on the type of food ingested. Food rich in carbohydrates leaves the stomach in a few hours. Protein-rich food leaves more slowly, and emptying is slowest after a meal containing fat. The rate of emptying also depends on the osmotic pressure of the material entering the duodenum. Since fats are particularly effective in inhibiting gastric emptying, some people drink milk, cream, or even olive oil before a cocktail party. The fat delays intestinal transport from the stomach where its absorption is slower. Hence alcohol enters the small intestine more slowly so that — theoretically, at least — a sudden rise of blood alcohol to a high level and consequent embarrassing intoxication are avoided. Fraser (1997) suggested that alcohol interacts with drugs and foods, delaying absorption and gastric emptying time. Therefore, it remains uncertain whether foods affect alcohol transit time or alcohol affects food transit time.

BIOPHARMACEUTIC CLASSIFICATION SYSTEM AND HUMAN DRUG ABSORPTION

In 1995, Amidon et al. devised a biopharmaceutics classification system (BCS) to classify drugs based on their aqueous solubility and intestinal permeability. The authors suggested that dissolution rate has a negligible impact on bioavailability of highly soluble and highly permeable (BCS Class I) drugs when the dissolution of a drug is sufficiently rapid (Kaus, et al., 1999). As a result, various regulatory agencies including the Food and Drug Administration (FDA) now allow bioequivalence waivers of formulations of BCS Class I drugs to be demonstrated by *in vitro* dissolution (often called a biowaiver). Definitive BCS classification is done when a potential Class I candidate enters human testing with classification according to methods outlined in the FDA guidance (2000; Table 12.2). For instance, solubility is determined at pH 1.2 and 7.5 and also at pH approximating the pKa (pKa – 1, pKa, and pKa + 1) of the agent.

TABLE 12.2
Biopharmaceutical Classification System

Biopharmaceutical Classification	Description	Examples
Class 1	High solubility, high permeability	Chlorpheniramine, cloxacillin
Class 2	Low solubility, high permeability	Clofazimine, gibenclamide
Class 3	High solubility, low permeability	Hydralizaine, methotrexate
Class 4	Low solubility, low permeability	Teophylline, trimethoprim

Sources: Food and Drug Administration, Guidance for Industry, etc., 2000; Amidon, G.L. et al., *Pharmaceut. Res.* 12: 413, 1995.

Kasim et al. (2004) undertook an analysis of approximately 260 oral immediate release drugs and compared the BCS classifications of these drugs based on partition coefficient (log P or CLogP) or dose number.* For a majority of the drugs examined, BCS classification was the same. About 67% of the drugs were classified as "high solubility" drugs.

For classification of drugs, preference is often given to data developed from clinical or preclinical studies with a preference given to data developed from renal excretion data in human studies or a human mass balance study with radiolabeled material. Human absolute bioavailability studies and preclinical permeability studies using rat intestinal perfusion or Caco-2 cells are also considered for classification. For immediate release dosage forms, a product is considered to be a rapidly dissolved substance when not less than 85% of a labeled amount of the substance dissolves within 30 min in acidic media (0.1 N HCl or simulated gastric media), pH 4.5 media, and pH 6.8 media or simulated intestinal fluid without enzymes.

Class 1 substances are well absorbed; the rate limiting step for absorption is dissolution of the agent. For immediate release dosage forms, i.e., those formulations that dissolve very quickly, gastric emptying time becomes rate limiting for absorption. Drug dissolution is the rate limiting step for the absorption of formulations that are Class 2 drugs. In this case, the *in vivo* dissolution profile will be a determinant for blood concentrations. Amidon et al. (1995) proposed that the dissolution profile should be determined over time and for at least 85% dissolution at several different pH values. This proposal has been incorporated into the FDA guidance (2000). For Class 3 drugs, absorption is limiting, and drugs of this class show large variations in permeability.

Monographs for several pharmaceuticals have been published in the open literature with an eye toward obtaining biowaivers from conducting *in vitro* or *in vivo* bioequivalence and bioavailability studies (Yu et al., 2002; Blume and Schug,

---

* Dose number (Do) was calculated as the highest dose strength divided by a predetermined volume (250 mL) and the result divided by the solubility. CLogP is an estimate of gastrointestinal permeability. (see Kasim et al., 2004).

1999; Kortejarvi et al., 2005). Without waivers, pharmaceutical companies would be mandated to undertake *in vivo* bioavailability and bioequivalence testing for newly formulated generic drugs or re-formulations of existing patented drugs. Such testing could have considerable cost ramifications. Class 4 drugs are difficult to formulate for oral dosage forms.

In vivo differences in the rate and extent of absorption of two equivalent solid oral products may be due to differences in drug dissolution. When the *in vivo* dissolution of a solid oral dosage form is rapid in relation to gastric emptying time, the drug has high permeability and the rate and extent of drug absorption are unlikely to be dependent on dissolution and/or gastrointestinal transit time. Under such circumstances, the FDA suggests that demonstrations of *in vivo* bioavailability or bioequivalence may not be necessary for products containing Class 1 substances. The BCS approach outlined by the FDA may be used to justify biowaivers for highly soluble and highly permeable drug substances (Class 1 agents) for immediate release, solid oral dosage forms.

A drug substance is considered highly soluble when the highest dose strength is soluble in 250 mL or less of aqueous media over a pH range of 1 to 7.5. The permeability class boundary is based on the fraction of dose absorbed in humans and on the rate of mass transfer across human intestinal membrane. A drug substance is considered highly permeable when the extent of absorption in humans is determined to be 90% or more of an administered dose based on a mass balance determination or in comparison to an intravenous reference dose. A drug substance is considered rapidly dissolving if 85% or more of the labeled amount dissolves within 30 min.

Lennernas (1998) examined several methods used to predicting human intestinal permeability. The authors suggested a good correlation exists between the measured human effective permeability values and the extent of absorption of drugs in clinical pharmacokinetic studies. Estimations of the absorption half-lives from the measured effective intestinal permeability (P_{eff}) agreed very well with the time to maximal amount of the dose absorbed. Human *in vivo* permeability can be predicted using preclinical permeability models such as *in situ* perfusion of rat jejunum, the Caco-2 model, and excised intestinal segments.

Prediction of passively transported compounds can be accurately predicted although evaluation of agents absorbed by carrier-mediated transport mechanisms requires a special degree of caution (Lennernas, 1998; Lennernas, 1997). Clearly, additional research is needed to further characterize the influence of active transport mechanisms, e.g., multidrug resistance transporters, and intestinal metabolism, e.g., Cytochrome P4503A4, on drug bioavailability observed with anti-cancer agents (Schellens et al., 2000).

XENOBIOTIC ABSORPTION

A xenobiotic, for the purposes of this chapter, is a natural or synthetic chemical substance that is foreign to the body — in other words, a chemical that is not a natural component of the organism exposed to it which in this case is a human.

With respect to intestinal absorption and metabolism, xenobiotics essentially must be (1) absorbed intact or unchanged, (2) combined or bound with some other substance that facilitates or enhances intestinal absorption by co-transport, (3) metabolized, then absorbed as some metabolite or metabolites, or (4) absorbed intact, then metabolized before the metabolites are absorbed into the blood or lymphatics.

In humans, as in most higher mammals and primates that have well developed intestinal tracts, a variety of means ranging from simple diffusion to energy-requiring, carrier-mediated transport systems (see Chapter 11) allow nutrients to be absorbed in the GI tract. These same absorption processes and transport systems are available to xenobiotics and, in general, the better the chemical similarity of a xenobiotic to the nutrient chemicals normally absorbed, the greater the likelihood of absorption.

Most absorption takes place in the first 1 to 2 m of the small intestine, the proximal region. This portion of the intestine contains gastric secretions, bile acids, and pancreatic secretions and for this reason has a relatively wide pH range. Absorption may occur all along the intestinal tract as well as the colon and, given the different conditions of regional pH as well as emulsifier, enzymatic, and microbial contents and the degree of motility, xenobiotic absorption occurs over a wide range of conditions. Most chemicals, nutrients, and xenobiotics absorbed in the GI tract are first transported to the liver, because all blood vessels surrounding the GI tract lead to the portal vein to the liver.

PRINCIPAL ROUTES OF XENOBIOTIC ABSORPTION

Diffusion

Permeation of xenobiotics across biological membranes occurs primarily by diffusion, with absorption into systemic circulation dependent on the concentration gradients across the gastrointestinal epithelium. Small molecules of molecular weight below 600 are readily absorbed across the epithelia through aqueous pores within the membrane, whereas larger molecules are absorbed across the gastrointestinal epithelium based primarily on the physiochemical properties of the agent, e.g., hydrophobicity. The degree of gastrointestinal absorption tends to increase with an increase in hydrophobicity. Estimation of absorption has historically been associated with an assessment of the octanol:water partition coefficient, Log P, and is the equilibrium ratio of the solute concentrations in the two solvents (see Chapter 10).

Active Transport

Although most xenobiotics will be absorbed across the gastrointestinal epithelium by simple diffusion, a number of compounds including many nutrients are absorbed via active transport mechanisms. Active transport is the movement of a molecule across a membrane, driven by energy in the form of expenditure of ATP and against a concentration gradient. In addition, specific proteins facilitate transport so that even large molecules can be moved across the membrane. Active transport results in greater concentrations of compounds within cells. Indeed, active transport of compounds into cells becomes particularly important when structurally related toxicants, e.g., 5-fluorouracil compete with a nutrient, for example, for the transporter protein. This competition can be used for therapeutic benefits.

In the last decade or more, a great deal of research has been reported on various protein transporters. Several gastrointestinal protein transporters have been identified. The multidrug-resistant protein (mdr) was one of the first family of protein transporters identified and was found to transport chemotherapeutic agents out of gastrointestinal cells and cells of other organs. Other gastrointestinal transporters that have been identified include nucleotide (nt), divalent-metal ion (dmt), and peptide (pept) transporters.

Filtration

Transport of molecules with molecular weights below 200 is carried through by the hydrostatic forces of water; this phenomenon is known as solvent drag (Blanchard, 1975). Although filtration is more common in the kidneys, it can occur to a limited extent in the gastrointestinal tract, e.g., calcium absorption.

Facilitated Diffusion

Facilitated diffusion is a carrier-mediated process of absorption similar to active transport. However, absorption does not occur against a concentration gradient, thereby distinguishing this process from active transport. The transport of glucose into the cell occurs with the Na^+–K^+ pump that generates a Na^+ gradient across the cell membrane. The glucose–Na^+ symport protein uses that Na^+ gradient to transport glucose into the cell.

Pinocytosis

Cells have the ability to transport macromolecules (proteins, polysaccharides, polynucleotides) to their interiors through endocytosis — a broad term that includes phagocytosis and pinocytosis. Phagocytosis is the process of enveloping a particle by modifying its membrane to form a phagosome around the particle. Phagosomes are then pulled by cytoskeleton motion of the cytosol into one or more lysosomes for digestion of the particles.

In contrast, pinocytosis transports liquid substances into cells. Pockets occur in a given area of a cell membrane, capturing the liquid and forming vesicles that are then pulled by cytoskeleton motion into the cytoplasm. Pinocytosis may be selective or non-selective. Selective pinocytosis occurs in two stages. The liquid substance adheres initially to membrane receptors and then the substance is transferred to vesicles that leave the membrane surface and transport their content to the cytoplasm. In non-selective pinocytosis, the vesicles envelop all the solutes eventually present in the extracellular fluid. Absorption of nutrient biomolecules occurs via this route, and various particles, e.g., cadmium, ferretin, are absorbed via the mechanism.

Properties of a xenobiotic also are significant factors determining whether absorption will occur and if so, where in the intestinal tract absorption is most likely. Examples of such factors include:

- Ability to withstand the harsh pH conditions of the stomach
- Physical properties of the xenobiotic: molecular structure, molecular size, ionization potential (pKa or pKb)
- Membrane solubility characteristics: hydrophilic, lipophilic

PARTITION THEORY

No discourse on the absorption of xenobiotics from the human intestine would be complete without a discussion of pH partitioning in the GI tract. To cross a membrane barrier, a drug must normally be soluble in the lipid material of the membrane; to enter and exit the membrane, it must be soluble in the aqueous phase. Many drugs have polar and nonpolar characteristics or are weak acids or bases. For drugs that are weak acids or bases, the pKa of the drug, the pH of the GI tract fluid, and the pH of the bloodstream will control the solubility of the drug and thereby the rate of absorption through the membranes lining the GI tract.

In general, it is recognized that non-ionized molecules can diffuse or be more readily absorbed across the lipophilic membrane surfaces of the GI tract than ionized xenobiotics, particularly those that are highly ionized. Xenobiotics that are prone to ionization typically have acid or base ionization or dissociation constants, pK_a or pK_b values, respectively, that can be determined experimentally. The pK_a of a xenobiotic can be defined as the pH at which the xenobiotic is 50% ionized, when $pK_a - pH = 0$; then the xenobiotic is 50% ionized and 50% non-ionized. Similarly, if $pK_a - pH = 0.5$, the solution is 24% ionized and 76% non-ionized. If $pKa - pH > 3$ then the solution is $\leq 0.1\%$ ionized. A useful relationship to calculate the percent ionization of a xenobiotic at any of the different pH levels that may be encountered in the human intestinal tract is as follows.

$$\frac{100}{1 + 10^x(pH - pK_a)}$$

where $x = -1$ for an acid drug and 1 for a basic drug. This relationship is based on the familiar Henderson–Hasselbalch chemistry equation:

$$pH = pKa + \log_{10} [A^-]/[HA]$$

or

$$pH = pKa \log_{10} ([base]/[acid])$$

that relates pH and pKa in terms of the log, base 10, proportions for a weak acid [HA] and its conjugate base [A⁻]. Hasselbalch originally used this relationship in his studies of metabolic acidosis 90 years ago but since then it has found more widespread use in toxicology and pharmacology in describing the membrane absorption characteristics of ionized substances including xenobiotics under different pH conditions such as are found in the stomach and intestinal lumen of the GI tract. Because the pH of the human GI tract including the intestines is variable along its length, this relationship is of value in predicting regions of the GI tract where a substance is most likely to be non-ionized and hence more readily absorbed (Henderson, 1908; Hasselbalch, 1916; de Levie, 2003). Most xenobiotics that can ionize represent either a weak acid or a weak base. For any weak acid–weak base conjugate pair and their respective ionization constants in aqueous solution:

$$Ka + Kb = Kw \quad \text{or} \quad pKa + pKa = pKw = 14$$

Weak acids are absorbed mainly in the stomach because they are present in non-ionized forms whereas weak bases are absorbed mainly in the intestine because of their non-ionized forms.

Brodie and colleagues (Shore, et al. 1957; Hogben et al. 1959) further developed the above relationships for application to the absorption of pharmaceuticals and proposed the pH partition theory to explain the influence of GI pH and drug pKa on the extent of drug transfer or absorption. Brodie and colleagues reasoned an ionized drug will not be able to get through the lipid membrane, but it can do so only when it is non-ionized and therefore has higher lipid solubility. They proposed the following general drug partition relationship that has since become known as "Brodie's D value."

$$D = \text{total concentration in blood/total concentration in GI tract}$$

stated in terms of ionized [I] and nonionized [U] drug in the blood (b) and GI (g) compartments where the ratio [U]/[I] is a function of the pH of the solution and the pKa of the drug, and can be estimated by the Henderson–Hasselbalch relationship as:

$$\log_{10} [I]/[U] = pKa - pH$$

When the pKa of the xenobiotic is known as are the pH values for the blood and region of the GI tract of interest, the relationship below can be used to estimate D values:

$$D = [U]_b + [I]_b/[U]_g + [U]_g$$

Originally Brodie determined D values experimentally and then reasoned that it should be possible to calculate a theoretical value if it is assumed that only non-ionized drug crosses the membrane and that net transfer of the drug stops when $[U]_b = [U]_g$. The result was that Brodie found an excellent correlation between the calculated D value and the experimentally determined values and that the calculation and use of D values are useful means of describing the relative concentration of ionized substances including xenobiotics in the GI tract and the blood. Table 12.3 shows a range of dissociation constants for various xenobiotics and calculated D values for the stomach (pH 2) and the intestine in the proximal region (pH 6.8) at a blood pH of 7.4. Note that due to the relative differential between the intestinal and blood pH values, the relative magnitude of the D value, even under the most favorable pKa or pKb conditions, is lower than the D values for the greater pH differential between the pH of the stomach and the blood. Even when absorption is favorable in the stomach for xenobiotics with low pKa values, the relative surface area for absorption is far less than that of the intestine such that conditions for greatest absorption can still be favorable even when D < 1 and are most favorable when D ≥ 1.

FACTORS AFFECTING GI ABSORPTION OF XENOBIOTICS

Even when the chemical and biochemical conditions for absorption of a xenobiotic are favorable, some general factors can affect the amount of absorption of any xenobiotic. Some of the principal factors are:

Gastric emptying time — Less time in the stomach means more time in the small intestine. Obstructions in the GI tract can affect gastric emptying time as can a number of other factors including gastric bypass surgery sometimes used as a treatment for morbid obesity.

Intestinal motility — Increased GI motility may facilitate absorption by more thoroughly mixing GI contents and bringing more toxicant in contact with mucosa. Decreased GI motility gives a toxicant more time to be absorbed.

Mucosal sloughing damage — Sloughing of the mucosal cells lining the intestines can be caused by toxic actions of a xenobiotic, ionizing radiation, and physical damage. Removal and scarring of this lining can result in poor absorption of xenobiotics and nutrients.

Diarrhea — This condition effectively dilutes and increases motility and can result in lowered absorption of a xenobiotic or absorption along a larger length of intestine than usual.

Disease — Malabsorption syndrome, gamma radiation, and toxic substances can all affect the GI tract in ways that can reduce xenobiotic absorption, especially if the condition causes mucosal sloughing and diarrhea as noted above.

Food — Generally, the presence of food reduces toxicant absorption. Certain xenobiotics can complex with Ca^{2+} ions in food or milk, leading to a reduction in absorption.

Splanchnic blood flow — This flow increases during eating and generally increases the rate of absorption of many substances including some xenobiotics.

Metabolism — Xenobiotics may be inactivated or activated toxicologically by GI enzymes or stomach acid before they are absorbed. GI microflora may also

TABLE 12.3
Xenobiotics with Different pKa or pKb Values and Estimated D Values[a]

Xenobiotic	Ionization Value	D Value (Stomach)	D Value (Intestine)
Acetamizin	pKa = 4.0	2490	3.98
Acetylsalicyclic acid	pKa = 3.49	7870	3.98
Aniline	pKa = 4.6	630	3.96
Atropine	pKb = 4.35	0.000004	0.252
Barbital	pKa = 7.8	1.4	1.27
Caffeine	pKb = 10.4 , 13.4	0.0245, 0.962	1, 1
Codeine	pKb = 5.8	0.00000461	0.28
Diclofenac	pKa = 4.5	793	3.97
Ephedrine	pKa = 9.6	1.01	1
Erythromycin	pKb = 5.2	0.00000414	0.259
Fentiazac	pKa = 3.6	6160	3.98
Hydromorphone HCl	pKa = 8.1	1.2	1.14
Ibuprofen	pKa = 5.2	159	3.91
Indomethacin	pKa = 4.5	793	3.97
Ketoprofen	pKa = 4.6	630	3.96
Morphine	pKb = 6.13	0.00000533	0.31
Penicillin V	pKa = 2.73	39400	3.98
Pilocarpine	pKb = 7.2, 12.7	0.0000198, 0.834	0.626, 1
Quinine	pKb = 6.0, 9.89	0.00000498, 0.00771	0.296, 0.998
Salicyclic acid	pKa = 2.97	24300	3.98
Sulfathiazole	pKa = 7.12	2.91	1.96
Tetracycline	pKa = 3.3, 7.68, 9.69	12000, 1.52, 1.01	3.98, 1.35,
Thiopental	pKa = 7.6	1.63	1.41
Tolbutamide	pKb = 8.7	0.000505	0.977
Tolmetin	pKa = 3.5	7700	3.98
Secobarbital	pKa = 7.9	1.32	1.22
Thiopental	pKa = 7.6	1.63	1.41

[a] pKa and pKb values at 25°C in water.

Sources: From Schanker, L.S., in *Fundamentals of Drug Metabolism and Drug Distribution*, Williams & Wilkins, Baltimore, 1971; Martin A., *Physical Pharmacy*, 4th ed., Lea & Febiger, Philadelphia, 1993; and Martinez-Pla, J.J. et al., http:www.biochempress;.com, 2003.

metabolize xenobiotics. Depending on the resulting metabolites, these actions would most likely improve absorption of the metabolite whether it is still potentially toxic or not. It is also possible that certain metabolic actions can hasten elimination, particularly those associated with the microbial flora in the lower GI tract.

Other Factors

Non-steroidal anti-inflammatory drugs (NSAIDs) — These drugs are associated with more adverse gastrointestinal effects than any other drug class. Roughly 20% of hospital admissions for bleeding ulcers in patients older than 60 years of age are the results of NSAID usage. In this population, death from upper GI bleeding is four times more likely in NSAID users than in non-users. Larger studies demonstrate similar findings in that the elderly have higher incidences of gastrointestinal hemorrhages, perforations, and fatalities as a result of NSAID therapy.

Thiefin and Beaugerie (2005) reviewed the effects of NSAIDs on the GI tract and found that the gastrointestinal toxicity of conventional NSAIDs is not confined to the stomach and proximal duodenum but extends to the rest of the small bowel, colon, and rectum. Long-term NSAID therapy usually induces clinically silent enteropathy characterized by increased intestinal permeability and inflammation. At the colon and rectum, NSAID use can result in *de novo* lesions such as non-specific colitis and rectitis, ulcers, and diaphragm-like strictures. In patients with diverticular disease, NSAID use increases the risk of severe diverticular infection and perforation. NSAIDs can trigger exacerbations of ulcerative colitis or Crohn's disease. With selective COX-2 inhibitors, the risk of gastrointestinal toxicity is reduced as compared to conventional NSAIDs but is not completely eliminated. Experimental studies suggest that long-term COX-2 inhibitor therapy may cause damage to a previously healthy small bowel. Similar to conventional NSAIDs, COX-2 inhibitors may be capable of triggering exacerbations of inflammatory bowel disease.

Erythromycin — Doses of 200 mg over 30 mins administered intravenously to mechanically ventilated patents increased indices of antral motility, accelerated gastric emptying, and altered the kinetics of acetaminophen absorption (Dive et al., 1995).

Wood creosote — This compound has been used as a gastrointestinal microbicide. However Ataka et al. (2005) found that the oral amounts usually administered were not sufficient to produce intraluminal antimicrobial activity. Wood creosote does apparently inhibit intestinal secretion induced by enterotoxins by blocking the Cl⁻ channel on the intestinal epithelium and also decreases intestinal motility accelerated by mechanical, chemical, or electrical stimulus by the inhibition of the Ca^{2+} influx into the smooth muscle cells. The antimotility and antisecretory effects of wood creosote are compared with those of loperamide.

Microbial effects — There are many examples of intestinal mucosal colonization by microbes leading to damage that allows increased penetration of xenobiotics in animal studies. In humans, it is known that impairment of blood flow and changes in gastric mucosa associated with *Campylobacter pylori* gastritis may predispose the elderly to NSAID-induced gastric damage (Gyires, 1994). Mucosal barrier defects in patients with irritable bowel syndrome also may allow the passage of luminal antigens of dietary and bacterial origin that then elicit the activation of mucosal immune responses involved in the generation of diarrhea (Barbara, 2006).

Radiation damage — It is well known from animal studies and human exposure studies that sufficient doses of ionizing radiation to the gastrointestinal tissues can result in damage to the intestinal mucosa termed gastrointestinal syndrome. This condition will surely affect the absorption of xenobiotics and nutrients and is a recognized concern when treating carcinoma patients with radiation in the vicinity of the GI tract (Lantz et al., 1984).

Penetration enhancers — The addition of substances to formulations can enhance the penetration of drugs through the intestinal wall. For example, gastrointestinal absorption of heparin is enhanced by lipidization or co-administration with penetration enhancers such as deoxycholic acid (Ross et al., 2005). It is therefore feasible that membrane penetration enhancers may also affect xenobiotic absorption.

Cellular efflux pump effects — Cellular efflux pumps such as P-glycoprotein (P-gp), serve as natural defense mechanisms and also influence the bioavailability and disposition of drugs and other xenobiotics. Efflux transporters in the intestine can hinder drug absorption. P-gp is a plasma membrane-bound drug efflux protein found primarily in drug-eliminating organs and presumably functions as a detoxifying transporter because it actively extrudes xenobiotics from the body (Ambudkar et al., 1999). In the small intestine, P-gp has been localized to the apical membranes of intestinal epithelial cells (Thiebaut et al., 1987), consistent with a role in effluxing compounds back into the intestinal lumen. Pharmacokinetic studies of paclitaxel, digoxin, and cyclosporine A (CsA) in knockout mice revealed the importance of intestinal P-gp in limiting the oral bioavailability of these drugs (Schinkel et al., 1995; Sparreboom et al., 1997).

In humans, intestinal P-gp contributes to the variability in the pharmacokinetic properties of CsA (Lown et al., 1997) and tacrolimus (Hashida et al., 2001; Fukatsu et al., 2001) in organ transplant patients. There is also evidence that these systems can be upregulated by environmental xenobiotics. Lecoeur et al (2006) analyzed the ability of diazinon to act as an efflux modulator in human Caco-2 cells and concluded that following repeated oral exposure, diazinon increased P-gp expression and activity. This suggests the involvement of P-gp in the transfer of diazinon that may lead to potential consequences for xenobiotic interactions.

XENOBIOTIC METABOLISM

There are many ways that xenobiotics can be metabolized before, during, and after intestinal absorption. For the sake of clarity, two different types of metabolism will be discussed with respect to intestinal metabolism: (1) intraluminal metabolism, referring to processes occurring inside the GI tract, and (2) extraluminal tissue metabolism, referring to processes occurring in the membranes and walls of the GI tract. Once absorbed into the portal blood and/or lymphatics, other forms of xenobiotic metabolism may occur. These will not be discussed here and are addressed in other volumes on hepatic drug metabolism and lymphatic function.

INTRALUMINAL METABOLISM

Inside the GI tract, a variety of enzyme systems are present and naturally act on food substances to prepare them for absorption. Much of this action is directed toward digestion and dissolution of food and nutrients in preparation for intestinal absorption. However some enzymes and processes in the intestinal lumen also metabolize xenobiotics and can make them either more or less prone to absorption. These may originate from normally secreted luminal substances or can be microbial.

The microbial flora within the human intestinal tract is particularly rich and contains species capable of xenobiotic metabolism and biotransformation (Zoetandal et al., 2006; Vaughan et al., 2002). The potential roles that various microbes may play in the metabolism, biotransformation (detoxification and toxification), and absorption of xenobiotics in humans have yet to be elucidated and further study is needed.

Humblot et al. (2005), for example, showed that 2-amino-3-methylimidazo [4,5-f] quinoline (IQ), a mutagenic/carcinogenic compound formed from meat and fish during cooking, may be biotransformed by human intestinal bacteria in addition to liver xenobiotic-metabolizing enzymes.

Animal studies indicate that flavonols are subjected to microbial metabolism in the porcine hindgut and that the glycosidic structure strongly influences the rate of metabolism (Cermak et al., 2006). This evidence suggests that intraluminal metabolism of flavonols also is likely to occur in humans.

EXTRALUMINAL TISSUE AND CELLULAR METABOLISM

Although we typically think of the liver as the principal site of xenobiotic metabolism of the digestive tract, the intestine also has the ability to metabolize some xenobiotics. Beginning with the gastrointestinal epithelium, metabolism is possible from the moment of absorption and both Phase I and Phase II metabolism reactions can occur. Cytochrome P450 metabolism is perhaps the most significant of the Phase I reactions that involve xenobiotics.

Phase I Drug Metabolism in Human Intestine

Cytochromes

Microsomal fractions can be prepared from the intestine just as they are prepared from the liver. The intestine in general possesses the same mechanisms of Phase I drug metabolism found in the liver, but the relative proportions are different: the N-oxide formation was predominant, followed by N-demethylation and hydroxylation.

Intestinal drug metabolism by cytochrome P450 3A (CYP3A) is increasingly recognized as an important determinant in limiting drug bioavailability (Cummins et al., 2002). CYP3A4 is the most prominent oxidative cytochrome P450 enzyme present in the human intestine (Wrighton et al., 1987; Voice et al., 1999) where it is localized to the columnar epithelial cells lining the intestinal lumen (Kolars et al., 1994). Despite the lower CYP3A4 content in the intestine relative to the liver, first pass metabolism in the intestine by CYP3A has conclusively been shown to be important in the disposition of midazolam (Paine et al., 1996) and cyclosporin (Kolars et al., 1991) in studies of anhepatic patients. Grapefruit juice that naturally contains grapefruit oil and two furanocoumarin constituents that are suicide inhibitors of intestinal CYP3A (Schmiedlin-Ren et al., 1997) were shown to be related to significant increases in the oral bioavailability of many CYP3A4 substrates including felodipine (Edgar et al., 1992).

Interestingly, most substrates of CYP3A4 are also substrates of P-gp, demonstrating the mutually broad selectivity of these proteins (Wacher et al., 1995). Co-induction of CYP3A and P-gp by rifampin was shown in human LS180 colon carcinoma cells (Schuetz et al., 1996) and human intestine (Kolars et al., 1992; Greiner et al., 1999). It appears that the nuclear receptor SXR/PXR, which can activate both CYP3A4 and P-gp, has species specific patterns of induction (Lehmann et al., 1998; LeCluyse, 2001; Synold et al., 2001).

The considerable overlap in substrate selectivity, tissue localization, and co-inducibility of CYP3A4 and P-gp led to the hypothesis that these two proteins work together to coordinate an absorption barrier against xenobiotics (Wacher et al., 1998; Zhang and Benet, 2001). In the enterocyte, the spatial separation of P-gp (located on the apical plasma membrane) and CYP3A4 (located on the endoplasmic reticulum) supports the idea that P-gp may control the access of drugs to intracellular metabolism by CYP3A4. Drugs absorbed into the intestinal epithelium can interact with P-gp and be actively extruded back into the intestinal lumen. If this process of diffusion and active transport occurred repeatedly, the circulation of the drug from the lumen to the intracellular compartment would potentially prolong the intracellular residence time of the drug, decrease the rate of absorption, and result in increased drug metabolism by CYP3A4 relative to the parent drug crossing the intestine (Ito et al., 1999; Hochman et al., 2000).

Epoxide hydrolase

Epoxide hydrolase (EH) is both cytosolic and peroxisomal in human hepatocytes and renal proximal tubules. In the human intestinal epithelium, it is exclusively cytosolic (Enayetallah et al., 2006).

Transglutamases

Transglutamases (TGs) are ubiquitous enzymes that have many functions. They are able to transform proteins by deamidation and/or transamidation that can crosslink proteins together (Malandain, 2005). Intestinal tissue TGs play an important role in immune reactions to wheat: celiac disease and wheat-dependent exercise-induced anaphylaxis. It therefore seems possible that some xenobiotics having amidated gluten or similar structural moieties may also be metabolized in similar fashion.

Phase II Metabolism in Human Intestine

Phase II metabolism, i.e., conjugation reactions, occurs to a large extent in the liver although there is a limited ability for these reactions to occur in GI cells. Multiple polymorphisms of the glucuronosytransferase (UGT) enzyme family have been demonstrated and various forms of UGT1 and UGT2 have been identified in the GI tract (Tukey et al., 2001). The best studies of polymorphisms involve UGT1A1, the enzyme responsible for bilirubin conjugation.

Some liver UGTs do not appear to be expressed in the digestive tract (e.g., UGT2B4). Some UGTs are expressed in the intestine but not in the liver (e.g., UGT1A8). The UGTs have been found primarily in the gastric tissue and the upper intestine, e.g., duodenum, but have also been identified in the lower GI tract (Tukey et al., 2001). The implications of UGT polymorphisms in drug metabolism are generally unknown although polymorphism in UGT1A6 may influence susceptibility to, for example, acetaminophen liver toxicity.

The glutathione transferase (GST) enzymes involved in liver and intestinal drug metabolism are cytosolic enzymes belonging to eight separate gene families and function primarily to detoxify electrophilic-reactive species (Hayes and Strange, 2000). The complements of GSTs present in liver and intestine are not identical. Some GSTs have greater activity in the intestine than in the liver, e.g., GSTA4, although most exert more activity in the liver. Children appear to have higher levels of intestinal GST1A1 activity, and this has been proposed as the basis for an increased dosing requirement of busulfan in young children (Gibbs, et al., 1999).

Bile contains millimolar concentrations of glutathione, and it is believed that this serves to prevent intestinal cells from becoming depleted of substrate for GSTs (Eberle et al., 1981). A recent study by Samiec et al. (2000) indicates that GSTs may exist outside enterocytes and within the overlying mucus. Polymorphisms in GSTs are common, and GSTM1 and GSTT1 are absent in 40% and 15% of whites, respectively (Hayes and Strange, 2000). Because depletion of hepatic cellular glutathione enhances susceptibility to the toxicity of electrophilic metabolites, polymorphisms or depletion of gastrointestinal GSTs may contribute also to susceptibility to certain types of drug-induced disease.

Cytosolic sulfotransferases also are polymorphic and are divided into five gene families. The human intestine expresses these enzymes (Nagata and Yamazoe, 2000) with catalytic activity showing considerable variation among individuals. Hepatic sulfotransferases are inducible, but induction of intestinal sulfotransferases has not been identified.

ENTEROHEPATIC CIRCULATION

Metabolism of most xenobiotics entering the portal blood after being absorbed from the intestines typically occurs in the liver; however, determinants of the bioavailability of xenobiotics are the degree of intestinal absorption and the hepatic first pass effect. As discussed above, xenobiotics must overcome several membrane barriers with various arrays of specialized transport proteins for xenobiotic uptake or efflux before reaching the systemic circulation. One of these, the P-glycoprotein MDR1 (multidrug resistance gene product, ABCB1) is expressed at the apical surfaces of enterocytes, where it mediates the efflux of xenobiotics into the intestinal lumen before they access the portal circulation. Increased expression of MDR1 reduces the bioavailability of MDR1 substrates such as digoxin, cyclosporin, and taxol.

Numerous xenobiotics can induce the MDR1 gene through activation of the nuclear pregnane X receptor (PXR). Some of these include PXR ligands such as rifampin, phenobarbital, statins, and St. John's wort. Other PXR-regulated genes include cytochrome P4503A4, the digoxin and bile salt transporter Oatp2 (organic anion transporting polypeptide 2, Slc01a4) of the basolateral hepatocyte membrane, and the xenobiotic efflux pump Mrp2 (multidrug resistance-associated protein 2, Abcc2) of the canalicular hepatocyte membrane. The constitutive androstane receptor (CAR) that induces Mrp2 and Mrp3 (Abcc3) can also interact with xenobiotics in a similar manner. Thus PXR and CAR are important "xenosensors" that mediate xenobiotic-induced activation of the detoxifying transport and enzyme systems in the intestine and liver (Kullak-Ublick et al., 2003).

Some xenobiotics can be absorbed into the portal circulation, transported to the liver, and excreted back into the intestine unchanged via the bile and may even be absorbed, transported to the liver, and again excreted via the bile. This enterohepatic circulation or cycling of some xenobiotics is not uncommon (Roberts et al., 2002). Xenobiotics that are typically excreted unchanged in the bile have the following characteristics:

- Molecular weight of 400 to 500
- Polarity: highly polar or capable of forming highly polar conjugates
- Degree of protein binding

Xenobiotics that are conjugated in the liver, typically as glucuronides, and then are excreted back into the intestinal lumen are valproic acid, chloramphenicol, digitoxin, and estradiol.

Some substances appear to be excreted unchanged in the feces. Balance studies comparing oral intake to fecal and urinary excretion indicate that they are entirely excreted via the feces in original molecular form. However, some of these xenobiotics are actually absorbed in significant amounts but are returned very rapidly and unchanged into the intestinal tract via the bile and then excreted in the feces. Imipramine is one such example (Dencker et al., 1976).

When enterohepatic cycling of a xenobiotic is interrupted by the administration of an intestinal binding agent such as activated charcoal or cholestyramine, there can be an impact on the plasma half-life of the xenobiotic. For example, the half-life of dapsone (approximately 20 hours) can be reduced by about 50% with the administration of activated charcoal. Activated charcoal administration also greatly accelerates the elimination of tricyclic antidepressants. Swartz et al. (1984) found that the apparent half-life fell below 10 hours for patients who had nasogastric administration of activated charcoal. Untreated patients exhibited extended half-lives averaging 36.8 hours and regularly over 60 hours.

METHODS FOR ASSESSMENT OF INTESTINAL XENOBIOTIC ABSORPTION AND METABOLISM

The three general classes of methods in current use to assess intestinal absorption of xenobiotics in humans are *in silico* computer modeling, *in vitro* procedures, and *in vivo* studies.

IN SILICO MODELS

These methods of modeling intestinal absorption of substances from the human GI tract were discussed in Chapter 11. In general, these models may be constructed using different approaches and software but all models seek to predict the amount of a substance absorbed into the bloodstream from the GI tract and most particularly from the intestinal tract. For this reason, the parameters necessary for constructing these models include chemical, physicochemical, and structural data of the substance to be absorbed and estimates of the biochemical and physiological parameters of the human GI tract for the regions of interest.

Models may be constructed using relatively rigid assumptions such as the biochemical and physiological parameters taken from normal or average values obtained from published literature. Alternatively, they may be more flexible and use physiological and biochemical parameters obtained from a population sample of the subjects who represent the exposed or potentially exposed population (i.e. diabetics, patients with a particular malabsorption syndrome, children, or subjects who follow a particular diet or activity regimen). Some quantitative structure–activity relationship (QSAR) models simply use structural data and *in vivo* outcome data, with or without additional physicochemical, physiological, or biochemical data, and predict qualitative absorption outcomes for substances for which preliminary risk estimates are needed quickly and obtaining actual human data is difficult or prohibitive.

IN VITRO PROCEDURES

In vitro procedures are often conducted with tissues from animals and to a lesser degree with human intestinal tissues or cells. Some studies using human intestinal tissue yielded useful results for isolating and studying specific phenomena, but results do not completely simulate actual conditions (Horikawa et al., 2005; Prabhu et al., 2003; Milovanovic et al., 2002).

Human Caco-2 (colon carcinoma) cells are used increasingly to study cellular transport phenomena and xenobiotic metabolism. Data from these studies are often useful in the construction of kinetic models of intestinal absorption (see Chapter 11).

While it can be argued that a cell line of this nature does not represent completely the biochemical and physiological characteristics of normal intestinal epithelial cells, data obtained from these models can be of value — particularly in understanding basic processes and xenobiotic biotransformations that would likely occur in normal cells or studying normal cells under particular conditions. Important data obtained *in vitro* can then be confirmed *in vivo* with human subjects.

There are many current examples of the use of this methodology to evaluate xenobiotic absorption and metabolism. Cummins et al. (2001) characterized the transport of [³H]-digoxin and the metabolism of midazolam in cells under different inducing conditions using sodium butyrate (NaB) and 12-O-tetradecanoylphorbol-13-acetate (TPA) inducers. Their results demonstrated that in the presence of both inducers, CYP3A4 protein levels were increased 40-fold over uninduced cells, MRP2 expression was decreased by 90%, and P-gp and MRP1 expression was unchanged. They also showed that midazolam 1-OH formation correlated with increased CYP3A4 protein, whereas [3H]-digoxin transport (a measure of P-gp activity) was unchanged with induction. P-gp and MRP2 were found on the apical membranes, whereas MRP1 was found perinuclearly within cells. CYP3A4 displayed a punctate pattern of expression consistent with endoplasmic reticulum localization and exhibited preferential polarization toward the apical sides of the cells.

In Vivo Procedures

In vivo measurement of gastrointestinal absorption has often been evaluated by the measurement of the substance in blood (see above discussion on BCS). Direct placement of the xenobiotic into the lumen of the stomach with serial sampling further gives a measurement of gastric absorption. In animal studies, this methodology is often used, particularly with ligation of the distal end of the stomach. Many of these procedures are used in animal studies; only limited numbers are conducted on humans.

Malabsorption methods in humans include gastroduodenal intubation and measurements of gastric juices, e.g., cholecystokinin and secretin (Chey and Chey, 2003). Malabsorption of nutrient substances also is measured in humans. D-Xylase and disaccharides are useful for determining altered absorption of nutrients from the intestine since these substances are often transported by active transport mechanisms (Walsh, 2001). Furthermore, measurement of excreted fats provides a limited measurement of absorption, but is useful as a diagnostic procedure prior to using more invasive methods such as endoscopy.

REFERENCES

Ambudkar SV et al. (1999). Biochemical, cellular, and pharmacological aspects of the multidrug transporter. *Annu Rev Pharmacol Toxicol* 39: 361–398.

Amidon GL, Lennernäs H, Shah, VP, and Crison JR (1995). A theoretical basis for a biopharmaceutics drug classification: correlation of *in vitro* drug product dissolution and *in vivo* bioavailability. *Pharmaceut Res* 12: 413–420.

Ataka K, Ito M, and Shibata T (2005). New views on antidiarrheal effect of wood creosote: is wood creosote really a gastrointestinal antiseptic? *Yakug Zasshi* 125: 937–950.

Barbara G (2006). Mucosal barrier defects in irritable bowel syndrome: who left the door open? *Am J Gastroenterol* 101: 1295–1298.

Blume HH and Schug BS (1999). The biopharmaceutics classification system (BCS): class III drugs: better candidates for BA/BE waiver? *Eur J Pharmaceut Sci* 9: 117–121.

Cermak R and Breves GM (2006). *In vitro* degradation of the flavonol quercetin and of quercetin glycosides in the porcine hindgut. *Arch Anim Nutr* 60: 180–189.

Chey WD and Chey WY (2003). Evaluation of secretion and absorption functions of the gastrointestinal tract, in *Textbook of Gastroenterology*, Yamada T, Ed., Lippincott Williams & Wilkins, Philadelphia.

Cummins CL, Jacobsen W, and Benet LZ. (2002). Unmasking the dynamic interplay between intestinal P-glycoprotein and CYP3A4. *J Pharmacol Exp Ther* 300: 1036–1045.

Cummins CL, Mangravite LM, and Benet LZ (2001). Characterizing the expression of CYP3A4 and efflux transporters (P-gp, MRP1, and MRP2) in CYP3A4-transfected Caco-2 cells after induction with sodium butyrate and the phorbol ester 12-O-tetradecanoylphorbol-13-acetate. *Pharm Res* 18: 1102–1109.

de Levie R (2003). The Henderson–Hasselbalch equation: its history and limitations. *J Chem Educ* 80, 146.

Dencker H et al. (1976). Intestinal absorption, demethylation, and enterohepatic circulation of imipramine. *Clin Pharmacol Ther* 19: 584–586.

Dive A et al. (1995). Effect of erythromycin on gastric motility in mechanically ventilated critically ill patients: a double-blind, randomized, placebo-controlled study. *Crit Care Med* 23: 1356–1362.

Eberle D, Clarke R, and Kaplowitz N (1981). Rapid oxidation *in vitro* of endogenous and exogenous glutathione in bile of rats. *J Biol Chem* 256: 2115–2117.

Edgar B et al. (1992). Acute effects of drinking grapefruit juice on the pharmacokinetics and dynamics of felodipine and potential clinical relevance. *Eur J Clin Pharmacol* 42: 313–317.

Enayetallah AE et al. (2006). Cell-specific subcellular localization of soluble epoxide hydrolase in human tissues. *J Histochem Cytochem* 54: 329–335.

Food and Drug Administration (2000). Guidance for Industry: Waiver of *in Vivo* Bioavailability and Bioequivalence Studies for Immediate Release Solid Oral Dosage Forms Based on a Biopharmaceutics Classification System, http://www.fda.gov/cder/guidance/3618fnl.htm

Fraser AG (1997). Pharmacokinetic interactions between alcohol and other drugs. *Clin Pharmacokinet* 33: 79–90.

Fukatsu S et al. (2001). Population pharmacokinetics of tacrolimus in adult recipients receiving living-donor liver transplantation. *Eur J Clin Pharmacol* 57: 479–484.

Gibbs JP et al. (1999). Up-regulation of glutathione S-transferase activity in enterocytes of young children. *Drug Metab Dispos* 27: 1466–1469.

Greiner B et al. (1999). Role of intestinal P-glycoprotein in the interaction of digoxin and rifampin. *J Clin Invest* 104: 147–153.

Gyires K (1994). Some of the factors that may mediate or modify the gastrointestinal mucosal damage induced by non-steroidal anti-inflammatory drugs. *Agents Actions* 41: 73–79.

Hashida T et al. (2001). Pharmacokinetic and prognostic significance of intestinal MDR1 expression in recipients of living-donor liver transplantation. *Clin Pharmacol Ther* 69: 308–316.

Hasselbalch KA (1916). Die Berechnung der wasserstoffzahl des blutes auf der freien und gebundenen kohlensaure desselben, und die sauerstoffbindung des blutes als funktion der wasserstoffzahl. *Biochem Zeitsch* 78: 112–144.

Hayes JD and Strange RC (2000). Glutathione S-transferase polymorphisms and their biological consequences. *Pharmacology* 61: 154–166.

Henderson LJ (1908). Concerning the relationship between the strength of acids and their capacity to preserve neutrality. *Am J Physiol* 21: 173–179.

Hochman JH et al. (2000). Influence of P-glycoprotein on the transport and metabolism of indinavir in Caco-2 cells expressing cytochrome P-450 3A4. *J Pharmacol Exp Ther* 292: 310–318.

Hoensch HP and Schwenk M (1984). Intestinal absorption and metabolism of xenobiotics in humans, in *Intestinal Toxicology*, Schiller CM, Ed., Raven Press, New York.

Hogben CAM et al. (1959). On the mechanism of intestinal absorption of drugs, *J Protocol Exp Therap* 125: 275–282

Horikawa N et al. Cyclic AMP-dependent Cl⁻ secretion induced by thromboxane A2 in isolated human colon. *J Physiol* 562: 885–897.

Humblot C et al. (2005). H nuclear magnetic resonance spectroscopy-based studies of the metabolism of food-borne carcinogen 2-amino-3-methylimidazo[4,5-f]quinoline by human intestinal microbiota. *Appl Environ Microbiol* 71: 5116–5123.

Hurwitz A et al. (2003). Gastric function in the elderly: effects on absorption of ketoconazole. *J Clin Pharmacol* 43: 996–1002.

Ito K, Kusuhara H, and Sugiyama Y (1999). Effects of intestinal CYP3A4 and P-glycoprotein on oral drug absorption: theoretical approach. *Pharm Res* 16: 225–231.

Kasim NA et al. (2004). Molecular properties of WHO essential drugs and provisional biopharmaceutical classification. *Mol Pharmacol* 1: 85–96.

Kaus LC et al. (1999). The effect of *in vivo* dissolution, gastric emptying rate, and intestinal transit time on the peak concentration and area-under-the-curve of drugs with different gastrointestinal permeabilities. *Pharmaceut Res* 16: 272–280.

Klaassen CD (2001). *Casarett and Doulis Toxicology: The Basic Scince of Poisons.* McGraw Hill, New York.

Kolars JC et al. (1991). First-pass metabolism of cyclosporin by the gut. *Lancet* 338: 1488–1490.

Kolars JC et al. (1994). CYP3A gene expression in human gut epithelium. *Pharmacogenetics* 4: 247–259.

Kolars JC et al. (1992). Identification of rifampin-inducible P450IIIA4 (CYP3A4) in human small bowel enterocytes. *J Clin Invest* 90: 1871–1878.

Kortejarvi H et al. Biowaiver monographs for immediate release solid oral dosage forms: ranitidine hydrochloride. *J Pharmaceut Sci* 94: 1617–1625.

Kullak-Ublick GA and Becker MB (2003). Regulation of drug and bile salt transporters in liver and intestine. *Drug Metab Rev* 35: 305–317.

Lantz B and Einhorn N (1984). Intestinal damage and malabsorption after treatment for cervical carcinoma. *Acta Radiol Oncol* 23: 33–36.

LeCluyse EL (2001). Pregnane X receptor: molecular basis for species differences in CYP3A induction by xenobiotics. *Chem Biol Interact* 134: 283–289.

Lecoeur S, Videmann B, and Mazallon M (2006). Effect of organophosphate pesticide diazinon on expression and activity of intestinal P-glycoprotein. *Toxicol Lett* 161: 200–209.

Lehmann JM et al. (1998). The human orphan nuclear receptor PXR is activated by compounds that regulate CYP3A4 gene expression and cause drug interactions. *J Clin Invest* 102: 1016–1023.

Lennernas H (1998). Human intestinal permeability. *J Pharmaceut Sci* 87: 403–410.

Lennernas H (1998). Human jejunal effective permeability and its correlation with pre-clinical drug absorption models. *J Pharm Pharmacol* 49: 627–638.

Lown KS et al. (1997). Grapefruit juice increases felodipine oral availability in humans by decreasing intestinal CYP3A protein expression. *J Clin Invest* 99: 2545–2553

Lown KS et al. (1997). Role of intestinal P-glycoprotein (mdr1) in interpatient variation in the oral bioavailability of cyclosporine. *Clin Pharmacol Ther* 62: 248–260.

Lui CY et al. (1986). Comparison of gastrointestinal pH in dogs and humans: implications of the use of the beagle dog as a model for oral absorption in humans. *J Pharmaceut Sci* 75: 271–274.

Malandain H (2005). Transglutaminases: a meeting point for wheat allergy, celiac disease, and food safety. *Allerg Immunol* (Paris) 37: 397–403.

Martin A (1993). *Physical Pharmacy*, 4th ed., Lea & Febiger, Philadelphia.

Martínez-Pla JJ et al. (2003). Chromatographic estimation of apparent acid dissociation constants (pKa) in physiological resembling conditions: case study. *Internet Electronic Conference of Molecular Design*, http://www.biochempress.com

Milovanovic DR and Jankovic SM (2002). A pharmacological analysis of the contractile effects of glutamate on rat and human isolated gut smooth muscle strips. *Methods Find Exp Clin Pharmacol* 24: 661–668.

Montrose MH, Keely SJ, and Barrett KE (2003). Electrolyte secretion and absorption: small intestine and colon, in *Textbook of Gastroenterology*, 4th ed., Yamada T, Ed., Lippincott Williams & Wilkins, New York.

Nagata K and Yamazoe Y (2000). Pharmacogenetics of sulfotransferase. *Ann Rev Pharmacol Toxicol* 40: 159–176.

Paine MF et al. (1996). First-pass metabolism of midazolam by the human intestine. *Clin Pharmacol Ther* 60: 14–24.

Prabhu R, Perakath B, and Balasubramanian KA (2003). Isolation of human small intestinal brush border membranes using polyethylene glycol and effect of exposure to various oxidants *in vitro*. *Dig Dis Sci* 48: 995–1001.

Roberts MS et al. (2002). Enterohepatic circulation: physiological, pharmacokinetic and clinical implications. *Clin Pharmacokinet* 41: 751–790.

Ross BP and Toth I (2005). Gastrointestinal absorption of heparin by lipidization or coadministration with penetration enhancers. *Curr Drug Deliv* 2: 277–287.

Samiec PS, Dahm LJ, and Jones D (2000). Glutathione S-transferase in mucus of rat small intestine. *Toxicol Sci* 54: 52–59.

Schanker LS (1971). Drug absorption, *Fundamentals of Drug Metabolism and Drug Distribution*, LaDu BN et al., Eds., Williams & Wilkins, Baltimore, chap. 2.

Schellens JHM et al. (2000). Modulation of oral bioavailability of anticancer drugs: from mouse to man. *Eur J Pharmaceut Sci* 12: 103–110.

Schinkel AH et al. (1995). Multidrug resistance and the role of P-glycoprotein knockout mice. *Eur J Cancer* 31A: 1295–1298.

Schmiedlin-Ren P et al. (1997). Mechanisms of enhanced oral availability of CYP3A4 substrates by grapefruit constituents: decreased enterocyte CYP3A4 concentration and mechanism-based inactivation by furanocoumarins. *Drug Metab Dispos* 25: 1228–1233.

Schuetz EG, Beck WT, and Schuetz JD (1996). Modulators and substrates of P-glycoprotein and cytochrome P4503A coordinately upregulate these proteins in human colon carcinoma cells. *Mol Pharmacol* 49: 311–318.

Shore PA, Brodie BB, and Hogben CAM (1957). Gastric secretion of drugs: a pH partition hypothesis, *J Protocol Exp Therap* 119: 361–369.

Sparreboom A et al. (1997). Limited oral bioavailability and active epithelial excretion of paclitaxel (Taxol) caused by P-glycoprotein in the intestine. *Proc Natl Acad Sci USA* 94: 2031–2035.

Swartz CM and Sherman A (1984). The treatment of tricyclic antidepressant overdose with repeated charcoal. *J Clin Psychopharmacol* 4: 336–340.

Synold TW, Dussault I, and Forman BM (2001). The orphan nuclear receptor SXR coordinately regulates drug metabolism and efflux. *Nat Med* 7: 584–590.

Thiebaut F et al. (1987). Cellular localization of the multidrug-resistance gene product P-glycoprotein in normal human tissues. *Proc Natl Acad Sci USA* 84: 7735–7738.

Thiefin G and Beaugerie L (2005). Toxic effects of nonsteroidal antiinflammatory drugs on the small bowel, colon, and rectum. *Joint Bone Spine* 72: 286–294.

Tukey RH and Strassburg CP (2001). Genetic multiplicity of the human UDP-glucuronosyltransferases and regulation in the gastrointestinal tract. *Mol Pharmacol* 59: 405–414.

Vaughan EE et al. (2002). Intestinal LABs. *Antonie Van Leeuwenhoek* 82: 341–352.

Voice MW et al. (1999). Effects of human cytochrome b5 on CYP3A4 activity and stability *in vivo*. *Arch Biochem Biophys* 366: 116–124.

Wacher VJ et al. (1998). Role of P-glycoprotein and cytochrome P450 3A in limiting oral absorption of peptides and peptidomimetics. *J Pharm Sci* 87: 1322–1330.

Wacher VJ, Wu CY, and Benet LZ (1995). Overlapping substrate specificities and tissue distribution of cytochrome P450 3A and P-glycoprotein: implications for drug delivery and activity in cancer chemotherapy. *Mol Carcinog* 13: 129–134.

Walsh JT (2001). Methods in gastrointestinal toxicology, in *Principles and Methods of Toxicology*, Hayes AW, Ed., Taylor & Francis, Philadelphia.

Wrighton SA et al. (1987). Purification of a human liver cytochrome P-450 immunochemically related to several cytochromes P-450 purified from untreated rats. *J Clin Invest* 80: 1017–1022.

Yu LX et al. (2002). Biopharmaceutics classification system: scientific basis for biowaiver extensions. *Pharmaceut Res* 19: 921–925.

Zhang Y and Benet LZ (2001). The gut as a barrier to drug absorption: combined role of cytochrome P450 3A and P-glycoprotein. *Clin Pharmacokinet* 40: 159–168.

Zoetendal EG, Vaughan EE, and de Vos WM (2006). A microbial world within us. *Mol Microbiol* 59: 1639–1650.

Index

A

Absorption, 5
  basic mechanisms of, 163
  definition of, 114
  distribution, metabolism, and excretion
    (ADME), 113
  GI transit times and, 98
  influences on degree of, 266
  parameters affecting, 44
  regional differences in, 273
Accessory pancreatic duct, 154
Acetaminophen absorption, 333
Acetazolamide, 306
Acetylcholine, 151, 184, 187, 191
Acetylcholinesterase enzyme, inhibition of, 196
Acid
  –base homeostasis, 165
  microclimate, 119
  secretion, histamine and, 323
ACTH, *see* Adrenocorticotropic hormone
Active absorption of bicarbonate ions, 219
Active transport, 120, 163, 221, 268, 286, 327
Adenosine triphosphate (ATP), 121, 193
  break-down of, 163
  expenditure, 268
ADME, *see* Absorption, distribution,
    metabolism, and excretion
ADP ribosylation factors, 193
Adrenocorticotropic hormone (ACTH), 259
Adventitia, 12
Aggregated lymphatic follicles, 15
Alcohol(s)
  common, 307
  dehydrogenase, 307
  interaction of food with, 324
Aldosterone, 168, 219
Alendronate, 61
Alkaline phosphatase, secretion of, 48
Alpha-adrenergic drugs, 41–42
Amanita phalloides, 305
Amatoxins, 305
Amino acid(s)

absorption of, 29
polypeptide, 152
protein formation from, 216
transport, 167, 169, 290
Amoxicillin, 221
Ampicillin, 221
Anal canal, 16
Analysis of gastrointestinal function, methods
    for, 35–51
  absorption, 44–46
  immune function, 46–48
    clinical chemistry analyses, 47–48
    gastrointestinal bleeding, 47
    pain, 48
  secretions, 42–44
  transit, 36–42
    esophageal transit, 36–38
    gastric emptying, 38–39
    motility of large intestine, 41–42
    motility of small intestine, 39–41
Anemia, 295
Ankyloglossia, 10
Antibody-secreting cells, development of, 95
Antidepressants, emetogenic activities of, 73
Antigen-presenting cells (APCs), 240
Antihistamines, side effects of, 254
APCs, *see* Antigen-presenting cells
Apical sodium bile acid cotransporter
    (ASBT), 131
Apoprotein, 291
Appendix, 16
Areae gastricae, 141
Arsenic-containing compounds, 192
ASBT, *see* Apical sodium bile acid
    cotransporter
Ascending colon, 145, 146
Ascites, 7
ATP, *see* Adenosine triphosphate
ATPases, 121
Atropine, 220, 257
Autacoids, 190
Autonomic nervous system, studies on, 56
Azathioprene, 189

M

T